Cancer and the Politics of Care

EMBODYING INEQUALITIES: PERSPECTIVES FROM
MEDICAL ANTHROPOLOGY

Series Editors
Sahra Gibbon, UCL Anthropology
Jennie Gamlin, UCL Institute for Global Health

This series charts diverse anthropological engagements with the changing dynamics of health and wellbeing in local and global contexts. It includes ethnographic and theoretical works that explore the different ways in which inequalities pervade our bodies. The series offers novel contributions often neglected by classical and contemporary publications that draw on public, applied, activist, cross-disciplinary and engaged anthropological methods, as well as in-depth writings from the field. It specifically seeks to showcase new and emerging health issues that are the products of unequal global development.

Cancer and the Politics of Care

Inequalities and interventions in global perspective

Edited by

Linda Rae Bennett, Lenore Manderson
and Belinda Spagnoletti

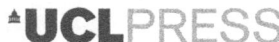

First published in 2023 by
UCL Press
University College London
Gower Street
London WC1E 6BT

Available to download free: www.uclpress.co.uk

Collection © Editors, 2023
Text © Contributors, 2023
Images © Contributors and copyright holders named in captions, 2023

Cover image credit: Good Traditions. 15 x 9 x 13 cm. Ceramic. 2019. Nicolás Rodriguez. Prior publication in: Nicolás Rodríguez (2021). Fresh water project [Agua Dulce Proyecto audio visual: Prácticas artísticas contemporáneas en territorio]. In Luxardo, N. and Sassetti, F. (eds.). In situ. Cancer as social injustice [El cancer como injusticia social]. Buenos Aires: Biblos Editorial, 939–952.

The authors have asserted their rights under the Copyright, Designs and Patents Act 1988 to be identified as the authors of this work.

A CIP catalogue record for this book is available from The British Library.

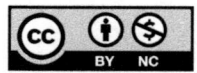

Any third-party material in this book is not covered by the book's Creative Commons licence. Details of the copyright ownership and permitted use of third-party material is given in the image (or extract) credit lines. If you would like to reuse any third-party material not covered by the book's Creative Commons licence, you will need to obtain permission directly from the copyright owner.

This book is published under a Creative Commons Attribution-Non-Commercial 4.0 International licence (CC BY-NC 4.0), https://creativecommons.org/licenses/by-nc/4.0/. This licence allows you to share and adapt the work for non-commercial use providing attribution is made to the author and publisher (but not in any way that suggests that they endorse you or your use of the work) and any changes are indicated. Attribution should include the following information:

Bennett, L.R., Manderson, L. and Spagnoletti, B. (eds.). 2023. *Cancer and the Politics of Care: Inequalities and interventions in global perspective*. London: UCL Press. https://doi.org/10.14324/111.9781800080737

Further details about Creative Commons licences are available at http:// creativecommons.org/ licenses/

ISBN: 978-1-80008-075-1 (Hbk.)
ISBN: 978-1-80008-074-4 (Pbk.)
ISBN: 978-1-80008-073-7 (PDF)
ISBN: 978-1-80008-076-8 (epub)
DOI: https://doi.org/10.14324/111.9781800080737

Contents

List of figures	vii
List of contributors	ix

1 Introduction: cancer ethnographies and the politics of care   1
Linda Rae Bennett and Lenore Manderson

2 Biomedical innovations, cancer care and health inequities: stratified patienthood in Brazil   23
Jorge Alberto Bernstein Iriart and Sahra Gibbon

3 'It just keeps hurting': continuums of violence and their impact on cervical cancer mortality in Argentina   42
Natalia Luxardo and Linda Rae Bennett

4 Laughing in the face of cancer: intersubjectivity and patient navigation in the US safety net   62
Nancy J. Burke

5 Morality tales of reproductive cancer screening camps in South India   83
Cecilia Coale Van Hollen

6 Intersections of stigma, morality and care: Indonesian women's negotiations of cervical cancer   109
Linda Rae Bennett and Hanum Atikasari

7 Untimely liver cancer and the temporalities of care in rural Senegal   130
Noémi Tousignant

8 Rehumanising illness: practices of care in a cancer ward in Athens, Greece   150
Falia Varelaki

9 Practices of containment in the 'south-within-the-north': women with breast cancer in southern Italy   171
   Cinzia Greco

10 Noisy bodies and cancer diagnostics in Denmark: exploring the social life of medical semiotics   190
   Rikke Sand Andersen, Sara Marie Hebsgaard Offersen and Camilla Hoffman Merrild

11 'Hard-to-reach'? Meanings at the margins of care and risk in cancer research   210
   Kelly Fagan Robinson and Ignacia Arteaga Pérez

12 Precarity and cancer among low-income populations in France: intractable inequalities   232
   Laurence Kotobi and Carolyn Sargent

Index   254

List of figures

5.1	Government cancer poster	84
5.2	Cervical cancer pamphlet cover	91
5.3	Breast cancer pamphlet cover	91
5.4	Cervical cancer pamphlet page on causes of cancer	92
5.5	Cervical cancer pamphlet page on causes of cancer	93
8.1	Moments in the cancer ward	153
8.2	Not alone	154
8.3	Touching hands – Dr A. during morning rounds	157
8.4	Fighting together	158
8.5	Dr A. and a patient, outpatient clinic	159
8.6	Monday morning, 9.50 a.m., outpatient clinic	162
8.7	'I'll be back . . .'	164
8.8	Preparing the patient for chemotherapy	165
10.1	Picture of a social housing association in Denmark	192
10.2	'Colon cancer detected in due time can be cured'	196

List of contributors

Rikke Sand Andersen is Professor MSO at University of Southern Denmark and Department of Anthropology, Aarhus University. For the past decade Andersen has conducted research on cancer diagnostics and general practice in Denmark. She is currently initiating research on the welfare state and family relations, exploring how people who live alone manage serious illness, and how notions of solitude may be understood through the diseased body.

Hanum Atikasari is a PhD candidate at the Institute of Cultural Anthropology and Development Sociology at Leiden University and is part of the 'Globalizing palliative care' project funded by the European Research Council. Her research explores how Indonesian women with breast and reproductive cancers, and their caregivers, navigate access to end-of-life care and what they perceived as a good care. Prior to joining Leiden University, she worked as a research assistant on the project 'Biographies of vulnerability and resilience: Indonesian women's experiences of living with cervical cancer'. The research was undertaken by the Nossal Institute for Global Health at the University of Melbourne.

Linda Rae Bennett is Professor of Medical Anthropology at the Nossal Institute for Global Health, the University of Melbourne. She is a global leader in research on sexual and reproductive health and rights in Indonesia, where she has over 25 years' experience. Her recent edited volume *Sex and Sexualities in Contemporary Indonesia: Sexual politics, health, diversity and representations* (2015) won the International Convention of Asia Scholars – Edited Volume Accolade (2017), and the Ruth Benedict Prize for the Most Outstanding Edited Volume (2015). Her current research explores the experiences of women affected by cervical cancer in Indonesia, including their resilience in navigating primary and secondary prevention, achieving diagnosis and negotiating treatment in a resource poor health system.

Jorge Alberto Bernstein Iriart is Associate Professor at the Institute of Collective Health of the Federal University of Bahia in Salvador, Brazil. He has a PhD in Anthropology from Université de Montréal, Canada. He develops research on personalised medicine and how new biomedical technologies are changing oncological clinical practice, the patient's illness experience and therapeutic pathways and its reflection upon health inequalities in Brazil.

Nancy J. Burke is Professor of Public Health and Anthropology at the University of California, Merced, and John D. and Catherine T. MacArthur Foundation Endowed Chair. She is also affiliated faculty in the Department of Anthropology, History and Social Medicine and member of the Helen Diller Comprehensive Cancer Center at the University of California, San Francisco. Her research addresses cancer care, clinical trial participation and recruitment and cancer survivorship in safety-net and community settings in the United States.

Sahra Gibbon is Professor in Medical Anthropology at UCL. She has carried out research examining the social and cultural context of cancer genetics in the UK, Cuba and Brazil and has long-standing interests in the interface between biomedical technologies, inequalities and public health.

Cinzia Greco is Wellcome Trust Research Fellow at the Centre for the History of Science, Technology and Medicine at the University of Manchester. She specialises in the study of cancer and has further research interests in medical innovation, inequalities in access to healthcare and gender and health. Her work has been published in journals such as *Medical Anthropology*, *Social Science & Medicine* and *Journal of Gender Studies*.

Laurence Kotobi is Professor and Chair of Social Anthropology at the University of Bordeaux (France) and member of the Bordeaux Population Health Research Centre (INSERM, UMR 1219). She is also Fellow of the French Collaborative Institute on Migration (2018–2021). Her research contributes to identifying the main social and cultural factors involved in health inequalities in France, especially in relation to migration trajectories, gender, economic precarity, religious observances (specifically Islam) and language issues. She is Scientific Coordinator of the qualitative study of the First Steps ANR project (2016–2021) 'Access to benefits, care trajectories and take-up of the Aide Médicale de l'Etat (AME) among undocumented immigrants in France'.

Natalia Luxardo is a social worker with a PhD in Culture, Society and Social Science. She is an independent researcher in Sociology and the Demography of Argentina at the National Scientific and Technical Research Council and Professor of Methodology at the University of Buenos Aires. Her primary expertise is in conducting collaborative projects with highly vulnerable communities and methodologies in critical medical anthropology. For the last two decades she has worked on cancer inequalities within the health system in Argentina. She is currently working on the everyday challenges for cancer prevention within communities of fishermen, farmers, rural women peasants and garbage collectors.

Lenore Manderson is Distinguished Professor of Public Health and Medical Anthropology at the University of the Witwatersrand, Johannesburg, South Africa, with professorial affiliations with Monash University (Australia). She is known internationally for her work on inequality, marginality and infectious and chronic diseases in Australia, South Africa and South-East and East Asia, and has published on cancer with Indigenous, immigrant and Anglo-Australian women. Her most recent book, with Nancy J. Burke and Ayo Wahlberg, is *Viral Loads: Anthropologies of urgency in the time of COVID-19* (2021).

Camilla Hoffmann Merrild is an anthropologist and Senior Researcher at the Center for General Practice at Aalborg University. She has worked extensively with social inequalities in health in the context of the welfare state, focusing on care-seeking practices and the experience of the body. She is currently conducting research on child maltreatment, exploring the significance of emotions and affect in making sense of suspicions of child neglect and abuse in the clinic.

Sara Marie Hebsgaard Offersen is an anthropologist and postdoctoral researcher at the Research Unit for General Practice and Research Centre for Cancer Diagnosis in Primary Care at Aarhus University, Denmark. Her research interests centre on everyday life perspectives on illness, and health and illness prevention in the context of the welfare state. She focuses on the moral, sensorial and uncertain spaces between being a person and being a patient. She is currently initiating a research project on the welfare state and family relations in Denmark.

Ignacia Arteaga Pérez is Philomathia Research Associate and Affiliated Lecturer at the Department of Social Anthropology, University of Cambridge. She is also a research fellow at Robinson College, Cambridge. Ignacia's current research concerns the practices of multiple stakeholders involved in the fields of cancer detection and care in the UK. She is the lead investigator of 'Represent: a community engagement roadmap to improve participant representation in cancer research early detection', a collaborative and comparative research project in the USA and the UK funded by the International Alliance for Cancer Early Detection (https://anthced.com).

Kelly Fagan Robinson is Leverhulme and Isaac Newton Trust Early Career Researcher Fellow and Affiliated Lecturer in the Department of Social Anthropology, University of Cambridge, and Fellow of Clare Hall. Her research focuses on the senses, communication and social connection. It foregrounds the ways that individual histories, bodies, sensorial hierarchies, education and experiences of formalised care can generate epistemic dissonances and injustices for British people. Her current research project, 'Faultlines on the frontlines' (2021–2024), tests the limits of testimony when attempting to ask for and prove need of support in the UK. This builds on her previous research, which investigated deaf people's visual–tactile communication resources, and the resistance that such practices confront in non-deaf spaces.

Carolyn Sargent is Professor of Anthropology, Affiliated Professor of Women, Gender and Sexuality Studies, and Global Health Faculty Scholar at Washington University in St. Louis. She has conducted field research in West Africa (Benin, Mali), in Jamaica and in France. Her recent interests centre on illness and sociality, immigration and health, the anthropology of cancer and the politics of reproduction. Her current research focuses on how West African immigrants living in France and in treatment for cancer conceptualise cancer and its management. Her most recent publication is *The Work of Hospitals: Global medicine in local cultures* (edited with William Olsen, 2022).

Belinda (Bel) Spagnoletti works for the Adelaide Primary Health Network, focusing on the integration, design and evaluation of primary mental healthcare and alcohol and other drug-commissioned services. Previously she coordinated an Australian Research Council-funded project focused on cervical cancer in Indonesia, as Research Fellow in Sexual and Reproductive Health at the Nossal Institute for Global Health at the University of Melbourne, Australia (2018–2021) and Visiting Researcher at Gadjah Mada University, Indonesia (2019–2021). Bel was awarded her PhD in International Health from the University of Melbourne in 2019.

Noémi Tousignant is Lecturer in Science and Technology Studies at UCL and currently holds a Wellcome Trust University Award. Her work explores intersections of scientific and health inequality in West Africa. Her current project looks at primary liver cancer as a case of inequality formed through the making of biomedical knowledge about carcinogenic exposures, the deployment of technologies for controlling these and the privatisation of care. She is co-editor of *Traces of the Future: An archaeology of medical science in Africa* (2016) and author of the award-winning monograph *Edges of Exposure* (2020).

Cecilia Coale Van Hollen is Professor in the Asian Studies Program of the School of Foreign Service at Georgetown University. She is a cultural and medical anthropologist specialising in social and cultural dimensions of health, medicine and global public health policy in India. She is the author of three books: *Birth on the Threshold: Childbirth and modernity in South India* (2003), *Birth in the Age of AIDS: Women, reproduction, and HIV/AIDS in India* (2013) and *Cancer and the Kali Yuga: Gender, health and inequality in South India* (2022). She is also the co-editor of *A Companion to the Anthropology of Reproductive Science and Technology* (forthcoming).

Falia Varelaki is a PhD candidate in Social Anthropology at the Department of Social Anthropology and History, University of the Aegean. Her research, conducted in Athens between 2016 and 2018, focuses on biopolitics of breast cancer in Greece, and examines the ways that the experience of breast cancer is constructed, not only through personal experience but also through state policies and medical discourses. Her thesis is concerned with practices of care, health inequalities, state policies and kinship. Her research was funded by an Ypatia scholarship.

1
Introduction: cancer ethnographies and the politics of care

Linda Rae Bennett and Lenore Manderson

In recent decades, growing attention has been paid to what is described as an 'epidemic' of cancer, the term used to reflect recorded increases in diagnosis, severe illness and mortality. It is likely, too, that with the increased longevity of populations worldwide, there is a rise in absolute incidence. Cancers develop with age, reflecting the slow development of many cancers, the accrued effects of exposure to carcinogens and infections and the decreased capacity of the body to eliminate damaged DNA. Increased visibility also reflects changes in technology and health systems that have resulted in improved diagnosis and reporting. Given this mix of circumstances, the language of epidemic is perhaps misplaced. But the rhetoric reflects growing awareness of the pervasiveness of multiple related diseases of organs, tissues, cell type, forms and progress. It's an explosion, an epidemic, of understanding cancer's complexity, its differences and the diverse populations who are affected. There are vast discrepancies in cancer prevalence, survival rates and responses between countries in the global south and global north, with disparities that reinforce the need to theorise cancer in local and global perspectives.

In summary, the number of new cases of cancer per annum has risen steadily this century. At time of writing, breast cancer is by far the most common cancer, and the leading cause of death globally among women regardless of income level. This is followed by lung, colorectal, prostate, stomach and liver (Global Cancer Observatory 2020). Some ten million deaths in 2020 were attributed to these six cancers worldwide, although the rankings vary by country status as determined by national income level and human development index. In low-income countries, for example, women are still most likely to die from breast and cervical cancer; men are most likely to die from prostate and liver cancer. Globally, around one-third of cancers are associated with so-called lifestyle factors (diet, smoking, alcohol use and body weight; see Manderson 2020 for critique), and almost as many again are from infections such as hepatitis and human papillomavirus (HPV). Poor access to screening, diagnosis and treatment, and so to technologies and health professionals, in low- and middle-income countries largely accounts for disparity in outcomes. Marissa Mika (2021), in her superb history and ethnography of cancer in Uganda, notes that for three decades – the 1980s, 1990s and 2000s – there was only one oncologist in the country, seeking to provide care to a population that increased from 12 to 33 million over this period. Although this may be an extreme example, in low-income countries especially, comprehensive care is not widely available and even basic drugs may be difficult to access.

A closer look at the epidemiology of cancer draws attention to the underlying unequal risk factors and outcomes within and between communities and countries. As noted by the Director of the International Agency for Research on Cancer (IARC), Christopher Wild (2019), cancer's incidence and outcomes highlight geographic differences, environmental conditions and changing practices associated with globalisation; they point to the unequal distribution of other health conditions, both infectious and non-communicable diseases, and to the material, social and political infrastructures that create the conditions for cancer's distribution.

Cancer mirrors inequalities. As analysed in the recent IARC report (Vaccarella et al. 2019), types of disease, their distribution, survival and mortality reflect social inequalities within and between countries. These inequalities are vast in: risk factors at community, household and personal levels; the capacity to embrace preventive behaviours, adhere to screening, and seek medical attention to enable early diagnosis and treatment; the quality and affordability of treatment, and access to extended care; and possible remission, quality of life and long-term outcomes. These all contribute to a sharp global cancer divide. IARC's report maps the social epidemiology of cancer and illustrates that education, income, class, geography, residence, race, ethnicity and gender are all predictive of disease. This attention to inequality shifts the focus from personal risk factors and direct risks, such as exposure to industrial carcinogens and air pollution, to structural vulnerabilities and barriers to care. Wild (2019: 4) argues that cancer is 'a universal illustration of inequality between human beings in terms of the risk of developing the disease, access to preventative measures, early detection, access to treatment and care . . . even hope'.

Other authors write of 'stark and consistent . . . remarkable inequalities in cancer incidence and mortality, both between countries and over time' and 'striking differences in mortality trends' (Vaccarella et al. 2019: 63, 65, 75). They attend too to the specific contours of inequality. Indigenous people worldwide continue to endure a 'legacy of colonisation, and ongoing marginalisation and disempowerment' (Garvey and Cunningham 2019: 79). Cancer's costs reflect 'worsening inequalities . . . whereby women, socio-economically disadvantaged groups, ethnic minorities, indigenous populations, and other vulnerable groups experienced poor outcomes' (Meheus, Atun and Ilbawi 2019: 137). Authors write in frustration and outrage of such national, state and local inequalities that strip contemporary technical advances from the majority of people worldwide, as a result of racism, sexism and social exclusion (Basu 2019: 217; Sarfati 2019: 16). This inequality extends to all aspects of life – the legal frameworks that govern access to and provision of care, income support, medical leave from work, insurance and loans, geopolitical status, structures of governance, the production, distribution, provision and flow of drugs and other technologies, and the training and support of specialities (Jemal and Siegel 2019; Liberman 2019; Livingston 2012; Mika 2021; Sullivan et al. 2019).

But cancer's specificities are lost even as the importance of attending to population and institutional differences are emphasised. Cancer is used loosely to cover a wide range of conditions: involving diverse organs; different cells and cell receptors; sometimes presenting as contained tumours, other times diffuse, elusive and disseminated; some acute, others chronic; some readily resolved, assuming timely care, others treatable but not curable (Manderson 2015, 2022, 2023). Social inequalities experienced by individuals and households, and nationwide structural inequalities, contribute to the likelihood or not of the prevention or development of cancer, and the events that unfold with the awareness of any kind of embodied anomaly. Diagnosis, treatment and death are all social facts.

We know that cancers develop in different ways, and their identification and treatment differs for biological, structural, economic and political reasons. But also, as Wild (2019: 4) notes, 'cancer is *lived* differently' (original emphasis). Yet in the IARC volume there is no space, nor perhaps disciplinary interest, to explain *how* cancer is 'lived' differently, nor is there the space or opportunity to tease out the complexities of inequality and its inherence in different social structures. Thus the IARC volume, like much other work on cancer, acknowledges the social divisions that determine cancer's likelihood and likely outcomes, but fails to engage with the work of anthropologists and other social scientists attending most closely to the differences that emerge within households, localities and states.

Ethnographies, in contrast, worry away at the differences that matter in relation to the disease and its history in individual bodies, the person and their social and material relations (McMullin 2016: 252), and the economics and politics that determine these differences. Anthropology attends to how cancer is lived, but also to the conditions of living that determine exposure to cancer's causes, and the likelihood of care, treatment and continuing life. It highlights the inequalities that explain the uneven outcomes of a person with cancer in India (Banerjee 2020), Kenya (Mulemi 2010) or Botswana (Livingston 2012), Brazil (Gregg 2003) or China (Lora-Wainwright 2013), for example, or as more extensively illustrated among US populations (see, among other works, Armin, Burke and Eichelberger 2019; Jain 2013; McMullin and Weiner 2008; Weiner 1999). It questions the skewed burden of deaths, and the meanings of life, caregiving, pain relief and death, in global and local terms.

Ethnographic research and anthropological theories therefore describe and help explain the contexts in which cancers develop, are identified and managed, as we explore in this volume. This project responds to the wider call to 'humanise' (Livingston 2012) our understandings of the global cancer divide (Knaul et al. 2021). In the contributing chapters, authors explore how peoples' experiences of different kinds of cancers, in different country contexts, are shaped by the institutions, social structures, politics and ordinary circumstances of their lives, and the inequalities inherent in these systems that pattern what we refer to as 'the politics of care'. Care is a human capacity, while inequity is an inherently political problem. Accordingly, by engaging the 'politics of care' as our theoretical terrain, the authors in this volume capture and interrogate the myriad intersections of care and inequity as they relate to cancer. Their critiques of the politics of cancer enable nuanced explorations of capacities for care, gaps in care, and the extraordinary ways in which individuals, families, health professionals, allied services and communities seek to fill these gaps. They offer great insight into how access to resources shapes capacities for care across highly varied carescapes (Bowlby 2012; Ivanova, Wallenburg and Bal 2016; Lau et al. 2021), among individuals and their families, to health systems and nation states, to the global economy with its entrenched economic stratification. At the same time, the authors remain aware that the suffering that cancer induces is not rendered irrelevant for those who do have access to adequate resources. They illuminate how the capacity to care for the suffering person as a human being, and not merely treat the afflicted body, is paramount for those living with and dying from cancer (see Chapters 7, 8 and 9 by, respectively, Tousignant, Varelaki and Greco, this volume). We are reminded that suffering is intrinsically relational and is not confined just to bodies marked by cancer – it is shared by loved ones, carers and health professionals, generating additional economies of care that are often multidirectional (see Chapter 6 by Bennett and Atikasari, and Chapter 9 by Greco, this volume).

We propose the politics of care as an alternative site for critical thought that can assist in overcoming simplistic categories such as those of the global south and global north. While the south/north dichotomy seeks to avoid allusion to the prior racist distinction of east and west, the binary still privileges the fiscal metrics of nation states over populations and individuals. As the IARC report documents, vast discrepancies exist within countries, and everywhere widening inequality sharpens the lived disparities of cancer risk, disease and consequence. Types of cancer, risks, access to healthcare and support all vary with implications at an individual level: a manual worker without valid papers, living in a high-income country, arguably faces greater barriers to care than a wealthy or even comfortably employed person in a low-income country (see Kline 2019; and Kotobi and Sargent, Chapter 12, this volume). These differences are not incidental. Political–economic relations and status, at individual and state levels, produce inequalities that are reflected in a politics of care, determining who has access to preventive health information and early interventions, influencing people's willingness to present for screening or diagnosis, and determining their ability to remain in care and, on an ongoing basis, to enable monitoring. We understand the form of these different relations – of people and risk, of patients and their health providers, and of patients and their treatment choices, for example – through the analysis of rich ethnography and by drawing on insights from our colleagues. Deploying the politics of care as a terrain for thinking on cancer enables analysis of the complexity of an extraordinary range of inequalities at multiple levels across overlapping carescapes.

In this volume, we generate new thinking on how social, economic, race, gender and other social and structural inequalities intersect, compound and complicate health inequalities; we work towards deeper understandings of how solutions to cancer-related inequalities need to take into account the complex dynamics of intersecting inequalities. As we have already noted, the distribution and lethal nature of different cancers varies globally for social, epidemiological and health-system reasons. To highlight this diversity here, we cover five continents – Africa, Asia, Europe, North America, Latin America – and eleven countries – Argentina, Brazil, Denmark, France, Greece, India, Indonesia, Italy, Senegal, United Kingdom and the United States – to be able to attend to local differences in disease and outcome, particularly among poor communities and low-income countries (see also Mathews, Burke and Kampriani 2015). Some contributors look at cancers as a group of diseases; others look at specific cancers (breast, cervical and liver), with the focus on women's cancers highlighting the current skewing in anthropological research (of itself, reflecting in part the strength of public advocacy). As we discuss later in this chapter, the various contributors to this volume engage with new, emerging and prior theoretical contributions in their context-specific analyses of the politics of care, so to untangle the contradictions, complexities and confluences of different cancers in different settings. The concept of 'interventions' for cancer and for other health conditions – measures and methods to divert a course – is under-theorised in medical anthropology. Cancer offers us new ways to think about the courses of different health conditions and the systems of prevention and care that are offered. As we describe, the contributing authors engage with and extend the idea of interventions by considering different approaches across cancers' trajectories to health promotion, vaccines (for HPV), prevention, screening, diagnosis, treatment, survivorship and end-of-life and palliative care, as well as noting the inequalities of their distribution and provision, access and affordability. Interventions, including diagnostics, treatment/care and formal support, are driven by governments and global bodies; they are offered to, withheld from, and accepted or rejected by different populations; they are made available to patients and populations at risk (and so, potential patients). Interventions are also initiated by patients to gain access to care; and they involve collaborative efforts between vulnerable communities and individuals, researchers and practitioners (that is, health workers, social workers, community-based organisations and ethnographers). Anticipating these contributions, in this introductory chapter we summarise different dimensions of the inequalities in patterns of care and access to and uptake of cancer technologies, including for prevention, diagnostics, screening and treatment. We suggest that gaps in access and uptake of interventions are intimately linked with people's social identities and economic means.

* * *

We are concerned in this volume with how social, economic, race, gender and other structures intersect in different locations to create the health inequalities that are imbricated in cancer disease and deaths. The first chapter following this introduction, by Jorge Alberto Bernstein Iriart and Sahra Gibbon, explores the stratification of patienthood in Brazil as a consequence of uneven access to biomedical innovations in cancer diagnostics and treatment, such as targeted medications, gene panel screening and immunological drug interventions. Brazil's three-tiered health system constitutes a structure of persistent inequity that provides those Brazilians with private health insurance plans access to the newest biomedical innovations and interventions, while three in four lack such access. As they illustrate, people are not necessarily complicit in this inequality. Rather, Brazil's constitutional commitment to the provision of universal healthcare has given rise to another intervention deployed by patients, the process of judicialisation, pursued in the hope of obtaining access to the best course of treatment by forcing the state to fund the cost of drugs and technologies not otherwise available in the public health system. Through positioning the courts as mediators of social justice in cancer care, Brazilian patients have expanded the institutional scope of local and national politics of care.

Chapter 2 also illuminates the contested positionality of Brazilian oncologists who are faced with the need to balance institutional and governmental pressures to keep costs down, while applying the medical code of ethics and protecting their patients' needs. Their decisions must be negotiated within the guidelines of the health system, and accordingly oncologists anticipate prescribing different regimes to patients with the same needs, depending on patients' level of insurance or the clinic they attend. For some physicians, this difference is ethically unacceptable, leading them to inform patients of the option of judicialisation and to support them to pursue this process. But as Iriart and Gibbon note, there are conflicting positions on and impacts of judicialisation as an intervention, from the perspectives of oncologists, patients and cancer care clinics. Doctors must confront the inflated cost of new innovations, including extremely high-cost treatments and diagnostic protocols, for those patients able to successfully negotiate the judicialisation process, while they struggle to treat other patients who lack access to resources. Doctors accordingly face the untenable choice of having to choose between offering the best care possible to single patients or maintaining services for the greatest number of patients, so perpetuating patient stratification regardless of what choice they make. The chapter demonstrates the dynamic and fraught nature of the politics of care, highlighting the ways in which structural inequalities require constant negotiation by those seeking and those providing care.

While doctors struggle with ethical dilemmas on a daily basis, as Iriart and Gibbon illustrate, so too do researchers. Ethnography is by practice relational, and various authors explore the nexus between ethnographic research and intervention in the lives and cancer trajectories of their research participants. This is most explicit in Natalia Luxardo's and Linda Bennett's chapter on the experiences of marginalised women living in Entre Ríos province, Argentina, who survive and support their families by waste picking. Recognising the failure of prior interventions to increase the uptake of cervical cancer screening among such marginalised women, the project conceived by Luxardo was implemented as a five-year community intervention aimed at reducing the structural and cultural drivers of health inequalities. The project was informed by both social work and critical medical ethnography. Collaborations with communities were developed to facilitate interventions to improve nutrition, education and livelihoods, and so address the conditions underlying poor health. Luxardo's fieldwork praxis demonstrates the ethical obligation to address the immediate needs of people in deprived and marginalised communities, in order to ensure supportive and sustained relationships; in this respect she anticipates Burke's arguments in Chapter 4, too, of the importance of 'trust' in women's adherence to cancer therapy. Robinson and Peréz, in Chapter 11, likewise address the ethical imperative of acknowledging the most pressing needs of their research participants. Luxardo's blended approach of social work and ethnography was crucial to building trust with women who too frequently were the targets of degrading and humiliating behaviour from people outside of their own communities. In this instance, the explicit coupling of intervention and ethnography supported a nuanced emic perspective on why women failed to engage with or disengaged from cancer screening. This insight could only be gained over time and through deep engagement with the multiple forms of structural violence that shaped women's vulnerability (Farmer 2004). As illustrated elsewhere too (Gregg 2003, 2011; McMullin 2016; Mika 2021; Wailoo 2011), extended histories of structural and direct personal violence, and legacies of racism, underpin how people engage with health providers and other professional workers, perpetuate emotions and actions of stigma and shame, and undermine women's motivation to participate in cancer interventions.

Nancy J. Burke in Chapter 4 attends to the experiences of patient navigation as an intervention designed specifically to counter barriers to access among disadvantaged communities within the context of the US safety-net system. Here, the focus is not on structural violence or vulnerability, nor the explicit violence that often characterises face-to-face interactions, although these are factors that influence cancer outcomes in the United States as elsewhere. Rather, she turns to the role of patient navigators, and their work in deflecting anxiety, awkwardness and fear through regular and often humorous interactions, including among cancer care staff and patients. Here Burke's use of the term 'improvisation' is not concerned with making do with lack, as is characteristic of patient care in Botswana (Livingston 2012) or in Uganda (Mika 2021), but in relational 'groundwork', intended to smooth over disharmonies for poor and disadvantaged patients attending public hospital breast clinics and cancer survivorship group meetings. These are women who live with continuing precarity, in insecure housing, on extremely low incomes, without health insurance and often without family support; they are women who recurrently face discrimination and stigma because of their lack of choice in how they must live. The patient navigators at the centre of Burke's chapter are charged with promoting access to timely diagnosis and reducing delays in treatment of cancer. In her study area, the intervention was initiated in an effort to redress women's late presentation with advanced disease, and at times their withdrawal from treatment, with resultant deaths at disproportionate high rates that made literal how poverty shapes outcomes. Laughter helped women overcome fear, anxiety and embarrassment. It helped them to address the side effects of treatment immediately and in the long term; this included in relation to the embodied effects of changing hormone levels for most women, for whom adjuvant therapy was a necessary treatment and precautionary measure to survival. Burke elucidates how successful interventions in cancer care depend on interpersonal relationality, and personal caring and kindness, as much as they do on commitments to resource allocation designed to close gaps in access and uptake of care.

Interventions directed at cancer prevention and control are diverse, although, as the authors in this volume illustrate, the predominant focus is still on individual behaviour and compliance, even when structural determinants of cancer and its inequities are acknowledged. Contributors significantly deepen our understanding of the politics of cancer-related interventions and innovations across multiple scales and engage with interventions both within and external to health systems. In Chapter 5, Cecilia Coale Van Hollen, for instance, critically engages with reproductive cancer screening camps conducted in Tamil Nadu in the south of India, which have the explicit objective of increasing the uptake of Pap smears and mammograms for the early detection of cervical and breast cancer.

The camps are redolent of the vasectomy and tubal ligation camps initiated from the early 1970s (Wilson 2017) and of later HIV testing camps (Nataraj 2011). These camps fall under the remit of health promotion, and are primarily directed at lower-class women, who are assumed by cancer educators to be ignorant. Yet the information provided to them relies on assumptions about their knowledge and behaviour, and is obscured by euphemisms, failing to adequately explain the biology of cancer risk and the direct relationship between HPV infection and cervical cancer. The public nature of these camps, and taboos that constrain discussions about sexuality and reproduction, inhibit women from addressing reproductive health issues with educators, so illustrating the inappropriateness of these public interventions.

By applying an ethnographic lens, Van Hollen reveals that cancer screening camps lack both efficacy and cultural resonance; they are out of place in terms of connecting with women's everyday lives, whilst they reinforce judgmental discourses of breast and cervical cancer causality that reflect dominant constructions of class, femininity and morality. Early marriage, high parity, poor hygiene, undergoing 'too many' abortions and tobacco use are all constructed as negative, morally undesirable and 'improper lifestyle choices' explicitly linked with cervical cancer causality. This is consistent with negative attitudes to cervical cancer, and so by association also screening tests, documented in Tamil Nadu as elsewhere in India and worldwide (see, for example, Gregg 2003, 2011; Hunt 2008; Martinez 2018; Pop 2022). Discourses also consistently tie these behaviours to lower-caste and lower-class Indian women, who in their failure to achieve the ideals of middle-class femininity are responsible for risk and consequent disease. Breast cancer risk, in contrast, is associated with behaviours linked with middle-class affluence in the Indian imaginary – delayed marriage, delayed childbearing, failure to breastfeed or breastfeed enough, fatty diets, lack of exercise, all of which are represented as the class-specific failures of middle-class women. Van Hollen draws attention to the highly contradictory messages around reproductive cancer causalities communicated in screening camps, while she also establishes how cancer education operates simultaneously as a public health intervention and as a social intervention that explicitly reproduces dominant gender and class norms. These morally loaded interventions rely on representations of cancer causality that lay the blame for both breast and cervical cancer with individual women, whilst ignoring the structural inequalities that drive high incidence and morality in India. This is despite increasing criticism of the tendency to ignore the structural drivers of cancer in favour of individual behaviour modification by those seeking to measure the relative impacts of individual versus structural interventions for cancer prevention (Martin-Morena, Ruiz-Segovia and Diaz-Rubio 2021).

A diagnosis of cervical cancer – a highly stigmatised disease in many societies – creates care work by compelling women to contain disclosure of the disease in order to prevent moral stigma directed towards their loved ones. Practices of containment become an important form of care that women living with cancer provide for others, with stigma and discrimination emerging as important barriers to accessing cancer screening, diagnosis and care. As many of the contributing authors illustrate, these barriers interact with disparities in health prevention and healthcare to shape cancer trajectories and outcomes among a range of vulnerable populations and across geographies and nation states. But these are not immutable. Linda Bennett and Hanum Atikasari, in their research in Indonesia documented in Chapter 6, like Natalie Luxardo, found themselves crossing between intervention and observation, even though they had chosen not to recruit women who were undergoing treatment or in the palliative stages of cancer. The reality of the field bore out the very real limitations of formal systems of cancer care available to women living with cervical cancer, most notably for women who were socially isolated, living without family support, without transport and with very limited income. Originally, their concern had been to avoid burdening women with research when they were at their most vulnerable, but women sought ongoing engagement with and support from members of the research team. As the research progressed, the researchers were willingly drawn into necessary informal interventions including providing women with emotional support and companionship, access to information and interpretation of diagnostic test results, facilitating transport to and from treatment and organising emergency financial assistance. In this respect, as researchers, they played the kind of role that Burke described of navigators in California, where non-family members are often essential brokers between patients and the healthcare system.

Insights into the forms, impacts and responses to cancer-related stigma in chapters on Argentina, Indonesia and India also highlight intersections between how blame for specific cancers is highly gendered and imbued with dominant and competing discourses of gendered and sexual morality. In Argentina, women who are routinely stigmatised within the health system, due to their marginal social identities, turn their moral gaze outward to criticise the morality of women gynaecologists in a discourse that morally condemns these female doctors. In Indonesia, Bennett and Atikasari observed that women often seek to deflect and contain the moral injury associated with cervical cancer diagnosis by forming new informal care networks, often constituted of fellow cancer survivors, that may replace prior personal relationships which, following their diagnosis, are no longer considered safe. This reflects Sophie Bowlby's (2012: 2110) thinking on the shifting temporalities of care and carescapes in which 'fellow travellers will change over time'.

The challenges to care relate to all forms of cancer and to caregivers as well as care recipients. Nursing care, Livingston (2012: 96) illustrates, is a 'moral endeavour' that involves hard labour. It includes the clinical work of medication, wound dressing and monitoring; the physical labour of toileting, cleaning and feeding; the 'sentimental' work of empathy, expressions of compassion and kindness; and expected constraint of the medical practitioners' own emotions that might variously include horror and disgust, pity and confusion, despair and sadness. These contradictions in care intensify when nurses must provide care to terminally ill people in settings where resources are severely limited. In rural Senegal, as Noémi Tousignant describes in Chapter 7, nurses' capacity to care is constrained by the immediate limitations of under-resourced rural health posts in which they work, including the unavailability of opiates to alleviate suffering, so leaving nurses with no option but to offer patients less potent and inadequate pain relief medications. Tousignant focuses on young people dying from liver cancer. Their poor prognosis is associated with very late diagnosis, reflecting a local history of systemic failures in prevention and early detection for both hepatitis B and liver cancer. As she describes, nurses were troubled by the young age of their liver cancer patients, their certainty that their patients' death was imminent and the speed at which their patients died. She conceptualises how these characteristics constitute 'untimely deaths', out of sync with the expected life span of young people, and divergent from normative globalised and locally embraced cancer temporalities.

When nurses were certain that further medical intervention would not prolong life and may reduce quality of life, Tousignant explains, some chose to strategically conceal and reveal prognostic knowledge to patients and their families to prevent wasteful and potentially harmful efforts to seek further diagnostic and therapeutic resources. In such cases revelation is carefully managed through the choice of an appropriate family member, who would ideally be resilient enough to cope with the knowledge of certain death, discreet enough not to disclose this information directly to the patient, and have sufficient authority to avert unnecessary therapies. Imminent death heightens nurses' perceptions of the need to maximise patients' quality of life by seeking to instil hope, calmness and continued social connection; they perceive that concealing terminal diagnosis acts to protect quality of life. Families support the strategic withholding from patients of the trajectory of the disease, and report the impact of hope in motivating patients to continue to eat, to practise self-care and to socially engage (see also Banerjee 2020; Gordon and Paci 1997; Kaufert 1999). This is not to suggest that all patients are ignorant of their diagnosis and prognosis. As Banerjee (2020: 42–48) describes in India, patients knowingly collude with non-disclosure to limit distress to others and to minimise stigma and isolation of one's self or family members. This chosen pathway of 'soft truth' (Bennett 1999) was aimed at containing the suffering inherent in diagnosis and prognosis. In Senegal, revelation and concealment therefore both constitute practices of care, directed at reducing suffering, maintaining quality of life, and providing expressed compassionate care in the absence of biomedical interventions, adequate palliative drugs and formal systems of institutional support. Tousignant's work further emphasises the relationality of care, through extending our understanding of the subtle negotiations involved in collaborations between family members and health workers seeking to ease the physical and emotional anguish and distress of terminally ill patients.

Attention to the practices of care enacted by health professionals is continued by Falia Varelaki in her hospital-based ethnography of a cancer ward in Athens, Greece, in Chapter 8. In this example, oncologists in 'Ward A' explicitly adopt 'improvisational practices' that enable them to reduce systemic barriers to timely access to care by subverting guidelines and engaging with their patients in the spaces between and outside of formal appointment times. Such improvisation is characteristic of medical care in any resource constrained environment, as Julie Livingston (2012) so powerfully illustrates for Botswana. But clinical practice is also one of testing and assessing, adapting knowledge to definable symptoms and accessible and affordable resources, titrating and adjusting, 'tinkering' (Mol 2008). As Varelaki describes, health professionals resist and seek to level the impact of inequalities within the health system. In working in Ward A, they explicitly understand care as necessary for mitigating the dehumanising effects of the corporeal suffering and bodily changes endured by their patients, and as a form of social healing protecting patients from social isolation and loneliness. In attending to the everyday interactions of patients and their care providers, Varelaki offers deep insight into the actions of health workers, including oncologists, residents and nurses who perceive their care practices as protecting the dignity, privacy and humanity of patients with advanced cancer. In describing the deeply humanising power of physical contact between cancer patients and their carers in 'Ward A', she highlights the ever-present physicality of end-of-life care, contributing another layer to the discourse on care and relationality that emerges in this volume.

In Chapter 9, Cinzia Greco is concerned with breast cancer in Italy, and the regional inequities that lead people throughout the country to regard southern Italy as the 'south-within-the-north'. In the poor provinces in which she conducted fieldwork, cancer is understood by women not as exceptional but as an additional hardship, compounding their chronic everyday experiences of marginality, limited personal resources, household and community poverty and their alienation within an ill-resourced health system. Women's resilience in living with cancer is an extension of their established coping mechanisms, in which family and community support are vital; personal connections and care fill the gaps that elsewhere might be met by higher-functioning health systems, patient navigation programmes or formalised community-based cancer care. How women managed breast cancer, Greco observes, depended on social relationships of reciprocity and ongoing care obligations, and subsequently women affected by breast cancer negotiated their own care and survival in relation to their everyday lives. In this context, she describes women who delayed diagnosis to avoid disrupting and distressing family members; deferred advising family members of a diagnosis while they proceeded with everyday family tasks; and who minimised the impact of surgery for the sake of others. At the same time, once cancer had been diagnosed, women described the importance of relationality in coping with the disease. While arguing that a positive and determined attitude might aid recovery, they also sought and were offered support from friends, neighbours, fellow congregants and the family members they regarded as most resilient. In this respect, Greco's analysis echoes Gordon and Paci's (1997) account from Tuscany, Italy, of the social 'embeddedness' of cancer narratives within a wider narrative of social unity and hierarchy. But also, women resisted catastrophising their diagnosis; they saw cancer as something 'we [the family] will get through together', one of the many health problems in the present and previously, along with other economic and interpersonal problems which they and other family members were experiencing or had experienced in the past.

In Chapter 10, on cancer in Denmark, Rikke Sand Andersen, Sara Marie Hebsgaard Offersen and Camila Hoffmann Merrild disrupt assumptions that 'welfare societies' such as Denmark are devoid of social inequalities. In their exploration of medical semiotics, they elucidate the inequalities of cancer risk and disease as experienced by low-income Danes living on the margins of the welfare state. They propose that individuals whose lives are scarred by constant stress and trauma over time have 'noisy bodies'. This 'noise' makes it difficult for clinicians to distinguish and attribute significance to subtle symptoms and bodily changes. But also, as they illustrate, entrenched discriminatory attitudes by doctors towards this population mean that people's accounts of bodily disease and distress are routinely underestimated and dismissed; it is all 'noise', not to be taken seriously.

In Denmark as in far less equitable settings, in high-, middle- and low-income countries, people with lower incomes and low levels of education may be less familiar with and so less attentive to bodily symptoms indicative of cancer or a similar serious condition – a persistent cough, blood in stools or unexplained pain, for example. Multiple health problems cloud people's capacity to differentiate and treat seriously some conditions but not others, such that their 'noisy bodies' were easily dismissed themselves and by others in their family, as well as by general practitioners and nurses. Those with least power, living in compromised economic and social circumstances, were also less likely to act on 'do not delay' messages and present to a clinic, both because of the logistic and financial difficulties of presenting for care and as a result of their anxiety about anticipated dismissive treatment by clinic staff on presentation. They were also mindful of public health advice to people not to overuse medical resources, part of a concerted effort by the government to drive down waiting times for specialist appointments, surgeries and continuing treatments (Andersen et al. 2010; Andersen and Tørring 2022).

We have observed the flow of support and engagement between researchers and research participants in Argentina (Luxardo and Bennett) and Indonesia (Bennett and Atikasari), and this is the case also in Kelly Fagan Robinson's and Ignacia Arteaga Pérez's research in the United Kingdom, as presented in Chapter 11. They proactively facilitated an 'economy of care' between themselves and research participants from underserved and marginalised communities, including Gypsy Roma Travellers. In this setting, redolent of the 'noise' about which Andersen, Offersen and Merrild write, cancer was situated in relation to other concerns that impacted people's everyday lives and livelihoods. 'It wasn't that cancer was silent', Robinson and Perez explain, but rather, it was 'ongoing white noise in a landscape of sonic-booms.' The 'economy of care' which the external researchers developed – providing food vouchers, paying for the use of community resources and compensating participants for their time – helped build trust with the research participants. In this chapter, the authors are concerned with local understandings of 'care' and 'risk' that help explain resistance to cancer screening. The people with whom they worked, labelled as hard-to-reach, were deeply suspicious of the care provided to them, and like other marginalised populations in other chapters in this volume, they brought to any care setting extensive experience of humiliation, structural and personal violence. Authoritarian relationships undermine care settings, and for Gypsy Roma Travellers and others forced to live on the margins of society, 'care' was consistently associated with the removal of children, incarceration and forced compliance with addiction recovery and probation regimes. For many participants, care was routinely experienced as coercive; and their experiences of discrimination when seeking healthcare and other social services reinforced deep suspicion and reluctance to present.

In Chapter 12, Laurence Kotobi and Carolyn Sargent further interrogate social and health disparities within high-income countries, through identifying and theorising the 'intractable inequalities' experienced by low-income migrant women of African origin who seek cancer care in France. Here as elsewhere, access to cancer care is largely tied to reliable livelihoods and stable residence, but immigration laws allow people without residential visas to stay in the country for medical care if indicated (Ticktin 2011). This includes African women with cancer diagnoses travelling to France on tourist visas, as well as women born overseas with residential permits living in France. Kotobi and Sargent highlight how structural vulnerabilities and inequalities complicate the ability of people to manage serious health problems concurrently with economic and social precarities; women, men and their families may live in over-crowded and poorly maintained dwellings, in deserted buildings without connected amenities or on the streets, seeking to avoid harassment while they ensure they survive. Women who present for cancer treatment are often unfamiliar with both legal and health systems, entitlements and treatment options. But their right to medical care is not supported by other structures of care, and in the context of limited multilingual skills of oncologists and the lack of reliable translators, Kotobi and Sargent found themselves compelled to act as interpreters to enable patients to engage satisfactorily with oncologists. In this study, their roles in interpreting were not simply translating, but ensuring women's comprehension of biomedical information that was not communicated in lay terms or had not been delivered in a patient-friendly manner. The researchers' presence as both translators and observers in patient–doctor interactions also provided social support for migrant women, who because of their migrant status had to negotiate cancer care without well-established social networks.

Kotobi and Sargent again illuminate how the informal intervention of ethnographers, as they facilitate medical care for cancer and provide other forms of care, can potentially impact on the health outcomes of participants.

* * *

Medical anthropologists routinely face ethical dilemmas in relation to access to and provision of care and the affordability of medication and other treatment. The study of illness places emotional demands on ethnographers as well as on those with whom they work, at times placing them in an awkward position of leaning on people with limited energy and few resources. The challenges of undertaking such research is perhaps especially true for cancer; depending on the type of cancer and its trajectory, those directly affected and others around them may have little energy to give; cancer takes up all their efforts. It is, as S. Lochlann Jain (2013) describes it, a total social fact, overwhelming individuals and their families.

Cancer, as an imagined single spectre, is still deeply feared. The language around cancer already portrays care as a multidirectional phenomenon occurring between people, anticipating extreme suffering, pain, distress and irreconcilable loss. This is not necessarily the case; for some of us, a diagnosis of cancer, at an early stage, with a health system that operates efficiently for those with resources and insurance, is promptly resolved (Manderson 2022). But elsewhere, as we illustrate, inequalities intersect, producing complexities that limit the effectiveness of interventions to prevent or promptly and effectively treat cancer. This points to the need for comprehensive action to address inequalities in order to address cancer's distribution and troubled consequences. In understanding these inequalities and the variations across time and space, we are faced with significant gaps in research into the experiences and meanings of cancer for those affected, as well as the suffering, strategies and resilience of people living with cancer.

The contributing authors in this volume provide evidence of the ways in which chronically unequal life circumstances flow into people's experiences of bodily anomaly, diagnostic processes, treatments and outcomes. At the level of health systems, worldwide people experience wide gaps in access to health and welfare services; nurses and others lack the ability to refer those in need to an appropriate support service when there are none, and patients have access only to services that are experienced as unsafe. The institutional violence experienced by Argentinian women, for example, the legacies of racism in the United

Kingdom, and the disregard of the powerlessness of immigrant African women in France and among poor Danes in Denmark, all draw attention to the need to address structural vulnerability in order to improve population engagement with cancer screening, people's willingness to present early for diagnosis, and their capacity to access and receive care.

In this context, researchers are embedded within the politics of care we seek to untangle, and so are necessarily part of the solution; as the authors note here, there is no way to document suffering and not act. Anthropology's ability to respond to real-life circumstances is reflected in these chapters, as authors pivot to meet the shifting priorities and needs of people living with cancer, so performing a practice of grounded ethics. While we began this chapter – and this book – with a sense of urgency for more anthropological studies of different cancers, in different settings, we conclude by advocating a reciprocal and grounded ethics as a necessary feature for ethnographers of cancer who wish to challenge the reproduction of cancer inequalities, and by doing so, engage explicitly with a 'politics of care' in which cancer research is acknowledged as an essentially political project.

Poverty creates the preconditions for pathologies and poor outcomes. The statistics that illustrate cancer's discrepancies make clear that social exclusion, economic precarity and political vulnerability predict the likelihood of developing cancer and late presentation for treatment, and those who live in such circumstances are also less likely to be able to access good quality of care. Achille Mbembe (2003, 2019), in articulating a theory of necropolitics, sets out the underlying ideologies, institutions and structures that determine who lives and who dies, in which vast numbers of people live and work under conditions that compromise their life chances in every respect. The global distribution of cancer instantiates this neglect, a disregard of the lives of some and the correlate privilege of other lives. Judith Butler (2004, 2010) defines this disregard in terms of grievability. Her example is of refugees, but the notion of grievability can be applied to any health problem. Cancer is particularly powerful in this respect including in Butler's own example: refugee status, internal displacement and statelessness all prevent the statistical accounting that points to people's health status and deprives them of care.

This does not mean that people who are poor are compliant or overwhelmed with hopelessness, and that they do not seek to find solutions to soften the challenges that they face. The chapters that examine cancer in Argentina (Luxardo and Bennett), the United States (Burke), Indonesia (Bennett and Atikasari) and the United Kingdom

(Robinson and Pérez) all provide evidence that people living in conditions of deprivation face compelling 'hierarchies of risk' on a daily basis, and that capacities for self-care are entwined with the care work of individuals living with cancer. Yet notwithstanding disadvantage, suffering and vulnerability, people routinely negotiate local carescapes. Individual resilience draws on the unique dynamics of reciprocity and community norms that help people gain perspective of their poor health and seek support through families, communities, healthcare and other support systems, and cancer peer and advocacy organisations. This points also to the multiple insights contributors offer on the nature of relationality in cancer care, and the efficacy that stems from relational practices which place people's humanity at the centre of interactions within and beyond the medical domain.

This volume establishes the 'politics of care' as a rich conceptual terrain for interrogating intersecting inequalities, and the diverse meanings and experiences of care, in relation to cancer. Contributors explore the nexus between interventions, care and inequality across a broad trajectory encompassing health promotion, cancer screening, diagnosis, judicialisation, treatment, patient navigation and navigators, and the provision of palliative care. In doing so, they demonstrate how ethnographic enquiry has the potential to inform appropriate modalities for cancer education that need to be grounded in local understandings of how people communicate about health and gender, their bodies, morality and notions of cancer causality. Moreover, contributors reveal why the design of cancer interventions must take into account both histories of marginalisation and structural violence, as well as the contextual realities of people's everyday existence that determine their ability and willingness to engage with interventions. These contributions have begun what must be a continuing challenge in response to the vast inequalities embedded in the social epidemiology of cancer, which is to understand in fine detail how cancer disparities function and thus how they can be ameliorated. In resource-poor settings, we need to know more about screening, treatment and care, and the implications of this in terms of life outcomes, for it is not enough to simply note the inequalities as numeric trends. We need more work, too, on understanding the topography of inequality, to understand the dynamics of personal income, power and privilege and financing systems. We need to better understand the structures and infrastructures that determine prevention, screening, treatment, palliative care and death, to provide insight into the different ways in which different cancers unravel. We need to continually trouble the global and local inequalities that influence cancer screening, diagnosis and care, and to support advocacy based on our work that addresses the politics in which human lives are differently valued. In short, anthropology must commit to a sustained radical interrogation of the 'politics of care' as a fundamental basis for informing real-world solutions to cancer inequalities both within and between different societies.

References

Andersen, Rikke Sand, Bjarke Paarup, Peter Vedsteda, Bro Fleming and Jens Soendergaard. 2010. '"Containment" as an analytical framework for understanding patient delay: A qualitative study of cancer patients' symptom interpretation processes', *Social Science & Medicine* 71(2): 378–385.

Andersen, Rikke Sand and Marie Louise Tørring, eds. 2022. *Cancer Entangled: Anticipation, acceleration and the Danish state*. New Brunswick, NJ: Rutgers University Press.

Armin, Julie, Nancy J. Burke and Laura Eichelberger, eds. 2019. *Negotiating Structural Vulnerability in Cancer Control*. Santa Fe: University of New Mexico Press.

Banerjee, Dwaipayan. 2020. *Enduring Cancer: Life, death, and diagnosis in Delhi*. Durham, NC: Duke University Press.

Basu, Partha. 2019. 'HPV vaccination and screening for cervical cancer'. In *Reducing Social Inequalities in Cancer: Evidence and priorities for research*, edited by Salvatore Vaccarella, Joannie Lortet-Tieulent, Rodolfo Saracci, David I. Conway, Kurt Straif and Christopher P. Wild, 217–221. Lyon, France: National Agency for Research on Cancer.

Bennett, Elizabeth S. 1999. 'Soft truth: Ethics and cancer in northeast Thailand', *Anthropology & Medicine* 6(3): 395–404.

Bowlby, Sophie. 2012. 'Recognising the time–space dimensions of care: Caringscapes and carescapes', *Environment and Planning A* 44(9): 2101–2118.

Butler, Judith. 2004. *Precarious Life: The powers of mourning and violence*. London: Verso.

Butler, Judith. 2010. *Frames of War: When is life grievable?* London: Verso.

Farmer, Paul. 2004. 'An anthropology of structural violence', *Current Anthropology* 45(3): 305–317. https://www.jstor.org/stable/10.1086/382250.

Garvey, Gail and Joan Cunningham. 2019. 'Social inequalities and cancer in Indigenous populations'. In *Reducing Social Inequalities in Cancer: Evidence and priorities for research*, edited by Salvatore Vaccarella, Joannie Lortet-Tieulent, Rodolfo Saracci, David I. Conway, Kurt Straif and Christopher P. Wild, 78–83. Lyon, France: National Agency for Research on Cancer.

Global Cancer Observatory. 2020. 'Estimated age-standardized incidence rates (world) in 2020, worldwide, both sexes, all ages'. Accessed 21 June 2022. https://gco.iarc.fr/today/online-analysis.

Gordon, Deborah and Eugenio Paci. 1997. 'Disclosure practices and cultural narratives: Understanding concealment and silence around cancer in Tuscany, Italy', *Social Science & Medicine* 44(10): 1433–1452.

Gregg, Jessica L. 2003. *Virtually Virgins: Sexual strategies and cervical cancer in Recife, Brazil*. Stanford, CA: Stanford University Press.

Gregg, Jessica L. 2011. 'An unanticipated source of hope: Stigma and cervical cancer in Brazil', *Medical Anthropology Quarterly* 25(1): 70–84.

Hunt, Linda. 2008. 'Moral reasoning and the meaning of cancer: Causal explanations of oncologists and patients in southern Mexico', *Medical Anthropology Quarterly* 12(3): 298–318.

Ivanova, Dara, Iris Wallenburg and Roland Bal. 2016. 'Care in place: A case study of assembling a carescape', *Sociology of Health and Illness* 38(8): 1336–1349.

Jain, S. Lochlann. 2013. *Malignant: How cancer becomes us*. Berkeley: University of California Press.

Jemal, Ahmedin and Rebecca Siegel. 2019. 'Social inequalities in cancer burden between Black and White populations in the USA'. In *Reducing Social Inequalities in Cancer: Evidence and priorities for research*, edited by Salvatore Vaccarella, Joannie Lortet-Tieulent, Rodolfo Saracci, David I. Conway, Kurt Straif and Christopher P. Wild, 89–93. Lyon, France: National Agency for Research on Cancer.

Kaufert, Joseph M. 1999. 'Cultural mediation in cancer diagnosis and end of life decision-making: The experience of Aboriginal patients in Canada', *Anthropology and Medicine* 6(3): 405–421.

Kline, Nolan. 2019. *Pathogenic Policing: Immigration enforcement and health in the U.S. South*. New Brunswick, NJ: Rutgers University Press.

Knaul, Felicia, Julie Gralow, Rifat Atun and Afsan Bhadelia. 2012. *Closing the Cancer Divide: An equity imperative*. Boston, MA: Harvard Global Equity Initiative.

Lau, Rosenlund, Marie Svensson, Natasja Kingod and Ayo Wahlberg. 2021. 'Carescapes unsettled: COVID-19 and the reworking of "stable illnesses" in welfare state Denmark'. In *Viral Loads: Anthropologies of urgency in the time of COVID-19*, edited by Lenore Manderson, Nancy J. Burke and Ayo Wahlberg, 324–343. London: UCL Press.

Liberman, Jonathan. 2019. 'The role of law in reducing global cancer inequalities'. In *Reducing Social Inequalities in Cancer: Evidence and priorities for research*, edited by Salvatore Vaccarella, Joannie Lortet-Tieulent, Rodolfo Saracci, David I. Conway, Kurt Straif and Christopher P. Wild, 167–173. Lyon, France: National Agency for Research on Cancer.

Livingston, Julie. 2012. *Improvising Medicine: An African oncology ward in an emerging cancer epidemic*. Durham, NC: Duke University Press.

Lora-Wainwright, Anna. 2013. *Fighting for Breath: Living morally and dying of cancer in a Chinese village*. Honolulu: University of Hawaii Press.

McMullin, Juliet. 2016. 'Cancer', *Annual Review of Anthropology* 45: 251–266.

McMullin Juliet and Diane Weiner, eds. 2008. *Confronting Cancer: Metaphors, advocacy and anthropology*. Santa Fe, NM: School of Advanced Research.

Manderson, Lenore. 2015. 'Cancer enigmas and agendas'. In *Anthropologies of Cancer in Transnational Worlds*, edited by Holly Mathews, Nancy J. Burke and Erin Kampriani, 241–254. London: Routledge.

Manderson, Lenore. 2020. '"Lifestyle" disease on the margins', *American Anthropologist* 122(3): 655–656. https://doi.org/10.1111/aman.13448.

Manderson, Lenore. 2022. 'Cancers' multiplicities: Anthropologies of interventions and care'. In *A Companion to Medical Anthropology*, 2nd edn, edited by Merrill Singer, Pamela Erickson and Cesar Abadia, 260–274. London: Wiley Blackwell.

Manderson, Lenore. 2023. 'Urgency, modernity and pace in cancer care'. In *Cancer Entangled: Anticipation, acceleration and the Danish state*, edited by Rikke Sand Andersen and Marie Louise Tørring. New Brunswick, NJ: Rutgers University Press.

Martin-Moreno, Jose, Natalia Ruiz-Segovia and Eduardo Diaz-Rubio. 2021. 'Behavioural and structural interventions in cancer prevention: Towards the 2030 SDG horizon', *Molecular Oncology* 15(3): 801–808.

Martinez, Rebecca. 2018. *Marked Women: The cultural politics of cervical cancer in Venezuela*. Palo Alto, CA: Stanford University Press.

Mathews, Holly, Nancy J. Burke and Eirini Kampriani, eds. 2015. *Anthropologies of Cancer in Transnational Worlds*. London: Routledge.

Mbembe, Achille. 2003. 'Necropolitics', *Public Culture* 15(1): 11–40.

Mbembe, Achille. 2019. *Necropolitics*. Durham, NC: Duke University Press.

Meheus, Filip, Rifat Atun and André Ilbawi. 2019. 'The role of health systems in addressing inequalities in access to cancer control'. In *Reducing Social Inequalities in Cancer: Evidence and priorities for research*, edited by Salvatore Vaccarella, Joannie Lortet-Tieulent, Rodolfo Saracci, David I. Conway, Kurt Straif and Christopher P. Wild, 137–149. Lyon, France: National Agency for Research on Cancer.

Mika, Marissa. 2021. *Africanizing Oncology: Creativity, crisis and cancer in Uganda*. Athens, OH: Ohio University Press.

Mol, Annemarie. 2008. *The Logic of Care: Health and the problem of patient choice*. London and New York: Routledge.

Mulemi, Benson A. 2010. *Coping with Cancer and Adversity: Hospital ethnography in Kenya*. Leiden, The Netherlands: Africa Studies Centre.

Nataraj, Shyamala. 2011. 'Consent is compulsory: Informed consent in HIV testing of pregnant women in India'. PhD dissertation. School of Public Health and Preventive Medicine, Monash University.

Pop, Cristina A. 2022. *The Cancer Within: Reproduction, cultural transformation, and health care in Romania*. New Brunswick, NJ: Rutgers University Press.

Sarfati, Diana. 2019. 'Why social inequalities matter in the cancer continuum'. In *Reducing Social Inequalities in Cancer: Evidence and priorities for research*, edited by Salvatore Vaccarella,

Joannie Lortet-Tieulent, Rodolfo Saracci, David I. Conway, Kurt Straif and Christopher P. Wild, 15–24. Lyon, France: National Agency for Research on Cancer.

Sullivan, Richard, Omar Shamieh, Tezer Kutluk, Adel Daoud and Adam P. Coutts. 2019. 'Inequality and cancer: The conflict ecosystem and refugees'. In *Reducing Social Inequalities in Cancer: Evidence and priorities for research*, edited by Salvatore Vaccarella, Joannie Lortet-Tieulent, Rodolfo Saracci, David I. Conway, Kurt Straif and Christopher P. Wild, 85–88. Lyon, France: National Agency for Research on Cancer.

Ticktin, Miriam I. 2011. *Casualties of Care: Immigration and the politics of humanitarianism in France*. Berkeley: University of California Press.

Vaccarella, Salvatore, Esther De Vries, Mónica S. Sierra, David I. Conway and Johan P. Mackenbach. 2019. 'Social inequalities in cancer within countries'. In *Reducing Social Inequalities in Cancer: Evidence and priorities for research*, edited by Salvatore Vaccarella, Joannie Lortet-Tieulent, Rodolfo Saracci, David I. Conway, Kurt Straif and Christopher P. Wild, 63–78. Lyon, France: National Agency for Research on Cancer.

Vaccarella, Salvatore, Joannie Lortet-Tieulent, Rodolfo Saracci, David I. Conway, Kurt Straif and Christopher P. Wild, eds. 2019. *Reducing Social Inequalities in Cancer: Evidence and priorities for research*. IARC Scientific Publications, No. 168. Lyon, France: National Agency for Research on Cancer.

Wailoo, Keith. 2011. *How Cancer Crossed the Color Line*. Oxford: Oxford University Press.

Weiner, Diane, ed. 1999. *Preventing and Controlling Cancer in North America: A cross-cultural perspective*. Westport, CT: Praeger.

Wild, Christopher P. 2019. 'Social inequalities and cancer: The imperative to act'. In *Reducing Social Inequalities in Cancer: Evidence and priorities for research*, edited by Salvatore Vaccarella, Joannie Lortet-Tieulent, Rodolfo Saracci, David I. Conway, Kurt Straif and Christopher P. Wild, 1–6. Lyon, France: National Agency for Research on Cancer.

Wilson, Kalpana. 2017. 'In the name of reproductive rights: Race, neoliberalism and the embodied violence of population policies', *New Formations* 91: 50–68.

2
Biomedical innovations, cancer care and health inequities: stratified patienthood in Brazil

Jorge Alberto Bernstein Iriart and Sahra Gibbon

> It is very exhausting, very stressful to do oncology in Brazil today, especially if you work in both scenarios [public and private], and I would say the vast majority of oncologists today, in one way or another, work in both scenarios . . . It is very frustrating . . . For people who live this every day it is revolting. It is very bad. We live in a schizophrenic system. In the morning I am one, in the afternoon I am another . . . because if I am in the public outpatient clinic, I have a portfolio of treatment [without access to many biomedical innovations], if I am in my private practice I have another, for the same patient. (Dr Estevão,[1] oncologist)

Dr Estevão shares this experience with many oncologists in Brazil who work in both public and private cancer clinics. Although the health system is underpinned by the principle of the universal right to health, Brazilian medical professionals face the daily ethical challenge of dealing with unequal access to genomic biotechnologies for their patients, including those linked to the promise and pursuit of personalised medicine.

Personalised medicine has raised expectations about the impact of developing so-called 'intelligent' drugs targeted at the patient's genetic makeup (Prainsack 2017; Tutton 2014). Oncology is considered at the forefront of this promise, with the potential for cancer treatment to be rapidly transformed by incorporating genomic biotechnologies, such as targeted medications, gene panel screening and immunological drug interventions (Cambrosio et al. 2018; Keating and Cambrosio 2011; Kerr and Cunningham-Burley 2015). Treatments with target drugs that act on genetic mutations and immunotherapies have in some cases generated significant improvement in the clinical results of certain types of cancer, resulting in less toxicity, fewer side-effects and increased overall survival (Gyawali and Sullivan 2017; Røe 2017). Some types of cancer, such as advanced melanoma and lung and kidney cancers, for which there were few or no effective treatments, now have therapeutic options that may positively impact patients' overall survival and quality of life. The high cost of these technologies, however, poses significant challenges concerning equity of access and benefits for all in the context of public health provision (Day et al. 2017), with emerging research suggesting that this is particularly problematic in low- and middle-income countries (Gyawali and Sullivan 2017; Iriart 2019; Røe 2017).

Drawing on ethnographic research in the field of oncology in Brazil's Northeast region, we discuss how oncologists and patients in public and private cancer clinics perceive, understand and negotiate strategies to address inequities in access to high-cost personalised technologies, such as targeted cancer drugs and immunotherapies. We describe and analyse the dilemmas faced by oncologists as they negotiate the challenges of newer and more expensive medical interventions in a context of inequitable and variable access and look at how strategies used in an arena of resource rationalisation create new patient stratifications that sit alongside and reproduce old inequities. The concept of inequities we employ in this context refers to inequalities that are unjust, systematic, unnecessary and preventable (Whitehead and Dahlgren 2006). We demonstrate how in Brazil inequities in accessing cancer prevention, diagnosis and treatment persist alongside emerging new inequalities, in a situation that both reflects and informs how precision oncology is being incorporated into the national health system. Building and extending engagement with the 'politics of care' in this collection, we argue that stratified patienthood in Brazil must be understood less as a product of global efforts to 'personalise' medicine and more as an outcome of dynamic, often disjunctured, social relations between the clinic, research and care. We observe how patients and health professionals engage in and are both the subjects and objects of diverse practices of 'improvisation' (Livingston 2012), 'pragmatism' (Lock, Kaufert and Harwood 1998) and 'containment' (Andersen et al. 2010) in constituting and traversing the uneven pathways of stratification at stake in Brazilian oncology.

Health technologies have a history and are embedded in a moral context. Their clinical applications are strongly influenced by cultural norms, politics and dominant scientific trends (Lock and Nguyen 2010). Innovations are embedded in a scientific 'imaginary' (Prainsack 2017; Tutton 2014) and are shaped by economic and political contexts and practices in 'local moral worlds' (Good 1995). Novel developments in cancer treatment in the United Kingdom and Europe are bringing about transformations in cancer patienthood (Kerr and Cunningham-Burley 2015), but are unevenly integrated across different fields of medical research and clinical practice and in the coordination of caregiving (Bourret, Keating and Cambrosio 2011; Day et al. 2017; Kerr et al. 2019). However, we know much less about these dynamics in lower-income and emerging economies in the global south. In examining how this is unevenly unfolding in the context of oncology in Northeast Brazil, we contribute to wider efforts to examine and theorise the shifting relationship between biological and social stratification in innovations in cancer treatment, research and care (Arteaga et al. 2019).

Brazilian public health, SUS and the 'right' to health

The 1988 Brazilian Constitution states that health is a citizen's right and that it is a duty of the state to promote health. That same year, Brazil established the Unified Health System or Sistema Único de Saúde – SUS) based on the principles of *equality* (providing access for all Brazilians, without any form of discrimination, to prevention and treatment services for patients with the same needs) and *comprehensive care* (providing access to preventive and curative interventions at all levels of the health system, from primary to tertiary care).

SUS has vastly improved access to primary and emergency care and helped Brazil to achieve universal vaccination, prenatal care coverage and reductions in infant mortality (Paim et al. 2011). However, in practice, the Brazilian health system is not unified but fragmented into public, private and supplementary health subsystems. SUS, or what is in practice a public subsystem, is financed by the state and serves approximately 75.6 per cent of the population (or 159 million people) (ANS 2019). The private subsector includes profitable and charitable institutions and receives financing from public and private sources. The supplementary health subsector covers various private health plans and is subsidised by the state (Paim et al. 2011).[2] There is wide variation in terms of private health plans with different levels of coverage, from basic plans to comprehensive and diverse services. Only 24.4 per cent of the population has health insurance (around 51 million people) (ANS 2019). As a result of the national economic crisis, from 2015 to 2019, 3.4 million people lost their healthcare plans and became dependent on the public subsystem (ANS 2019). The relationship between the public, private and supplementary subsectors is under constant strain due to competition for public resources and chronic underfinancing of the public system (Paim et al. 2011). Since 2016, the intensification of government austerity led to public spending cuts, with funding of the public subsystem worsening, as reflected in the queues and long waiting times for medical consultations and procedures. While patients are free to move through the different subsystems, in practice this depends on their ability to pay privately for a medical consultation, procedure or a private health plan.

Methods

In this chapter, we draw on research conducted with three oncology centres (a charitable hospital, a private clinic and public clinic) in Salvador, the capital city of Bahia state in Brazil. Cancer is an important health problem in Brazil and the National Cancer Institute (INCA 2019b) estimated that 625,000 new cases of cancer would occur in Brazil in 2020, with 32,580 in the state of Bahia. Bahia state has a population of approximately 14.8 million, of whom 2.8 million live in Salvador, the state capital (IBGE 2019a). According to the National Survey by Continuous Household Sample, 44.8 per cent of the state's population live below the poverty line, receiving up to USD 5.50 per day on average (IBGE 2019b). The population coverage rate per health plan in Bahia is only 11.3 per cent, rising to 30 per cent in the city of Salvador (ANS 2019).

The private clinic was attended only by patients who had private health insurance plans or who had paid for the consultation directly.[3] The charitable hospital received patients with health insurance plans, direct payment and SUS patients. Private patients were treated in the oncology section in the hospital's main building. The waiting room was well decorated with comfortable armchairs. The offices were spacious and the chemotherapy was provided in individual private rooms with relaxing decor. SUS patients were received in another building, farther from the main hospital. The waiting room and the offices were simple and smaller but well maintained. The chemotherapy room was communal, with no private rooms. The physicians nevertheless referred to the SUS service associated with the hospital as '*SUS plus*' (a service superior to the average in the public subsystem) because patients had easier access to doctors and to hospital infrastructure used by private patients (including, for example, complementary exams).[4] The facilities of the private clinic were similar to the private sector of the charitable hospital. Both are considered high-level centres for cancer treatment in Salvador.

The public cancer centre serves SUS patients and is financed exclusively by the state. The public waiting rooms and offices are simple but well maintained and chemotherapy is provided in communal rooms. The volume of patients in the waiting room, however, is considerably higher than that observed in the private clinic or in the private section of the charitable hospital. Hospitals that serve SUS patients have a huge demand for cancer treatment, receiving patients from the whole state of Bahia. This results in significant waiting times for patients needing treatment.

Between November 2017 and February 2019, we observed scientific seminars and clinical case discussions and talked to patients and physicians before and after consultations and in waiting rooms. Semi-structured interviews were performed with 17 physicians (16 oncologists and one oncogeneticist), two pharmacists, two nurses and one social worker. Of the 17 doctors interviewed, 13 worked both in the public and private subsectors. Three doctors worked only in the private subsector and one doctor only in the public subsector. Seven doctors had more than one job and worked in other institutions, in addition to that where they were contacted by the researchers. We also interviewed 39 patients, of whom 27 were women and 12 men. Patients had the following types of cancer: breast (15 patients), colorectal (9), gastrointestinal (7), lung (6), melanoma (2), ovarian (2) and liver (1). Twenty-one attended the private subsystem and they had, in general, higher education levels and higher incomes than the 18 SUS patients. Twenty-six lived in Salvador city and 13 in the interior of Bahia, the majority SUS patients (10). Some had to face several hours of travel by public transport to access treatment in the capital.

The incorporation of new biotechnologies and the process of judicialisation

The approval process for drugs and genetic testing in Brazil is complex as different institutions evaluate and determine what will be available in the public, private and supplementary subsystems. The incorporation of new medications is regulated by the Agência Nacional de Vigilância Sanitária (National Agency of Sanitary Surveillance) (ANVISA); once approved by ANVISA, in the private and supplementary subsystems, the drug then needs approval from the Agência Nacional de Saúde Suplementar (National Supplementary Health Agency) (ANS) for it to be prescribed by physicians. After receiving ANS approval, all private health insurance companies must pay for the drug if prescribed. However, ANS updates its list of covered procedures at two-year intervals, leading to delays for clinicians in incorporating new drugs into treatment plans. In the public subsystem, following ANVISA approval, new medical technologies must then be approved by the Comissão Nacional de Incorporação de Tecnologias no Sistema Único de Saúde (National Commission for the Incorporation of Technologies) (CONITEC). Due to their high cost, few drugs or genetic tests related to precision oncology have been incorporated into SUS. Sometimes, they are approved by CONITEC, but the amount transferred by the Ministry of Health to a public cancer centre to treat a patient with a specific diagnosis is usually insufficient to cover their costs.

Several targeted drugs have been approved for availability in SUS, including Trastuzumab for breast cancer in patients expressing HER2 protein, Imatinib for chronic myeloid leukaemia and Gefitinib and Erlotinib for metastatic cancer with EGFR mutation. Medicines such as Gefitinib and Erlotinib, although approved for SUS, are effectively not available, as the resources allocated by the Ministry of Health to reimburse the cancer centre are well below actual costs. Trastuzumab was approved by ANVISA for prescription in Brazil in 2000, but it was not included in the SUS list of medicines until 12 years later and only as an adjuvant treatment (Ferreira et al. 2016). Few new immunological drugs are available in public health settings. Predictive genetic tests like those for BRCA1 and 2 that can inform treatment pathways elsewhere are also unavailable in public settings (MCG 2020).[5]

Inequalities in access to biomedical innovations are not confined to the public subsystem. Private health plans also have varying coverage and patients may experience refusals by insurers for the payment of medical procedures and medications. The Ministry of Health publishes Therapeutic Guidelines for various types of cancer in an attempt to establish a common standard of treatment and diagnosis in Brazil and subsequently, in theory, cancer centres should draw up their own local guidelines (Kaliks et al. 2017). In practice, the inability to provide the same protocol for patients with similar needs leads to frustration and embarrassment among physicians. When we asked a doctor if there were local therapeutic guidelines at the cancer centre where he works (which receives both private and SUS patients), he told us that it was 'simply impossible', as that would mean having an official record that treatment protocols differed depending on whether the patient had a private health plan or the resources to pay for the treatment.

We also observed differences in access to high-cost drugs in the city of Salvador, even among SUS units, as described also for other states of Brazil (Kaliks et al. 2017). Some hospitals had access to high-cost medicine through research trials. Others had succeeded in establishing a direct agreement with the pharmaceutical industry to reduce prices for some medicines and make them available to SUS patients, as one oncologist described:

> We have now added the Iressa (Gefitinib) [in agreement with the pharmaceutical industry], before we only could get it judicially. Immunotherapy is very, very, very expensive. The target therapy you can get depends on, for example, if it is a laboratory that already has other medications in the hospital, then it tries to lower [the price]. We have now introduced Temozolomide, or Temodal that is for the central nervous system. This is an orphan disease, we did not offer anything in SUS, nothing, just radiotherapy. Temodal is the only medicine that makes a difference for central nervous system patients. The Pharmaceutical Industry was interested in reducing the cost, because the patent was broken and another company is producing it but with a very high cost. It is not a value that fits our budget. (Dr Debora, oncologist, public cancer centre)

In this context, a phenomenon known as judicialisation has become the primary means for those seeking access to medications that are currently unavailable in the public health system or which private health plans have refused to fund. Based on the constitutional commitment to universal healthcare as a citizen's right, patients seek access to high-cost drugs through judicial actions, a system of seeking and obtaining access to health resources which has dramatically expanded in Brazil since the 1990s. This initially focused on accessing drugs for people living with HIV and has since extended to other medications, both basic and specialist healthcare services and interventions for a wide range of conditions including cancers and rare genetic diseases (Aureliano and Gibbon 2020; Biehl 2013; Diniz, Medeiros and Schwartz 2012; Gibbon and Aureliano 2018). This scenario reveals, even as it reproduces, the intersection between old and new health inequalities in collective efforts to access cancer treatment. We illustrate this now through the therapeutic journey of Edvania, one of our research participants.

Biomedical innovations in cancer care: old and new health inequities

Edvania is 52 years old and lives in a small town in the Bahia countryside, 82 km from the capital. She completed secondary school and works as a cleaner. She lives with her partner, a blacksmith; her family income is low and she has no health insurance. In 2015, Edvania noticed a lump in her breast. It would have taken a long time to get a specialist appointment in the public system; a mammogram and biopsy through the SUS would also have taken months. With her sister's encouragement, she raised money through her extended family to cover the cost of a consultation with a private oncologist and to pay for the necessary examinations in private clinics and laboratories. Edvania was diagnosed with breast cancer, but without a health plan she was dependent on the public subsystem for her treatment, to be undertaken in the capital. Through contact with a doctor in her city, who knew an oncologist at a charitable hospital in Salvador, she was referred for treatment in a SUS oncology centre recognised for its above-average quality of care and resources. To travel between her city and Salvador, she depended on the free transport service provided by her municipality. However, she was twice left stranded when the transport returned to her home city before she had completed her consultation. The oncologist informed her that the medicines Trastuzumab and Pertuzumab would be most appropriate for her cancer (she was diagnosed with HER2-positive metastatic breast cancer),[6] but these were expensive and not available in SUS.

Edvania's therapeutic pathway illustrates old and new inequities in obtaining a diagnosis and treatment for cancer in Brazil. Like other patients we talked to, she faced difficulties in accessing a GP, an oncologist and diagnostic exams. She did not experience significant delay with her treatment because her relatives pooled their resources to cover the costs of private doctors, a mammogram and a biopsy. Poorer patients without similar support and resources would likely have to wait at least a few months more before they could start treatment. Many SUS patients face difficulties in accessing screening (mammography, cervical cancer cytology and colonoscopy) and diagnostic exams (ultrasonography, tomography, endoscopy and magnetic resonance), making it difficult for oncologists to effectively stage the disease and make appropriate treatment decisions.[7] One oncologist works in an SUS hospital, and explained:

> ... the problem is the volume [of patients]. The hospital is an open door and the physical structure is limited, because there is no office to put more doctors. The chemotherapy room is probably the largest room in Bahia but it does not fit anybody else. If I picked up an extra [patient] today, he will only start chemotherapy in 20 days because he has no chemotherapy chair to sit down [in]. (Dr Maria, oncologist)

The incorporation of high-cost oncology drugs adds another layer of inequity, with poor people often excluded from these treatments. However, patients such as Edvania, and the oncologists treating them, seek care via avenues of judicialisation. For example, Edvania's oncologist prescribed Trastuzumab and Pertuzumab, gave her a report and instructed her to seek a public defender (*defensoria pública*),[8] since she did not have the resources to pay a lawyer. The court ruled favourably for Edvania and the state was obliged to provide her with the medicines. Four months after the start of the process, in December 2015, she received Trastuzumab at her home and, two months later, Pertuzumab. When we met Edvania in 2018 this had succeeded in keeping the disease under control for two years.

Judicialisation and the ethics of practising oncology

For oncologists, advising patients to go through a process of judicialisation is sometimes the only option to obtain the possible best treatment regimen to increase overall survival and improve quality of life for patients, although this is not guaranteed even when a judicial action to obtain novel treatments succeeds. However, pursuing a pathway of judicialisation is a significant bureaucratic burden for doctors, who must fill out reports. It also causes stress and exhaustion for patients who must go through the justice system and so experience substantial delays, often of several months, until a judicial outcome is determined and the patient receives the medication:[9]

> It is a situation where we are on the one hand pressured not to judicialise. On the other hand there is a patient where I know what the treatment is. I know that the treatment exists, but the Ministry [of Health] anyway, the institutions do not want to provide this. I have a commitment to always offer the patient the best, so I am between the cross and the sword. (Dr Meyer, oncologist)[10]

Doctors working in public institutions are under increasing pressure from state and municipal governments to not prescribe high-cost drugs currently unavailable in the public subsystem and are also under threat of being penalised for doing so by having the expense of any successful judicial action for treatment transferred to their cancer centres. The cancer centres, in turn, pressure doctors not to prescribe drugs that are unavailable or for which the federal government has provided insufficient funding to cover the treatment costs. Further, as suggested above, the use of judicialisation generates significant unease and discomfort among oncologists. Some perceive that it is their obligation to inform the patient about existing treatments, but not encourage legal prosecution of the state to obtain new drugs. Doctors opposed to judicial proceedings fear that spending on expensive drugs for a single patient could lead to a lack of basic drugs for hundreds of others in a chronically underfunded public subsystem. Other doctors stated that their primary commitment was with the patient in front of them and that it was not their responsibility to deal with funding issues. Judicialisation, from their perspective, was an imperfect way to guarantee the constitutional right to health. One oncologist we met argued that the state had already failed the patient when it did not provide access to a means of prevention, early diagnosis and rapid initiation of treatment and that it failed the patient a second time when it denied the person access to a drug that could potentially increase survival or quality of life.

The controversies concerning judicialisation in Brazil have generated much debate (Oliveira 2019). Arguments against judicialisation include the financial impact for the state that must pay drugs without prior planning and at a much higher cost than if there was a purchase after an agreement to reduce costs with the pharmaceutical company manufacturing them (Aureliano and Gibbon 2020; Menicucci and Machado 2010). The costs of judicialisation have been increasing; municipalities, the states and the federal government spend an estimated BRL 7 billion (around USD 1.75 billion) per year to comply with judicial decisions (Crepaldi and Moraes 2018). Critics of judicialisation also argue that it generates inequities as it guarantees access to high-cost medicines to wealthier people with best access to the legal system (Chieffi and Barata 2010; Vieira and Zucchi 2007). Advocates or proponents of judicialisation, however, point to notable successes, with some drugs now incorporated into the public subsystem because of the pressure generated by the high number of lawsuits (Oliveira 2019; Oliveira and Noronha 2011).

The pharmaceutical industry is an important actor because it has significant interest in selling new, high-cost drugs in a huge market such as Brazil. To do so, it offers free genetic testing to facilitate the stratification of patients who will benefit from the targeted drugs. The industry's intention is to retain the doctor's commitment to prescribing the medications produced by companies by paying for the genetic tests. The tests are offered by the industry for all patients, opening up the possibility for those who would not have access to the drugs to go to court to request them. Some critics of judicialisation point to the pharmaceutical industry's marketing and lobbying of social (researchers, patients, doctors) and governmental sectors for the incorporation of new drugs in the health system, arguing that this stimulates the judicial demand for new drugs (Ventura et al. 2010).

An important point related to access to precision medicine is its cost–benefit ratio. Some drugs make a difference in increasing overall survival and quality of a patient's life and not making them available to all patients who can benefit means increasing health inequity. The World Health Organization (WHO) has included some target drugs (Trastuzumab, Gefitinib, Erlotinib, Imatinib) and immunotherapies (Nivolumab and Pembrolizumab) in its list of essential medicines based on their proven benefits (WHO 2019). Many drugs that enter the market, however, bring marginal benefit at an extremely high cost. Fojo, Mailankody and Low (2014) show that the average improvement in overall survival of 71 new drugs approved by the FDA for cancer treatment between 2002 and 2014 was only 2.1 months. Another study that evaluated cancer drugs approved between 2009 and 2013 by the European Medicines Agency concludes that 52 per cent of drugs that entered the market lacked evidence of overall survival or quality of life (Davis et al. 2017). The supply of these high-cost drugs through the courts in Brazil provide few benefits while compromising the limited resources available for therapeutic alternatives.

In 2016, in order to reduce the expense of lawsuits, the government of Bahia issued a decree regulating the prescriptions of therapies outside the list available in the public subsystem. The decree made it difficult to prescribe medicines outside this list, requiring justification by the doctor and approval from the director of the cancer centre to which the physician was attached, and raised the possibility that the cost of the prescribed treatment would be passed on to the cancer centre through the retention of financial transfers. Commenting on this likely impact, the coordinator of a public cancer centre told us that if the service provided Pertuzumab (see Edvania's case, above)[11] for five patients the service would have to close its doors. There would be no resources for the remaining patients.

As a result, the doctor is at the centre of an ethical conflict between the imperative to do the best for their patient and the institutional and governmental pressures to reduce the costs of high-cost drugs through legal action. On the one hand, the code of medical ethics and the principles of equality and comprehensive care are upheld by the Brazilian Constitution and embedded in the SUS. According to this ethical framework a patient cannot be discriminated in their right of access to the best available treatments suitable to attend his or her need. On the other hand, there is concern about the high cost of these medicines and the consequences for cancer centres, while the public subsystem and its limited resources may be unable to provide basic exams and treatments.

Biological and social patient stratifications

Most physicians saw the different protocols to treat patients with equal needs as a source of stress and frustration. For some, it was even a reason to stop working in the public subsystem:

> It is very difficult to work in the morning in a place where you have to work with protocols and treatments from three decades ago and in the afternoon, you come to another place and treat very similar patients in a totally different way. (Dr Anália, oncologist)

The ethical dilemmas and feelings of frustration among health professionals are greater in the case of diseases such as kidney cancer, melanomas or central nervous system cancers that lack effective alternative treatments in the public subsystem. In these cases, judicialisation would be justified, as Dr Rosa explained: 'for central nervous system, Temodal for glioblastoma, is the only drug that gives overall survival gain for the patient. In my point of view, it is unethical not to provide Temodal for this patient.'

Melanoma, in which the prognosis of patients is strongly determined by access to new biomedical technologies, illustrates this inequity. A recent study shows that more than 98 per cent of patients treated for these cancers between 2015 and 2017 in the public subsystem received minimally effective treatments with an overall survival of six months (Kaliks et al. 2019). Patients with access to a combination of two immunotherapy drugs (Nivolumab and Ipilimumab)[12] had an overall survival of over 48 months. However, the cost of treatment with Ipilimumab is around USD 18,200 per month per patient.

Oncologists are at the centre of these ethical dilemmas, balancing the institutional and governmental pressures that sit in tension with judicialisation, the code of medical ethics, the principles of SUS and the needs and interests of patients. Their reluctant and conflicted 'activism' in facilitating judicialisation must be seen as an expression of what Biehl (2013) describes as the 'ambiguous political subjectivities' that provide a context for and which arise from the process of health judicialisation in Brazil (see also Aureliano and Gibbon 2020). Such actions also reference a politics of care that is subject to pragmatic strategies not only of 'improvisation' (Livingston 2012) but also, as we explore below, forms of 'containment' as health professionals make informal and tacit decisions about for whom judicialisation may prove a viable means of obtaining treatment and/or further care options.

Although oncologists believe that there is an ethical obligation for the physician to inform patients about the existence of new biotechnologies that might be useful, even if they are not available, this does not always happen. Considering the consequences for the institution and for the system that can come from judicialisation, this option is sometimes neither mentioned nor offered. Most patients in the public subsystem are poor and have a lower educational level and generally do not question the treatment offered. They are effectively denied the right to information about the existence of more effective treatments. In some cancer centres, oncologists are forbidden to help patients to judicialise and are told to prescribe only the medicines available at their institution. Several oncologists commented that there was a significant reduction in the prescription of medicines by judicial means in their institutions following the 2016 decree regulating the prescriptions of drugs outside the list available in the public subsystem. However, one strategy used by oncologists to help patients gain access to high-cost drugs is to ask another oncologist who works in a private institution to provide the prescription and report for the patient, making it possible for them to pursue a demand for the high-cost medication in court.

Thus, an informal stratification of patients is performed based on a series of often unspoken and implicit criteria that select those considered most likely to succeed in the process of judicialisation and treatment. Rather than simply prescribing the most appropriate treatment, the oncologist is required to make a cost–benefit assessment, taking into consideration the financial impact that a particular prescription might have for their institution and the health system and the patient's capacity to carry out and see through the judicial process.

In selecting patients eligible to 'judicialise', some oncologists mention the ability to be proactive. In Portuguese to *'correr atras'* or 'chase after' refers to patients with the capacity to understand their illness and the necessary ability to request medicines by going through the judiciary. This persistence is generally associated with patients with a higher educational level, a support network to help them navigate the judicialisation process, minimal resources for good nutrition and transport to attend consultations. Two oncologists reflect on the complex dynamics of these decisions:

> Since the profile of our patients is very different, I have an illiterate patient who does not know what he is doing there. So usually I end up offering, I say that there are other medications for those who can really get it and understand. (Dr Maria, oncologist)

> I even communicate to the patient that there is such a drug that is the first line [treatment] that responds well, but that it is not available on SUS. I try to explain in some way for him to understand, but I cannot come and say: 'go there go into justice and everything' . . . But when I see that really if he chases after ('*correr atras*'), we can really get a real benefit out there, then I really insist to go through the justice system. We make a report and such . . . it's very complicated to decide that. It's complicated to explain this to the patient, because at that moment the one who is responsible for the patient is the doctor, not the one who is in the Ministry of Health . . . (Dr Ieda, oncologist)

Stratification and differentiation in novel oncology interventions in Brazil is therefore not limited to the bio-clinical information determining treatment protocols for individual patients; it is already reproduced and sustained through informal stratification undertaken by oncologists, who make decisions about whether to suggest or encourage judicialisation. Patients from the most disadvantaged backgrounds – with low education, who are illiterate, poor and often from rural backgrounds – are less likely to have the opportunity to access high-cost drugs through prosecution. The Brazilian state's failure to develop a policy with clear criteria to introduce new technologies in the health system and that take into account benefits and cost-effectiveness, in accordance with SUS principles, means that such decisions end up being delegated to oncologists and judges. These decisions, many health professionals feel, should have been debated and agreed upon by society.

Some oncologists help patients to judicialise to obtain high-cost drugs because they perceive that it is unfair not to give them medicines that could improve their overall survival or quality of life. The perception of inequalities as inequities by oncologists, patients and communities is important to the formulation and support of social policies and political actions directed towards achieving health equity (Barreto 2017). At the same time, decisions concerning resources to provide precision oncology for everyone, as indicated, should not be left to the discretion of individual oncologists or judges. A cost–benefit assessment by regulatory agencies, including the state, is fundamental because the inclusion of high-cost drugs with small benefits in SUS or its delivery by judicialisation could contribute to increasing health inequities using scarce resources that could be better applied to other health needs. The government needs also to negotiate with the pharmaceutical industry to reduce the prices of drugs so as to incorporate them into the public subsystem.

On 11 March 2020, the Brazilian Supreme Court of Justice ruled that the government was no longer required to be forced to pay for high-cost medications that are not on the SUS list, making it even harder to access these resources by judicial means. However, there continue to be exceptional cases, such as when the patient and family are unable to afford the drug or when no similar treatment is available. It is too early to know how this recent decision will affect the number of judicial actions for high-cost cancer medications in Brazil, but given growing social and economic inequalities in the country the stratified inequities in oncology treatment will likely persist.

Conclusion

Brazil has a universal health system based on values such as the right to health, equality and comprehensive care, in which all citizens should have access to the means of promotion, prevention and treatment appropriate to their needs. Nevertheless, in an underfunded and fragmented healthcare system with public, private and supplementary subsystems, these principles are not easily fulfilled. As we have illustrated, there are sharp inequities in the protocols for cancer treatment and access to the new biomedical technologies, depending on the institution where the patient is being treated and the type of health insurance they have (or do not have). At the same time, old inequities persist and are sometimes reinscribed in new ways. The inclusion of new high-cost technologies in Brazilian cancer care creates new inequities by increasing the gap between those who have and those who do not have access to their benefits. The high costs of new target and immunotherapeutic drugs restrict the possibility of the public subsystem making them available; here there are already difficulties in providing basic medical technologies. Given that just over three-quarters of the Brazilian population are dependent on the public subsystem, most technological innovations in cancer care are accessible to only one in four Brazilians who have health insurance plans.

The incorporation of so-called precision oncology in Brazil, at least in its current form, will not have a public health impact. For this, it would be necessary to address long-standing inequities in health promotion, in improving access to preventive exams, in increasing the percentage of patients with early diagnosis and in guaranteeing the start of treatment with minimum delay. From the point of view of the clinics, however, the Brazilian health system needs to make those drugs that would cause a difference in overall survival and quality of life available to all patients. Inequity in access to technologies that represent the difference between life and death, as in the case of advanced melanoma and other cancers, is morally unacceptable.

For oncologists, inequities in access to new technologies pose ethical dilemmas concerning the existence of different treatment protocols for patients with the same needs. Judicialisation is one strategy used by physicians to address unequal access to high-cost medicines, but this generates other forms of social stratification. As a result, the new biomedical technologies being incorporated into oncological practice in Brazil currently contribute to an increase of health inequities.

Acknowledgements

We thank the National Research Council of Brazil for funding the research and the editors of this volume for their generous feedback and commentary.

Authorship

Jorge Iriart participated in the conception of the research project, fieldwork, analysis and writing of the chapter. Sahra Gibbon participated in data analysis and chapter writing.

Notes

1. Pseudonyms are used throughout this chapter.
2. The difference between the private system and the supplementary system is that in the first the patient pays for medical consultations and procedures by direct disbursement. The patient does not receive reimbursement for the amount paid. They may, however, have part of these costs deducted in their income tax. In the supplementary system, a person signs up to a health insurance plan with a monthly payment that allows them access to consultations and medical procedures in partner institutions. Part of the amount paid may also be deducted in income tax.
3. The private clinic and the charitable hospital only accept health plans that have an agreement with them.
4. This included examinations such as X-ray, ultrasonography, tomography, endoscopy and magnetic resonance.
5. Genetic tests for BRCA1 and 2 mutations are indicated to assess the risk of developing breast and ovarian cancer, but are also used in ovarian cancer to determine treatment pathways (MCG 2020). Many genetic tests are not available in the public or supplementary subsystems. Oncotype DX, for example, which enables identification of breast cancer patients who may not need to undergo chemotherapy, is not available in both subsystems. The pharmaceutical industry offers free genetic tests but only for those associated with commercialised drugs.

6   Studies show that the association of these drugs has an increase in overall survival of approximately 15.7 months (CONITEC 2017). Some 15 per cent of breast cancer cases present HER2 protein overexpression.
7   Aiming to reduce the time between diagnosis and treatment, in 2012 a law was approved, establishing that the initial cancer treatment in the SUS should begin a maximum of 60 days after the signing of the patient's pathological report. Despite the law, according to Instituto Nacional de Câncer (INCA) (2019a), 48.8 per cent of patients diagnosed with breast cancer in Brazil between 2013 and 2015 did not start their treatment within that time period.
8   According to the Brazilian Constitution, every citizen has the right to seek justice whenever they suffer a threat or violation of their rights. When citizens are unable to pay for a lawyer, they may rely on the Public Defender, a state-funded institution, which incurs no personal cost to them.
9   According to oncologists, in actions that request medicines approved by ANVISA the patient usually has their lawsuit approved.
10 'Entre a cruz e a espada' is a Brazilian expression that refers to a dilemma. It is similar to the English expression: 'between a rock and a hard place'.
11 In 2017, a CONITEC (2017) report considered that treatment with Pertuzumab was not cost-effective compared to chemotherapy. After a public consultation, however, the committee reconsidered its recommendation and approved the incorporation of Pertuzumab in the public subsystem for the treatment of metastatic HER2-positive breast cancer as first-line treatment conditional on price negotiation with the pharmaceutical industry. The medication, however, became available for prescription in SUS in the second half of 2020.
12 Drugs often need to be combined to achieve the best clinical results, thus contributing to increases in the cost of treatments.

References

Andersen, Rikke Sand, Bjarke Paarup, Peter Vedsted, Flemming Bro and Jens Soendergaard. 2010. '"Containment" as an analytical framework for understanding patient delay: A qualitative study of cancer patients' symptom interpretation processes', *Social Science & Medicine* 71(2): 378–385. https://doi.org/10.1016/j.socscimed.2010.03.044.

ANS (Agência Nacional de Saúde Suplementar) 2019. 'Dados Gerais. Beneficiários de planos privados de saúde, por cobertura assistencial (Brasil – 2008–2018)'. Accessed 30 March 2020. http://www.ans.gov.br/perfil-do-setor/dados-gerais.

Arteaga, Ignacia, Cinzia Greco, Henry Llewellyn, Emily Ross and Julia Swallow. 2019. '(Dis)continuities in cancer care: An ethnographic approximation to practices of disease stratification', Somatosphere. Accessed 1 June 2020. http://somatosphere.net/2019/discontinuities-in-cancer-care-an-ethnographic-approximation-to-practices-of-disease-stratification.html/.

Aureliano, Waleska and Sahra Gibbon. 2020. 'Judicialisation and the politics of rare genetic disease in Brazil: Rethinking activism and inequalities'. In *Critical Medical Anthropology: Perspectives in and from Latin America*, edited by Jennie Gamlin, Sahra Gibbon, Paola M. Sesia and Lina Berrio, 248–269. London: UCL Press.

Barreto, Mauricio Lima. 2017. 'Desigualdades em Saúde: uma perspectiva global', *Ciência & Saúde Coletiva* 22: 2097–2108.

Biehl, João. 2013. 'The judicialization of biopolitics: Claiming the right to pharmaceuticals in Brazilian courts', *American Ethnologist* 40(3): 419–436. https://doi.org/10.1111/amet.12030.

Bourret, Pascale, Peter Keating and Alberto Cambrosio. 2011. 'Regulating diagnosis in post-genomic medicine: Re-aligning clinical judgment?' *Social Science & Medicine* 73(6): 816–824. https://doi.org/10.1016/j.socscimed.2011.04.022.

Cambrosio, Alberto, Peter Keating, Etienne Vignola-Gagné, Sylvain Besle and Pascale Bourret. 2018. 'Extending experimentation: Oncology's fading boundary between research and care', *New Genetics and Society* 37(3): 207–226. https://doi.org/10.1080/14636778.2018.1487281.

Chieffi, Ana Luiza and Rita de Cassia Barradas Barata. 2010. 'Legal suits: Pharmaceutical industry strategies to introduce new drugs in the Brazilian public healthcare system', *Revista de Saude Publica* 44(3): 421–429. https://doi.org/10.1590/S0034-89102010000300005.

CONITEC (National Committee for Health Technology Incorporation). 2017. 'Relatório de recomendação pertuzumabe trastuzumabe'. Accessed 28 March 2019. http://conitec.gov.br/images/Relatorios/2017/Relatorio_PertuzumabeTrastuzumabe_ CA_Mama.pdf.

Crepaldi, Thiago and Claudia Moraes. 2018. 'Judicialização da saúde. Juizes passam a ditar políticas públicas no setor'. Consultor Jurídico. Accessed 28 March 2019. https://www.conjur.com.br/2018-ago-15/judicializacao-saude-juizes-passam-ditar-politicas-publicas-setor.

Davis, Courtney, Naci Huseyin, Evrim Gurpinar, Elita Poplavska, Ashlyn Pinto and Ajay Aggarwal. 2017. 'Availability of evidence of benefits on overall survival and quality of life of cancer drugs approved by European Medicines Agency: Retrospective cohort study of drug approvals 2009–13', *British Medical Journal* 359: j4530. https://doi.org/10.1136/bmj.j4530.

Day, Sophie, Charles Coombes, Louise McGrath-Lone, Claudia Schoenborn and Helen Ward. 2017. 'Stratified, precision or personalised medicine? Cancer services in the "real world" of a London hospital', *Sociology of Health & Illness* 39(1): 143–158. https://doi.org/10.1111/1467-9566.12457.

Diniz, Debora, Marcelo Medeiros and Ida Vanessa D. Schwartz. 2012. 'Consequências da judicialização das políticas de saúde: custos de medicamentos para as mucopolissacaridoses', *Cadernos de Saúde Pública* 28: 479–489.

Ferreira, Carlos Gil, Maria Isabel Achatz, Patricia Ashton-Prolla, Maria Dirlei Begnami, Fabricio K. Marchini and Stephen Doral Stefani. 2016. 'Brazilian health-care policy for targeted oncology therapies and companion diagnostic testing', *The Lancet Oncology* 17(8): e363–370. https://doi.org/10.1016/S1470-2045(16)30171-1.

Fojo, Tito, Sham Mailankody and Andrew Low. 2014. 'Unintended consequences of expensive cancer therapeutics – the pursuit of marginal indications and a me-too mentality that stifles innovation and creativity: The John Conley Lecture', *JAMA Otolaryngology Head & Neck Surgery* 140(12): 1225–1236. https://doi.org/10.1001/jamaoto.2014.1570.

Gibbon, Sahra and Waleska Aureliano. 2018. 'Inclusion and exclusion in the globalization of genomics: The case of rare genetic disease in Brazil', *Anthropology and Medicine* 25(1): 11–29. https://doi.org/10.1080/13648470.2017.1381230.

Good, Mary-Jo Delvecchio. 1995. 'Cultural studies of biomedicine: An agenda for research', *Social Science & Medicine* 41(4): 461–473.

Gyawali, Bishal and Richard Sullivan. 2017. 'Economics of cancer medicines: For whose benefit?' *The New Bioethics* 23(1): 95–104. https://doi.org/10.1080/20502877.2017.1314885.

IBGE (Instituto Brasileiro de Geografía e Estatística). 2019a. 'Salvador, população estimada. 2018'. Accessed 30 March 2019. https://cidades.ibge.gov.br/brasil/ba/salvador/panorama.

IBGE (Instituto Brasileiro de Geografía e Estatística). 2019b. 'Sintese dos indicadores sociais 2018'. Accessed 30 March 2019. https://www.ibge.gov.br/estatisticas-novoportal/sociais/populacao/9221-sintese-de-indicadores-sociais.html?=&t=o-que-e.

INCA (Instituto Nacional de Câncer). 2019a. 'A situação do câncer de mama no Brasil: Síntese de dados dos sistemas'. Accessed 30 April 2020. https://www.inca.gov.br/sites/ufu.sti.inca.local/files/media/document/a_situacao_ca_mama_brasil_2019.pdf.

INCA (Instituto Nacional de Câncer). 2019b. 'Estimativa 2020. Incidência de câncer no Brasil'. Accessed 9 November 2020. https://www.inca.gov.br/sites/ufu.sti.inca.local/files/media/document/estimativa-2020-incidencia-de-cancer-no-brasil.pdf.

Iriart, Jorge Alberto Bernstein. 2019. 'Precision medicine/personalized medicine: A critical analysis of movements in the transformation of biomedicine in the early 21st century', *Cadernos de Saúde Pública* 35(3): e00153118. Accessed 16 September 2022. https://www.scielo.br/j/csp/a/MDnkgxSFz89BSRM45zhNM3D/?lang=en.

Kaliks, Rafael Aliosha, Tiago Farina Matos, Vanessa de Araujo Silva and Luciana Holtz de Camargo Barros. 2017. 'Differences in systemic cancer treatment in Brazil: My public health system is different from your public health system', *Brazilian Journal of Oncology* 13(44): 1–12.

Kaliks, Rafael Aliosha, Andre Marques Santos, Tiago Farina Matos and Luciana Holtz. 2019. 'How is advanced melanoma treated in the public health system in Brazil: A call for change', *Brazilian Journal of Oncology* 15: 1–7. https://doi.org/10.5935/2526-8732.20190020.

Keating, Peter and Alberto Cambrosio. 2011. *Cancer on Trial: Oncology as a new style of practice*. Chicago: University of Chicago Press.

Kerr, Anne and Sarah Cunningham-Burley. 2015. 'Embodied innovation and regulation of medical technoscience: Transformations in cancer patienthood', *Law, Innovation and Technology* 7(2): 187–205. https://doi.org/10.1080/17579961.2015.1106103.

Kerr, Anne, Julia Swallow, Choon Key Chekar and Sarah Cunningham-Burley. 2019. 'Genomic research and the cancer clinic: Uncertainty and expectations in professional accounts', *New Genetics and Society* 38(2): 222–239. https://doi.org/10.1080/14636778.2019.1586525.

Livingston, Julie. 2012. *Improvising Medicine: An African oncology ward in an emerging cancer epidemic*. Durham, NC: Duke University Press.

Lock, Margaret and Vinh-Kim Nguyen. 2010. *An Anthropology of Biomedicine*. Oxford: Wiley-Blackwell.

Lock, Margaret, Patricia Kaufert and Alan Harwood. 1998. *Pragmatic Women and Body Politics*. Cambridge, UK: Cambridge University Press.

MCG (Mainstreaming Cancer Genetics). 2020. 'What was the Mainstreaming Cancer Genetics Programme?' Accessed 5 April 2020. https://www.mcgprogramme.com/.

Menicucci, Telma Maria Goncalves and Jose Angelo Machado. 2010. 'Judicialization of health policy in the definition of access to public goods: Individual rights versus collective rights', *Brazilian Political Science Review (Online)* 5(1). Accessed 5 April 2020. http://socialsciences.scielo.org/scielo.php?script=sci_arttext&pid=S1981-38212010000100002.

Oliveira, Vanessa Elias de. 2019. 'Caminhos da judicialização do direito à saúde'. In *Judicialização de políticas públicas no Brasil*, edited by Vanessa Elias de Oliveira, 177–200. Rio de Janeiro, Brazil: Editora Fiocruz.

Oliveira, Vanessa Elias de and Lincoln N. T. Noronha. 2011. 'Judiciary-executive relations in policy making: The case of drug distribution in the state of São Paulo', *Brazilian Political Science Review* 5(2): 10–38.

Paim, Jairnilson, Claudia Travassos, Celia Almeida, Ligia Bahia and James Macinko. 2011. 'The Brazilian health system: History, advances, and challenges', *The Lancet* 377(9779): 1778–1797. https://doi.org/10.1016/S0140-6736(11)60054-8.

Prainsack, Barbara. 2017. *Personalized Medicine: Empowered patients in the 21st century?* New York: New York University Press.

Røe, Oluf Dimitri. 2017. 'The high cost of new cancer therapies: A challenge of inequality for all countries', *JAMA Oncology* 3(9): 1169–1170. https://doi.org/10.1001/jamaoncol.2016.6335.

Tutton, Richard. 2014. *Genomics and the Reimagining of Personalized Medicine*. Farnham: Ashgate Publishing.

Ventura, Miriam, Luciana Simas, Vera Lucia Edais Pepe and Fermin Roland Schramm. 2010. 'Judicialização da saúde, acesso à justiça e a efetividade do direito à saúde', *Physis* 20(1): 77–100.

Vieira, Fabiola Sulpino and Paola Zucchi. 2007. 'Distorções causadas pelas ações judiciais à política de medicamentos no Brasil', *Revista de Saúde Pública* 41(2): 214–222.

Whitehead, Margaret and Göran Dahlgren. 2006. 'Concepts and principles for tackling social inequities in health: Levelling up Part 1'. Accessed 25 April 2020. https://www.euro.who.int/__data/assets/pdf_file/0010/74737/E89383.pdf.

WHO (World Health Organization). 2019. 'World Health Organization model list of essential medicines: 21st list 2019'. Accessed 25 April 2020. https://apps.who.int/iris/bitstream/handle/10665/325771/WHO-MVP-EMP-IAU-2019.06-eng.pdf.

3
'It just keeps hurting': continuums of violence and their impact on cervical cancer mortality in Argentina

Natalia Luxardo and Linda Rae Bennett

Mirta: We're discriminated against for having a social plan. Last month we were in a public demonstration and the ones passing through the streets, some very rich ladies said, 'These fucking negros, go to work.' We're always somebody's fucking negros, because we're poor, because we have a social plan, because we live in shitty places . . .

Lina: They pass judgement on you before they meet you. What bothers me is that they say 'Shitty negro go to work,' because it's not that I want to come here every day [to work at a social organisation for financial assistance], many days I'd rather stay at home.

Silvia: I've already gotten used to it . . . but it just keeps hurting.

(Informal conversation, January 2020)

Focusing on cervical cancer, in this chapter we examine the structural and cultural drivers of health inequalities experienced in the everyday social worlds of persistently poor Argentinian women and how these contribute to increased probability of cancer death. We focus on women who are marginalised within the health system and who, as shown by statistics and prior qualitative studies, fail to screen at all or on a regular basis for cervical cancer, delay attending hospitals and die as a result of advanced cancer (Luxardo and Manzelli 2017). Through situated ethnography we explain women's disengagement with cancer prevention practices within the broad social, economic, cultural and political structures of

Entre Ríos province in Central Argentina. Our core argument is that socially and economically vulnerable women are consistently subject to racist and class violence in their daily lives and rendered as other in the national imaginary, within the health system as elsewhere. This results in their disengagement or inconsistent engagement with cancer prevention.

The women of whom we write live in informal settlements that have arisen around an open-pit garbage dump. In this locale, garbage trucks overturn collected waste from more affluent neighbourhoods; this waste provides livelihoods for those who are excluded from the formal economy. Within these neighbourhoods the air is stale and smoky from garbage being continually burnt, water is polluted and the streets are impossible to walk along when it rains. Housing is rudimentary and unsupported by city infrastructure. Many informal settlements arise on the edge of rivers or streams surrounding the garbage dump, so providing dwellers with access to water, albeit unsafe for drinking. Homes are overcrowded and households are supported by whatever means available. Overcrowding and violence mean that women and their children are at times homeless and must sleep on the streets or in car parks.

These communities were initially formed by migrants from small towns and cities, looking to the provincial capital for an exit from local financial crises. Most arrived in the city with few resources and no formal qualifications. In this chapter, we refer to both women and their communities at times as marginalised, including in reference to social, racial, class and economic marginalisation. We discuss how the overlapping forms of violence which women must negotiate are gendered, as are women's acts of resistance. Our ethnographic lens allows us to consider how cancer outcomes for women are shaped by their everyday and cumulative experiences of disadvantage and deprivation and how these experiences are the product of structural inequalities.

Cervical cancer prevention in Argentina

According to the National Cancer Institute (NCI), cervical cancer is the third most commonly diagnosed cancer among women and is a significant public health issue in Argentina, with an estimated 4,500 diagnosed cases and 2,000 deaths each year (NCI 2020) and with deaths skewed towards women living in poor areas (Martínez and Guevel 2013; Tumas, Pou and Días 2017). The Early Cervical Cancer Detection Subprogram was launched in 1998; a decade later the National Cervical Cancer Program within the Ministry of Health was established and reflects strategies developed by organisations such as the World Health Organization and the Pan American Health Organization. In the early 2000s, a common health agenda was established for the Americas, supported by loans granted by the Inter-American Development Bank and the World Bank to several countries in the region, including Argentina (Iummato 2020). In this context, research was conducted in 2007 to identify the cervical cancer prevention activities carried out in 24 Argentine provinces and to analyse their organisational framework, coverage of Pap smears, organisation of cytology labs and follow-up and treatment of women with precancerous and cancerous lesions (Arrossi, Paolino and Sankaranarayanan 2010). Findings indicated that screening was usually opportunistic, conducted with excessive frequency on women who had good access to the health system and rarely among socially vulnerable women (poor, uneducated women with no health insurance). There were no clear guidelines for target populations or on the recommended frequency of screening. Other limitations included a lack of quality assurance controls for testing, insufficient lab personnel and inadequate equipment for diagnosis and treatment. Each province was found to follow different screening policies; none followed the national recommendation that women aged 35–46 undergo a Pap smear once every three years (Arrossi, Paolino and Sankaranarayanan 2010).

This preliminary study led to the development of a National Cervical Cancer Prevention Program in 2008 aimed at reducing cervical cancer incidence and mortality rates. Key programme goals were to reach high coverage of target populations, increase use of high-quality screening tests and encourage the adoption of treatment by and follow-up strategies with women with precancerous lesions and cancer. Low coverage was identified as a particular issue, as the resources available were focused on very young women who use sexual and reproductive health services, although they are the lowest-risk group. In the programme, the word 'detection' was replaced with 'prevention', which in turn was defined as a *process* including the administration of Pap smears, adequate reading of tests and treatment of women 35 to 64 years old. The prevention strategy included primary prevention through human papillomavirus (HPV) vaccination and secondary prevention through free screening in the public sector for those without private health insurance.

Argentina is a federation and provinces adopt national guidelines depending on their application criteria, budgets and logistics. In the province of Entre Ríos, the Cervical Cancer Prevention Program targets women between the ages of 25 and 65 and prioritises screening coverage as a quality indicator for prevention programmes. The data published in the National Risk Factor Survey in 2019 conducted in Entre Ríos showed a gradual increase in the percentage of women ever receiving a Pap smear from 2005 onwards: 53 per cent in 2005, 62 per cent in 2009, 69 per cent in 2013 and finally 72 per cent in 2018. Despite this gradual increase, cervical cancer incidence and mortality rates remain unacceptably high, especially among socially and economically vulnerable women. The research on which we draw specifically aimed to understand why marginalised women were at higher risk of cancer mortality in these communities.

Within Entre Ríos province, gynaecological services are offered free of cost through community health centres, which are encouraged to provide routine Pap smears. Pap smears are the most frequently used screening method; visual inspection with acetic acid is less common. Colposcopies are theoretically available at community health centres, but are more commonly conducted in a hospital setting (Palermo, Sassetti and Luxardo 2021). Following screening, there is wide heterogeneity of clinical practices for delivering results. Some clinics wait for the woman to return; others follow up more proactively. In this chapter, we focus on women's experiences of seeking gynaecological care as they narrated them, rather than the clinical issues identified by healthcare workers (see Luxardo and Manzelli 2017).

Methodological and theoretical approaches

In March 2016, we established a collaborative ethnographic study including health workers, local researchers and community members, and focused on a research site of 50 km^2 serviced by ten primary health centres. During the first year of research, we decided to focus on communities within the selected healthcare zones whose livelihoods were linked with an open-pit garbage dump that had existed for over a hundred years on the outskirts of a city in Entre Ríos. A significant number of people in Argentina resort to informal survival practices and structural inequality results in sectors of the population living in deep poverty for generations, often excluded from social security and social integration mechanisms and facing multiple underemployment issues linked to informal subsistence activities (Salvia 2012). The women in our research were part of this group living in extreme poverty and while some were able to access welfare payments, these payments were insufficient to address their structural exclusion.

Women participants were involved in multiple subsistence activities, including scavenging in the garbage dump for items they could use directly (including food) or could reclaim and market. They have been increasingly affected by illegal drug-dealing activities impacting on the community's social fabric, reinforcing negative stereotypes of marginal areas and the people who live there. The highly derogatory term often used to refer to these women and their communities by more affluent members of Argentinian society is *negros del volca*, literally 'dump niggers'. The term *negros de alma* (black souls) is another offensive euphemism used to describe non-white Argentinians and refers to an identity inscribed based on the ways that people speak, dress, interact and take care of their own health and the health of their loved ones. These terms highlight the specificity of racial vilification of this group, not simply based on skin colour (that is, being non-white) or having indigenous heritage, but also incorporating class and cultural identities.

This ethnography focused on understanding women's well-being in the context of their everyday lives, viewing cancer risk as one component of a range of risks and hardships women are required to negotiate (Manderson and Warren 2016). Overall, Luxardo, the first author and principal ethnographer, formed close links with a total of 35 women aged 28–62 and conducted prolonged participant observation of their daily routines and conversations. Most women were Catholic or from other Christian denominations; many were first-, second- or third-generation migrants from rural areas. The data generated through this ethnography included fieldnotes of participant observations and everyday conversations with and between women, data from formal interviews, audio-visual records, audio messages and homemade videos created by and exchanged with women. This corpus of data provided a multilayered understanding of women's rejection of and disengagement with cervical cancer screening. This was linked to their everyday experiences and identities as lower-class, racially vilified women, who, according to the mainstream Argentinian imagination, live on the margins of 'respectable society'. What emerged as 'data' relevant to cervical cancer was embedded in women's own frameworks about their sexual and reproductive health concerns and their health-seeking practices.

Discussions on cervical cancer were typically linked with gynaecological tests, including Pap smears. No women in this research had check-ups within the recommended intervals and some had never had a Pap smear. Most had had one, but abandoned repeat screening, even when they continued to visit health centres for other reasons, such as accessing contraceptives, receiving antenatal care or in connection with their children's health. They knew they were at risk of developing cervical cancer because they had known women who had suffered and died from it. They knew that Pap smears were free, the days on which they were available and how to make an appointment and they lived in close proximity to public health centres. They had also engaged with cancer prevention and/or detection tests such as mammograms or HPV vaccinations for their daughters and many were aware that cervical cancer was preventable and treatable if detected early. Hence common barriers to access cervical cancer screening observed in other lower-resourced communities, such as information, logistics and economic barriers (Islam et al. 2017), were not significant in explaining women's low engagement with services.

In initial conversations, women explained their disengagement with cervical cancer screening through such responses as 'Just because', 'Because I didn't want to', 'Because I didn't feel like it'. Some women referred to barriers to access such as feelings of embarrassment if the health professional was a man or pressure from male partners not to see male doctors (Afsah 2017; Islam et al. 2017), but these issues were partial and ambiguous explanations. This suggested that something more complex was at play, requiring that we explore everyday social practices (not limited to health) and the historic reality of these structurally vulnerable communities.

Quesada, Hart and Bourgois (2011) have argued for greater attention to structural factors (such as gender inequality and racism) to understand health inequities, since these factors are clearly linked to material forces determining class oppression and economic inequalities. Given this, we deploy the concept of *continuums of violence* as an analytical framework for theorising the complex intersections of different forms of ongoing structural disadvantage that shape women's vulnerability to cervical cancer in these communities. In applying the concept of continuums of violence, we also drawn on conceptualisation of *structural violence* (Farmer 2004; Galtung 1969), Foucault's (1978) notion of *biopower* and Bourdieu's (2000) theorising of *symbolic violence*. The concept of continuums of violence enables us to identify the unique consequences of oppressive structures, while also recognising their specific manifestation in the local worlds in which these inequalities play out in women's everyday lives. Conceptualising overlapping continuums of violence that coexist at multiple levels allows us to investigate the salience of violence generated from both within and outside of these communities. Our analysis also highlights how multigenerational cycles of poverty and marginalisation produce continuities of violence over time, of which there is no local memory of a beginning point or a perceptible end point; rather women experience persistent oppression, marginalisation and ongoing suffering. Thus, our conceptualisation of continuums of violence specifically acknowledges these continuums as ongoing, perpetuated through repeated cycles of violence, which differs from notions of continuums as necessarily having polarised end points along a fixed numeric continuum. The overlapping continuums we explore below include: continuums of everyday violence occurring in women's immediate physical environment, their intimate relationships and their communities; continuums of institutional violence that occur within the health system and include obstetric violence; and continuums of racist and class violence that are pervasive in wider Argentinian society.

Continuums of everyday violence

Local conditions in the research setting were shaped by and acted to perpetuate interpersonal and structural violence. The harsh realities of survival in heavily degraded environments compromised the physical safety of women and their families. For instance, the constant smoke emitted by the garbage dump caused severe respiratory problems that worsened according to the season. Common infectious diseases were unavoidable due to seasonal water shortages (for example, more drinking water is available in winter than in summer, when wealthy households fill their swimming pools and these neighbourhoods, the most peripheral of the city, receive less water, sometimes none during certain hours). In conditions of material deprivation, women cannot avoid unsafe working conditions, as failure to scavenge results in no income or food for themselves and their children. Women attend to the embodied realities of food insecurity and routine infections for themselves and their families before considering preventative care.

Serious injury among children was frequent in these communities, stemming from environmental hazards and lack of local council attention to safety guidelines. Accidents recorded during fieldwork included children falling down an uncovered manhole, being electrocuted from contact with uninsulated utility pole wires and being crushed by a truck while they were waiting for garbage to be dumped. Women focused on the immediate survival of their children, setting aside their own health and preventive measures to ensure they met the immediate needs of others (Ponce 2013). In these communities, where the conditions of daily life are precarious and subsistence is not guaranteed, the burden of care on women is much higher than it is for middle-class and elite women with access to wider networks of social and economic capital.

Women commonly discussed their concern regarding their children's engagement with drugs and the lack of alternative activities and livelihoods for youth in these settlements. Throughout the fieldwork, youth suicides were frequent, with at least six young lives so lost over the four-year research period. In everyday conversations, youth suicide was linked with drug use, mental health crises and the lack of any imagined future beyond these settlements. Legal and illegal drug consumption and marketing cycles influenced women's daily lives, regardless of whether they directly participated in drug use or distribution, because of the eminent risks these issues posed for their children. Risks for children also included increasingly violent street culture and sporadic spikes in gun violence from both community members and outside forces. This attracted intervention by security forces, with excessive responses that threatened the lives of adolescent boys. Women were unable to protect their children from gun and other violence.

Gender-based violence and domestic violence were routine in women's lives. Women described living with violence within their intimate social circles, including as perpetrated by their male partners, their parents during their childhood and, to a degree, their own adolescent sons and daughters. Domestic violence was triggered by factors including police reports and (breached) injunctions, separations, changes of residence, temporary relocations with trusted families and reconciliations or resignations. Some women made sense of this violence through the lens of belonging to a traumatised community, which to an extent normalised domestic, community-level and structural violence. Women's resignation is reflected in the following excerpt:

> She [Nora] didn't feel like talking this time . . . she said 'if I told you everything I've been through you'd have enough material for a book, but I can't while he's close by' . . . When she accompanied me to the bus stop, she told me that some years ago she had to call the police because he broke two of her ribs. An injunction was issued but then he came back to the house and 'I let him, he's old and sick now, so he can't hurt anyone anymore.' (Fieldnotes, Anacleto Medina 2017)

However, other traumatised women did not accept the violence and sought to avoid vulnerability, as described by Ludmila:

> My first partner was violent . . . [he] kidnapped me . . . he pointed a gun at me, like this, and threatened to kill me . . . he would beat me

up, or kick me . . . I used to be one of those who think 'Screw her if they beat her up' . . . Because, as a girl, after my first partner, who used to beat me up, I never let anyone beat me again. That is why I was very aggressive. With everyone. If they yelled at me I reacted by beating them. (Group discussion, January 2020)

Casual conversations with women also revealed the prevalence of sexual violence against women and girls. As Patricia noted, this was a threat that women had to negotiate on a daily basis: 'We must also talk about cases of sexual abuse, because they are very common but they never mention them – which is something that also . . . affects me a lot. It is very common.' Although women acknowledged that sexual violence was pervasive, they were also concerned that it was tolerated or suppressed, adding to the unspoken burden of violence women were expected to endure:

> Some girls are raped by their own relatives, beaten; they give birth when they're 13, 14 years old . . . and ask me for advice . . . Sometimes we file a report, as in the case of a 20-year-old woman who had been raped by her father since she was four. But her stepmother threatened her and she had to withdraw the report. The stepmother said, 'it was only because he was drunk or drugged at the time'. (WhatsApp chat, May 2020)

Women continually strived to negotiate everyday violence. Their life choices were seriously constrained by structural violence and its material deprivations. Their own health and safety, and that of their families, were shaped by the toxic physical environment they live in and by pervasive community-level and interpersonal violence. Cycles of violence are self-perpetuating and women's role in shouldering the burden of both survival and care in this context was paramount to the survival of the community. The burden of collective care and survival on these women, living with everyday violence, was such that preventative healthcare for 'the self' was rarely perceived as an immediate priority.

Continuums of institutional violence

The routine nature of women's engagement with reproductive health services, coupled with the 'normality' of structural and symbolic violence directed against them within the public health system, resulted in enduring institutional violence. The continuing nature of this violence deters women from attending screening, even though most women were aware of its importance to prevent cervical cancer or identify early signs of disease. Women were familiar with appointment systems, the physicians in charge at local health centres and mechanisms for receiving free care. Many were ambivalent about having Pap smears and others avoided them altogether, although they often insisted their daughters, granddaughters and nieces should be screened to protect their health. Women expressed their ambivalence in various ways:

> Natalia: What about a Pap smear?
> Nora: I never had one. They did an EKG of my ovaries and everything's ok. My last kid was born by C-section.
> Natalia: Is that free?
> Nora: Yes, the gynaecologist does it.
> Natalia: Did she explain to you what a Pap smear is?
> Nora: Yes.
> Natalia: Why do you think you've never had one?
> Nora: Just because . . . I didn't want to. I just don't want to. My mom [never had one] either. 'I won't show my coochie to anyone!' [she said]. 'But mom', I said, 'how many children did you have?' I have 13 siblings. She never had one either. But yes, yes, I must have one. I have to get an appointment. It's right here [three blocks away]. Doctor Laura does it and then she gives you the results. It doesn't take long, just one or two weeks. I know that because my daughters already had one, I send them . . . They always have them . . . I just don't want to. I have a sister who died from [uterine] cancer, she never saw a gynaecologist. (Home interview with Nora, July 2016)

As Nora explained, and in Nancy's and Mirta's conversation below, women may reject Pap smears, but this does not mean that they dismiss their importance for other women to have Pap smears or receive HPV vaccination:

> Mirta: I had a Pap smear some seven years ago. I used to have one every year. My daughter was vaccinated against HPV when she was 11.
> Nancy: When I got pregnant they asked me if I wanted one and I said no.
> Natalia: Why did you say no?

> Nancy: Just because. I didn't feel like it. They also asked me to have ... that [mammogram]. It was a long time ago, because I had a small thing here [breast], a small lump ... And it hurt, It hurt all the time ... that is why they ordered the test.
> (Group conversation, Mirta and Nancy, October 2018)

As fieldwork extended and engagement with women deepened, their reasons for avoiding Pap smears beyond the catch-phrase of 'just because' became increasingly apparent. Women's experiences of reproductive healthcare were at times too traumatic for them to want to engage further with a system they did not trust for a health problem they had not yet experienced. Women's ambivalence towards Pap smears was closely linked with negative experiences in which relationships with obstetricians/gynaecologists and health services were revealed as unsafe. A recurrent theme was situations in which women felt uncomfortable, intimidated or disrespected. This took many forms, including what doctors considered 'jokes' – humiliations reinforcing power asymmetries that caused women to feel anxious about interacting with the health system. Laura's experience, below, illustrates why women may choose not to return to health services at which they felt disrespected and disempowered:

> Laura: During my first pregnancy my doctor was [name removed]. He was a gynaecologist. I started with a female gynaecologist but she left and was replaced by another woman. Then she left and I got a man ... I had a colposcopy eight years ago, before I got pregnant, and I had it done by him. That fucking bastard scared me, because he explained to me how everything worked and he said: 'See the camera? [the instrument used for a colposcopy] well, out there [the television in the waiting room] they will see everything I see here ... ' I said, 'Are you kidding me?'
> (Group conversation, Laura, February 2019)

Many health centres have a television for people to watch while waiting for appointments, meaning that according to his 'humorous' remark, which Laura did not identify as such, the people in the waiting room could watch her gynaecological examination.

Women frequently discussed their experiences of local health services during pregnancy and childbirth and recounted details of other women's experiences. Premature births and stillbirths in this community are common. For instance, whenever Luxardo met with Nora, she talked about her children and grandchildren as she went about her daily tasks and in this context Nora regularly mentioned her stillborn son. Nora had experienced no complications until the day of his birth, when she endured unnecessary delays; no beds were available and the midwife insisted that they wait before calling the obstetrician despite Nora's insistence to do so. Nora explained that no one had listened to her and that they would not allow her elder daughter to be with her during the birth. She shared her intimate memories of her loss and trauma: 'they showed him to me . . . he was fat, with curls . . . he was beautiful . . . they killed him [at the hospital]'. To Nora it did not matter that it was over ten years ago. The pain was there, as fresh as the day it happened, and the gynaecological and obstetric services of the public health system were clearly identified as the party responsible for her loss.

Other women also disclosed traumatic experiences of miscarriages that they attributed to a doctor's refusal to listen to them and/or believe they were pregnant. One woman was disbelieved and assumed not to be pregnant simply because she was 44 years old; she recalled the doctor 'laughing in her face'. Another woman was told that she could not be pregnant because she had been using oral contraceptives, despite the fact that oral contraceptive failure is common; she later miscarried. Miscarriages were thus attributed to both the failure of doctors to listen to and treat women when they were pregnant and unwanted interventions, as described by Patricia:

> Patricia: My sister, for example, saw her (gynaecologist) for her first pregnancy and I told her: 'Don't see her, don't see her . . .' She did and she had her do a colposcopy. They kept telling her she was fat . . . I told her she should not go to have the test . . . She had it, they broke her water and she miscarried. After that I don't trust that woman . . . She's on trial . . . for doing abortions. (Group conversation, Patricia, February 2019)

Women openly criticised doctors' denial of their voices, as people with legitimate knowledge of their own bodies. They described how they were ignored, mocked and ridiculed and constructed as ignorant when attempting to explain what was happening to them. As Dora explained: 'They treat you as an ignorant. You keep telling them, because they are your children and you know them, but . . . "No, I am the doctor, I know"' (Fieldnotes, February 2019). This devaluation of women's knowledge and refusal to hear their concerns and preferences was particularly prevalent in the context of pregnancy care and in childbirth, and clearly constituted obstetric violence contributing to the continuing violence these women lived with (Quattrocchi 2020; Tobasía et al. 2019). When interruptions and discontinuations of cervical screening are viewed within this context of obstetric violence, women may well opt for strategies that avoid forms of violence already known to them, rather than seeking to avoid cancer screening per se.

The ethnographic data further revealed a stark contradiction between what biomedicine says will happen in the context of cervical cancer screening and prevention, and what women empirically experienced. According to these women biomedicine continually errs, produces bad diagnostics, poor or ineffective treatments, false negatives and positives and heterogeneous treatment paths. These failures, based on women's personal experiences, negate the dominant view of biomedical interventions as necessary, reliable and infallible and signify screening procedures as uncertain. When women view the public health system as unreliable and unsafe, they lose confidence in the efficacy of screening procedures and avoid health services. The institutional violence that women experience, in the course of seeking out reproductive healthcare within the public health system, is aptly described as a form of structural violence precisely because it is institutionalised, and acts to reproduce and deepen health and social inequalities (Farmer 2004). This institutional violence is experienced as continuous across women's life course from their earliest engagement with reproductive health services and into middle and older age, and is concurrent with everyday violences that women endure in their working and personal lives.

Continuums of racial and class violence

> My only hope is that this [COVID-19] pandemic makes the ethnic cleansing that we [respectable white Argentinian people] deserve ... with five or six million negros less ... less social plans ... maybe this country finally starts up. (Radio interview with a local politician, 8 April 2020)

> All South Americans are descendants of Europeans. (Mauricio Macri, Argentina's former president, 25 January 2018)

These quotes are from powerful public figures in Argentinian society who are invested with legitimate authority and represent a dominant cultural worldview that reproduces stigmatisation and racialisation directed towards marginalised women (Hicken et al. 2018). The opening quotes from women in this chapter illustrate the ongoing impact of racist and stigmatising discourses: 'we are discriminated against because we are poor, because we have social plans, because we live in shitty places'. As noted, the women in this study and their families are frequently referred to by the derogatory term 'dump negros', a racialised and class-based insult which causes great distress to women and their families. Women whose livelihoods depend on garbage picking and/or social plans (welfare payments) are dehumanised in the dominant Argentinian imagination to the extent that the value of their lives is publicly negated by the suggestion that society would be better off without them – as asserted, ethnic cleansing of the 'undesirables' via the COVID-19 pandemic was described as of benefit to the wider society.[1]

Blatant, systematic racism and class discrimination are a constant in women's lives, they constitute an inescapable continuity of violence reinforced by offensive stereotypes. These stereotypes are often directed at women's parity and involve an implicit questioning of the legitimacy of motherhood within the context of poverty. Common assumptions include that poor women have lots of children so they can 'live off welfare', 'because they are ignorant' and because 'they are promiscuous'. When the institutional and obstetric violence that women experience is viewed through the wider lens of society-level discrimination, which explicitly questions women's legitimacy as mothers and their rights to have children, subtle and explicit eugenics appears to influence women's decisions to avoid screening or seeing gynaecologists.

Women commonly felt afraid and uncomfortable when interacting with middle-class healthcare providers with power over their bodies and with morals and values contrary to their own. Many women shared experiences (of their own or of others close to them) in which doctors intervened in their sexual and reproductive health, sometimes through 'manipulations' aimed at convincing women of the validity of doctors' views regarding tubal ligation or abortion. Women viewed doctors' attempts to constrain their reproductive potential as consistent with a different (middle-class and biomedical) value system. Within the communities where women live, abortion was often viewed as abhorrent, as was infanticide:

> Luis: Once I was walking with my children over there, where we go down, and . . . when I came near they told me there was a dead baby . . . I couldn't see what was going on from the

>   dump, so I started looking carefully and I saw him, his little face . . . But it was a baby that had been born . . . the way in which his life was taken from him, poor guy, they stuck cotton up his mouth and nostrils . . . He was maybe 2 or 3 months old. I couldn't see him because he was very white . . .
> Mary: You have to be a bitch to do that . . . An innocent creature who can't defend himself . . . Most of us here are against abortion, yes. (Group conversation, August 2019)

This study was conducted within a historically significant period, as public advocacy for women's right to safe, legal and free abortion within the public health system became increasingly visible in Argentina.[2] Most women in this study claimed to be against abortion and some identified the struggle for access to safe abortion as the fight of 'women of a different class'. While sharing opinions about the national abortion debate, women highlighted the sacred value of their children, especially in contexts in which their lives were frequently at risk and their very existence was deemed almost 'a miracle'. Women's frequent experiences of miscarriage, premature birth, negative neonatal care and raising children in a neighbourhood environment of multiple risks enhanced the personal and symbolic value of children. Moreover, the high incidence of unintentional injury, suicide and homicide among youth was keenly felt by mothers, who understood their children's chances of surviving to adulthood were compromised within this high-risk environment. Women felt a need to defend their children, not only because they were at risk due to material deprivation and constant everyday violence, but also from an ontological viewpoint embedded in the frequent insistence of mainstream society that poor people should not have so many children.

Persistent, multiple and overlapping forms of violence shape and constrain these women's everyday lives and their screening practices. However, there were spaces and contexts in which the women defended their dignity and openly resisted values that negated their identities. This typically involved the rejection of and refusal to engage with doctors known to perform abortions or who were themselves childless. Casual discussions between women friends would often include rumours about the personal lives of gynaecologists and obstetricians. Women questioned whether or not they had children, where they had worked previously and how they had ended up in these locales, what their lives were like and whether or not they were heterosexual. These kinds of conversations, mockery and jokes frequently arose as explanations by women of why these doctors mistreated others:

> Lina: I think she [a female obstetrician] doesn't have any [children], or maybe she can't have children and that's why she has a . . . something personal against pregnant girls. She told me that thing about the dogs, that they are like her children . . . I didn't see her for my second pregnancy.
>
> Gabriela: There's another doctor I don't want, because I don't like her, she has a million lawsuits for abortions, so I don't like her. I want nothing to do with her. (Informal group discussion, 2019)

Persistent racial and class violence projected at women creates structural asymmetries in terms of women's ability to openly express their viewpoints with doctors in healthcare encounters, as illustrated above in relation to institutional violence. In the context where women's voices are unlikely to be heard or respected, the choice to avoid a particular doctor can be interpreted as a pragmatic strategy (Lock and Kaufert 1998) that enables women to avoid unwanted interventions and to escape imposed values pertaining to reproduction, sexuality and motherhood. Many women found ways to access the resources they needed (such as contraceptives) without participating in the recommended gynaecological check-ups and controls imposed through the health system:

> Laura: Once I took my daughter for a check-up and they gave me a Pap smear, about seven years ago . . . That was it, I never had another one. Actually, you reminded me that I have to pick up some [birth control] pills. They always ask you to have a check-up before giving you the birth control pills or an injection, but I won't do it. I have been getting the pills without seeing the doctor for seven years now.
>
> Sonia: Yeh, I've been having injections for nine years now and I don't see the doctor either. (Informal group discussion, 2019)

Women's evasions of the recommended protocols are a pragmatic form of resistance (Scott 2007) that arises in circumstances when the social and symbolic power differences between women and their doctors preclude direct confrontation. Continuums of racial and class violence underpin the avenues available to women to exercise agency in pursuit of their own health and that of their children. Another layer of understanding emerges as to why women avoid, interrupt or discontinue cervical cancer screening when we read these choices as a form of intended resistance that protects women from vulnerability and/or obstetric abuse.

Continuities of violence, cervical cancer mortality and possibilities for a politics of care

Throughout this chapter, we have situated women's choices to reject or interrupt cytological screening, despite their knowledge of its importance in cancer prevention, as embedded within their everyday lives and shaped by overlapping continuums of violence. These continuums operate within women's most intimate relationships, at the community level, in healthcare institutions and interactions with healthcare providers and within an overarching politics of racial and class discrimination. The entrenched nature of these continuums has been illustrated through our analysis of the multiple forms of violence that are the direct result of ongoing, multigenerational structural inequalities. For these women, the significantly higher risk of dying from cervical cancer, due to the failure to regularly screen, can be viewed as both a consequence of women's responses to intersecting forms of structural violence, as well as constituting a form of structural violence. Health interventions seeking to increase the uptake of screening among vulnerable women are unlikely to be successful if they fail to address the structural violence that deters women from accessing cervical cancer screening and reproductive healthcare more generally.

Our analysis of women's experiences of reproductive healthcare demonstrates the profound lack of cultural safety that marginalised women experience within the Argentinian public health system. Women spoke consistently of being ignored, silenced, laughed at, ridiculed and receiving substandard technical care, that is – poor medicine for the poor (Broom and Doron 2011). Thus, women's choice to not screen or not to undergo repeat screening can be interpreted as preventive (Menéndez 2008), precisely because they view such avoidance as a strategy of self-protection against the negative impacts of engaging with an unsafe health system. Lack of respect and safety in reproductive healthcare is driven by both race and class discrimination and a distinct mismatch between the values of women and healthcare providers. For cancer care to achieve cultural safety these entrenched politics of discrimination within the health system must be directly addressed.

Self-care for marginalised women must be negotiated in the context of their available resources and existing burdens of care. In communities where everyday life is precarious, and the overall health status of children and communities is poor, the immediate health and safety concerns of women receive greater attention than practices of prevention. Within these communities the gendered construction of women's roles as the primary carers of their families often translates into patterns of care where women focus their care outwards, away from themselves and onto children and other female kin. While self-care receives less attention, practices of care that focus on the well-being of family and community have greater resonance. Understanding how wider practices of care are shaped within these communities holds potential for interventions that draw on collective notions of well-being and care, and are less focused on the compliance of individual women with screening programme targets.

Our efforts to understand the complex causes of avoidable cancer deaths among Argentinian women who endure intersecting continuums of violence illuminates the importance of ethnographic enquiry into the politics of cancer care. The multilayered ethnographic data collected in these communities has enabled a lens that captures the impacts of racism, poverty, sexism and other forms of structural violence on women's practices of self-care. However, understanding women's screening choices in the context of their everyday social worlds is essential but insufficient. Far-reaching structural transformations, requiring considerable time and resources, are essential to redress current disparities in cervical cancer morbidity. Our intersectional analysis has allowed us to see how the smallest of failed interventions can have terrible effects in these communities, because of women's amplified vulnerability, the continuity of violence they experience and the persistence of their suffering. When women live with mounting trauma throughout their lives, layers of suffering can be easily activated with any misstep in the context of health system interactions. The retraining of health providers to facilitate cultural safety in cervical cancer screening should begin with the recognition of women's vulnerability as stemming from the continuity of the violence they must negotiate, as well as recognition of their values, rights and resilience.[3]

Acknowledgements

We thank the National Council of Scientific and Technical Research, the NCI (Argentina), the University of Buenos Aires and the Faculty of Social Sciences and Gino Germani Research Institute for the financial and academic support given to the project. We especially thank the women and men belonging to the Casa de Atención y Acompañamiento Comunitario 'José Daniel Rodríguez' for their warm welcome and support and thank also Lenore Manderson. The study was approved by the Bioethics Committee (Ministry of Health of Entre Rios), December 2015 and December 2017. Natalia Luxardo conceptualised and conducted the fieldwork; Luxardo and Linda Rae Bennett conducted the data analysis and theoretical framework for the chapter; Bennett cowrote and undertook the final edits of the chapter.

Notes

1   For further discussion of the evolution and intersection of racism and class discrimination in Argentinian society, see Frigerio (2006) and Geler (2016).
2   On 30 December 2020, the Voluntary Pregnancy Interruption Act No. 27,610 of Argentina was passed by the National Congress and enacted on 14 January 2021. The law establishes the right to abortion in all cases up to and including week 14, maintaining the validity of the right to abortion in cases of rape and risk to the life or health of the mother, with no time limit.
3   For additional ethnographic analysis of women's choice not to undertake cervical cancer screening, published in Spanish, see Luxardo (2021).

References

Afsah, Yusi Riwayatul. 2017. 'Perceived barriers of cervical cancer screening among married women in Minggir, Godean, Gamping Sub-Districts, Sleman District Yogyakarta', *Indonesian Journal of Nursing Practices* 1(2): 75–82. Accessed 16 September 2022. https://journal.umy.ac.id/index.php/ijnp/article/view/3441.

Arrossi, Silvina, Melisa Paolino and Rengaswamy Sankaranarayanan. 2010. 'Challenges faced by cervical cancer prevention programs in developing countries: A situational analysis of program organization in Argentina', *Revista Panamericana de Salud Pública* 28(4): 249–257. Accessed 16 September 2022. http://www.scielosp.org/scielo.php?script=sci_arttext&pid=S1020-49892010001000003.

Bourdieu, Pierre. 2000. *Cosas dichas*, 2nd edn. Barcelona, Spain: Gedisa.

Broom, Alex and Assa Doran. 2011. 'The rise of cancer in urban India: Cultural understandings, structural inequalities and the emergence of the clinic', *Health* 16(3): 250–266. https://doi.org/10.1177/1363459311403949.

Farmer, Paul. 2004. 'An anthropology of structural violence', *Current Anthropology* 45(3): 305–317. https://www.jstor.org/stable/10.1086/382250.

Foucault, Michel. 1978. *Historia de la sexualidad*. Buenos Aires, Argentina: Siglo XXI.

Frigerio, A. 2006. '"Negros" y "Blancos". Buenos Aires: Repensando nuestras categorías raciales'. In *Temas de Patrimonio Cultural*, edited by L. Maronese, 77–98. Buenos Aires, Argentina: Gobierno de la Ciudad de Buenos Aires.

Galtung, Johan. 1969. 'Violence, peace and peace research', *Journal of Peace Research* 6(3): 167–191.

Geler, L. 2016. 'Categorías raciales en Buenos Aires', *RUNA, Archivo Para Las Ciencias Del Hombre* 37(1): 71–88.

Hicken, Margaret T., Nicole Kravitz-Wirtz, Myles Durkee and James S. Jackson. 2018. 'Racial inequalities in health: Framing future research', *Social Science & Medicine* 199: 11–18. https://doi.org/10.1016/j.socscimed.2017.12.027.

Islam, Rakibul M., Baki Billah, Md Nassif Hossain and John Oldroyd. 2017. 'Barriers to cervical cancer and breast cancer screening uptake in low-income and middle-income countries: A systematic review', *Asian Pacific Journal of Cancer Prevention* 18(7): 1751–1763. https://doi.org/10.22034/APJCP.2017.18.7.1751.

Iummato, L. 2020. 'Saber experto, intereses y políticas de salud: el caso del Programa Nacional de Cáncer de Mama'. Master's thesis, Universidad Nacional de Lanús, Buenos Aires.

Lock, Margaret and Patricia A. Kaufert. 1998. 'Introduction'. In *Pragmatic Women and Body Politics*, edited by Margaret Lock and Patricia A. Kaufert, 1–27. Cambridge, UK: Cambridge University Press.

Luxardo, Natalia. 2021. '"Porque no quise": descifrando qué hay detrás de los rechazos o discontinuidades en los tamizajes de cuello de útero'. In *In Situ. El cáncer como injusticia social*, edited by Natalia Luxardo and Fernando Sassetti, 873–921. Buenos Aires, Argentina: Editorial Biblos.

Luxardo, Natalia and Hernán Manzelli. 2017. 'Blurred logics behind frontline staff decision-making for cancer control in Argentina', *Health Sociology Review* 26(3): 224–238. https://doi.org/10.1080/14461242.2017.1298973.

Manderson, Lenore and Narelle Warren. 2016. '"Just one thing after another": Recursive cascades and chronic conditions', *Medical Anthropology Quarterly* 30(4): 479–497. https://doi.org/10.1111/maq.12277.

Martínez, María Laura and Carlos Gustavo Guevel. 2013. 'Desigualdades sociales en la mortalidad por cáncer de cuello de útero en la Ciudad Autónoma de Buenos Aires, 1999–2003 y 2004–2006', *Salud Colectiva* 9(2): 169–182. https://doi.org/10.18294/sc.2013.30.

Menéndez, Eduardo L. 2008. 'Epidemiología sociocultural: propuestas y posibilidades', *Región y Sociedad* 20(2): 5–50.

NCI (National Cancer Institute). 2020. 'Estadísticas – Mortalidad. Ministerio de Salud, Argentina'. Accessed 24 December 2020. https://www.argentina.gob.ar/salud/instituto-nacional-del-cancer/estadisticas/mortalidad.

Palermo, María Cecilia, Fernando Sassetti and Natalia Luxardo. 2021. 'Estrategias para el control del cáncer y rol de los sistemas de información en salud en el Primer Nivel de Atención', *La Revista Argentina de Salud Publica* 13: 1–7.

Ponce, Marisa. 2013. 'La prevención del cáncer de cuello de útero y de mama en servicios de salud y organizaciones no gubernamentales de la Ciudad Autónoma de Buenos Aires', *Salud Colectiva* 9(2): 215–233. https://doi.org/10.18294/sc.2013.33.

Quattrocchi, Patrizia. 2020. 'Violencia obstétrica desde América Latina hasta Europa: similitudes y diferencias en el debate actual'. In *Violencia obstétrica en América Latina: conceptualización, experiencias, medición y estrategias*, edited by Patrizia Quattrocchi and Natalia Magnone, 195–201. Remedios de Escalada, Argentina: Universidad Nacional de Lanús.

Quesada, James, Laurie Kain Hart and Philippe Bourgois. 2011. 'Structural vulnerability and health: Latino migrant laborers in the United States', *Medical Anthropology* 30(4): 339–362. https://doi.org/10.1080/01459740.2011.576725.

Salvia, Agustín. 2012. *La Trampa Neoliberal. Un estudio sobre los cambios en la heterogeneidad estructural y la distribución del ingreso en la Argentina: 1990–2003*. Buenos Aires, Argentina: Eudeba.

Scott, James C. 2007. *Los dominados y el arte de la resistencia. Discursos ocultos*. Mexico City: Ediciones Era.

Tobasía-Hege, Constanza, Mariona Pinart, Sofia Madeira, Alessandra Guedes, Ludovic Reveiz, Rosario Valdez-Santiago, Vicky Pileggi et al. 2019. 'Irrespeto y maltrato durante el parto y el aborto en América Latina: Revisión sistemática y metaanálisis', *Pan American Journal of Public Health* 4: 36. https://doi.org/10.26633/RPSP.2019.36.

Tumas, Natalia, Sonia Alejandra Pou and María del Pilar Díaz. 2017. 'Inequidades en salud: análisis sociodemográfico y espacial del cáncer de mama en mujeres de Córdoba, Argentina', *Gaceta Sanitaria* 31(5): 396–403. https://doi.org/10.1016/j.gaceta.2016.12.011.

4
Laughing in the face of cancer: intersubjectivity and patient navigation in the US safety net

Nancy J. Burke

Everyone was laughing, including Morgan, the Nurse Practitioner. Jen, the patient navigator, sat on the filing cabinet next to the desk with the computer monitor and patient Emilia looked around incredulously, with a smile that extended across her face, from the edge of the bed where she sat. Her daughter shook her head, giggling at her mother's responses, and added more context and detail to the stories. The exchange seemed casual and light, but it took place at the end of a discussion of how to keep at bay, to the largest degree possible, a recurrence of Emilia's breast cancer. She was in the safety-net breast clinic for a check-up, having completed her surgery and about to begin long-term endocrine treatment with aromatase inhibitors.

Emilia's visit is one of many in which patient navigators work with patients and providers to create easeful conversations in which patients are seen as people, not simply as patients. As I illustrate, relational groundwork underlies the ease of this exchange. I posit laughter and intersubjective connection as central to the work of cancer patient navigation in a safety-net public hospital breast clinic treating un- and underinsured patients in northern California. Rather than proscribed or heavily scripted, I show that the skilled work of patient navigation in this clinic serves as an example of what Bourdieu (1977: 5) has referred to as the 'artful improvisations' that characterise human practices.

I draw upon the many different settings and spaces in which navigators work in their care of patients, and highlight exchanges in the public hospital breast clinic, cancer patient navigator training sessions and breast cancer survivorship group medical visits. The ethnographic examples explored detail moments that occurred in the course of over 15 years of fieldwork. During that time the navigation programme has grown, positions have changed and staffing has shuffled while key components of the programme have remained consistent.

Patient navigation

Women cared for in the breast cancer clinic at Urban Hospital (pseudonym) are largely un- or underinsured. Many are bilingual in English and Spanish, Mandarin, Cantonese, Ukrainian or Tagalog; they struggle with English and rely on bi- and trilingual patient navigators for interpretation, or the AT&T (telephone) language line when a patient navigator is not available. A large proportion are marginally housed or unhoused and suffer from stress associated with precarious or uncertain income. Biomedical research has documented the associations between ethnicity, income, education status and employment with a later stage of cancer diagnosis and cancer survival rates (Clegg et al. 2009; Simard et al. 2012; Tannenbaum et al. 2013; Thuret et al. 2013; Ward et al. 2004; Whitman, Orsi and Hurlbert 2012). While some of these disparities have been linked to biology, the majority have been shown to stem from lack of timely access to appropriate care (Rodday et al. 2015). Breast cancer patient navigation programmes were developed in the United States in an effort to address this, to help un- and underinsured women complete interdisciplinary cancer treatment. They were designed to bridge some of the structural inequalities underlying the US safety-net system of healthcare by assisting underserved or 'vulnerable' patients better navigate complex systems to get the treatments they need (Burke 2019; Gabitova and Burke 2014). Safety net in this context refers to healthcare centres that serve patients regardless of their ability to pay. In the United States, the safety-net system supports the working poor and precariously housed.

Harold Freeman created the first patient navigation programme in Harlem, NY, in 1990, in an effort to expand access to cancer screening and follow-up after abnormal results for African American women living in the area; in doing so, he successfully improved survival in women with breast cancer (Freeman 2006; Oluwole et al. 2003). He defined patient navigation as a community-based service delivery intervention designed to promote access to timely diagnosis and treatment of cancer and other chronic diseases by eliminating barriers to care (Freeman 2013). Elimination of these barriers has been shown to have exactly this effect.

A study of five of ten centres from the US National Cancer Institute's Patient Navigation Research Program found that employment, housing status and marital status were associated with delays in diagnostic resolution and that patient navigation eliminated these disparities for those receiving it (Rodday et al. 2015).

In recognition of the role of patient navigation in addressing disparities, the US Congress passed the Patient Navigation Outreach and Chronic Disease Prevention Act in 2005 and described patient navigation as an effective intervention to improve health outcomes by reducing delays to quality care through the use of a person guide throughout the healthcare system (Griggs et al. 2012). At the same time, the US Congress (2005) created a funding mechanism designed to support research on the impacts of patient navigation. In 2010 the Patient Protection and Affordable Care Act identified patient navigation as a strategy to facilitate insurance access (Centers for Medicare and Medicaid Services, n.d.) and provided federal funding for navigators to assist in confirming eligibility and enrolling in coverage through marketplaces. This was an important intervention as lack of insurance is associated with worse cancer outcomes (Pulte, Jansen and Brenner 2018) and financial toxicity is associated with cancer treatment (Chebli et al. 2020). Since then, several policy initiatives have supported the implementation of patient navigation programmes. For example, the American College of Surgeons Commission on Cancer (COC) in 2012 required all COC-accredited organisations to have a cancer patient navigation programme (Dixit, Rugo and Burke 2021).

The Breast Cancer Patient Navigation Program at Urban Hospital was initiated in mid-1997 to serve women in the local area who were appearing with late-stage disease, were not following through with treatment and were dying at higher rates than would occur with timely treatment. The design of the programme emerged from discussions in town halls conducted throughout the city. Milly, who would become Director of the Cancer Patient Navigation Program, led the discussions, which highlighted a desire for more accessible and personal care, recognition of the barriers to completing treatment for poor and non-English-speaking patients and a call for community concerns to inform clinical care. While patient navigators were originally conceived as clinic outreach workers whose role was to interface with the community surrounding the hospital, raise awareness about breast cancer risk and screening modalities and improve communication between the hospital and non-English-speaking populations in the hospital's catchment area, the town hall discussions pushed the breast clinic director and outreach staff to reconsider the roles the navigators should play. Rather than focus on outreach, they decided to turn to 'in-reach', providing support to women who were making it to the hospital to ensure that they had the support they needed to make it through the treatment process.

The breast clinic director designed the patient navigation programme to be managed by a nurse practitioner but delivered by women with no particular medical training. This was a conscious decision to try to break down communication barriers and power dynamics providers experienced with their patients and to promote the opportunity for relational connection with women 'like them' (Vargas et al. 2008). The primary qualifications each navigator brings to their position include prior experience in a hospital setting, strong communication skills and the ability to work in a complex, multicultural setting with complex patients with high social needs. Bi- or multilingualism is essential for a subset of navigators. This linguistic and cultural expertise distinguishes this programme from those elsewhere that utilise nurses, cancer survivors, social workers or volunteers to navigate patients. In many of these programmes, patient navigators come from the community or are socially/culturally/ethnically similar to the population they serve. Prior research highlights their role in empowering and educating patients and offering support and guidance, particularly to 'vulnerable communities' (Freund et al. 2008). Patient navigators do this by helping patients with instrumental tasks, such as facilitating access to benefits and providing interpretation at medical appointments. Some, including those at Urban Hospital, provide support throughout the continuum of care from diagnosis to survivorship (Paskett, Harrop and Wells 2011). Research on the effects and processes of navigation has highlighted the relationship and trust-building activities that navigators engaged in with breast cancer patients as central to their abilities to better integrate patients into care (Holmes et al. 2012; Natale-Pereira et al. 2011).

In the Urban Hospital breast clinic, every breast cancer patient is assigned a navigator the first day she enters the clinic, at times prior to her diagnostic resolution. There are usually five patient navigators on staff. They provide services in English, Spanish, Cantonese and Mandarin, and work with medical interpreters to fulfil the needs of patients speaking languages other than English. A key element of patient navigator support is their access to providers and their understanding of the way the safety-net healthcare system works. They field questions from patients and can often get answers for them in between clinic visits. This seemingly simple task can keep a patient from going to the emergency room or urgent care. Without responsive patient navigators, patients can spend frustrating hours trying to find the right phone number, waiting on hold endlessly only to be told they have reached the wrong part of the hospital. Patient navigators make appointments on behalf of patients, remind them of upcoming appointments, participate and take notes in clinic visits, remind patients to ask questions of providers while in clinic, assist with medication questions and at times triage patient concerns between appointments. They build trusting relationships with providers and become important sources of information about patients' broader social context that might impact their ability to adhere to chemotherapy or radiation regimens. They also build and maintain relationships with community-based organisations that provide financial, nutritional and emotional resources for their patients. Their willingness and ability to leverage these relationships and institutional knowledge on behalf of their patients constitutes an essential aspect of their value, both to patients and providers. While these aspects of navigational work have been noted elsewhere (de la Riva et al. 2016; Dudley et al. 2012; Krok-Schoen, Oliveri and Paskett 2016; Paskett, Harrop and Wells 2011), the contribution laughter makes to their delivery, and the intersubjective connection it supports, has yet to be explored.

Laughter

The role of laughter in the provision of medical care and healing has been subject to debate in US healthcare largely since the publication of Norman Cousins' 1976 article 'Anatomy of an Illness (As Perceived by the Patient)' in the *New England Journal of Medicine* and, subsequently, the book by the same name (Cousins 1976, 1979). Cousins' reflections on his recovery from what was thought to be a progressive and incurable illness of ankylosing spondylitis, a painful degenerative joint disease, highlighted the biological impacts of the laughter he engaged in, particularly its direct relationship with pain-free sleep and eventual cure. Cousins identified the failures of the hospital and medical system to foster a healing environment – by creating a stressful atmosphere where undisturbed sleep was nearly impossible, through lack of coordination between specialists resulting in over-testing or multiple specimens being taken and through providing poorly balanced meals including processed foods filled with preservatives – as inhibiting his ability to fight the disease (Cousins 1976). He challenged medical providers by asking if feelings of physical and mental distress can damage the body's chemistry, then couldn't positive feelings, such as those generated by laughter, rehabilitate it? This question has been taken up in a national movement of laughter yoga led by Laughing Guru Madan Kataria (Khatchadourian 2010).

Kataria promotes the physical benefits of laughter and distinguishes laughter from humour. This is important, as his laughter clubs, now an international phenomenon, are based in the practice of the physical experience of laughter without jokes. When promoting his approach, he cites William James' 1884 supposition that emotions are created *by* the body, not simply manifest within it, and argues that mirthful laughter can have a 'liberating, transformative effect – one that momentarily erases all practical concerns, fears, needs, and even notions of time' (Khatchadourian 2010: 7). He tells his followers that 'laughter is a divine vehicle for empathy and compassion' (Khatchadourian 2010: 7) and contends that laughter boosts immunity and is of particular benefit for cancer patients. He has urged members of his laughter group to 'go and give some sessions with cancer self-help groups' (Khatchadourian 2010: 10).

Early research on laughter focused on its effects on breathing and muscle tone and suggested that laughter's 'favorable impact on the mind influences various functions of the body and makes them healthier' (Walsh 1928, cited in Khatchadourian 2010: 10). Psychologists and neuroscientists have explored this insight more recently and found that even forced laughter can affect one's state of mind. Neuhoff and Schaefer (2002), for example, found that forced laughter and smiling were associated with elevated mood, even when performed alone, not in social settings. Berk and colleagues (1989: 395) found that laughter 'can reverse or attenuate' hormonal changes brought on by stress, and Morishima and colleagues (2019: 11) found that 'laughter therapy may improve specific domains of QOL [quality of life] and symptoms in cancer survivors'. They recommend that it be implemented 'as a complementary therapy for cancer patients, even if the beneficial effects are subtle' (Morishima et al. 2019: 11). Studies such as these are not definitive, but like Norman Cousins, they suggest the positive effects of laughter. They are enough to inform practice, however, as 'certified laughter trainers' have proliferated and laughing clubs can be found in hospitals and cancer centres around the world.

In the following discussion, I explore three contexts in which laughter emerged in the work of patient navigation. My goal is not to posit the centrality of laughter, but rather to detail its discursive contours and its multivalence. Laughter is not always natural, positive or appropriate. But sometimes it is. The malleability of this artful improvisation (Bourdieu 1977: 5) in practice reflects the flexible responsiveness that characterises, and underlies, the power behind patient navigation to soften the edges of care for women who are often neglected or marginalised.

Approach

Research reported here includes data from over 15 years of ethnographic engagement with the patient navigation programme at Urban Hospital. In that time, I conducted interviews with breast cancer surgeons, oncologists, patient navigators, social workers, nurse practitioners and oncology patients and have taken detailed fieldnotes from over 350 clinic days in outpatient oncology clinics. I have also observed and taken detailed fieldnotes in patient education sessions, support groups, survivorship group medical visits, grand rounds, pre-clinic staff meetings, patient navigation education sessions and tumour boards.

My process for conducting observations in the breast clinic included asking a resident, fellow, nurse practitioner, oncologist or patient navigator if I could shadow them during clinic times and take notes in a small notebook I kept with me. Throughout the clinic day I followed these providers into spaces where cases were presented to attendees, pathology reports discussed and treatment plans outlined. Prior to each patient visit, I approached the patient and asked if she minded if I observed the visit, ensuring her, in accordance with a verbal consent script approved by the University Committee on Human Subjects Research, that refusing to do so would in no way influence the care given. Because these clinics took place in a teaching hospital, it was common to have a number of people in the exam room, oftentimes taking notes. Therefore, the addition of the anthropologist was less disruptive than it may have been in a different care setting. I followed similar processes when observing patient navigator training or group medical visits.

Patient navigator training: laughter yoga

While Urban Hospital providers describe patient navigators as valued members of the care team, their 'lay' status and lack of official training can undermine their perceived legitimacy. As I have discussed elsewhere (Burke 2019), this can, at times, inhibit a patient navigator's ability to advocate on behalf of a patient. In 2010, Breast Cancer Disparities Program Director, Marjorie, instituted monthly patient navigator education training to aid professional development and provide continuing education opportunities. In a sense, the training was envisioned as a way to 'bring navigators up to speed' and to empower them with knowledge. In other words, the training was in part an attempt to address the legitimacy issue.

Marjorie constructed the training as an opportunity for learning and to foster communication between the broader network of community-based organisations providing support to breast clinic patients with the patient navigators coordinating their care. The meetings were open to community-based navigators – those working for non-profits in the area who specialised in providing wellness opportunities for patients and linked them to rental and nutrition assistance – as well as staff from those non-profits providing hot meals and food boxes, transportation, breast cancer support groups and housing assistance. The meetings were an opportunity to check in across organisations, to informally share information about patients supported by multiple staff and from different non-profits and the hospital navigators and to engage in a form of continuing education. Sessions addressed clinical trial participation (Burke 2019), treatment updates such as nipple-preserving surgery, nipple tattooing (Burke et al. 2015), grief management and research updates on the value of nutrition and stress management. The value of the training courses, and their purpose, shifted in response to the needs of the programme and direction received from Director of Medical Oncology. For example, the sessions on cancer clinical trials and treatment updates were designed to ensure that patient navigators who were interpreting for oncologists had the necessary information not only to interpret correctly but also to answer follow-up questions (Robinson-White et al. 2010; Vargas et al. 2008). Oncologists and nurse practitioners were well aware of the trusting relationship that patient navigators cultivated with their patients and that they often fielded questions on the providers' behalf. Other sessions focused more on the health and well-being of the navigators themselves, in attempts to provide them with skills to deal with the grief of losing long-term patients and with the emotional toll of providing support to family members left behind. Still others focused on administrative changes in the hospital and building connections with non-profit staff working outside the hospital. The expanse of the training reflected the comprehensive services provided by patient navigators; they assisted with everything from immigration papers, to insurance, to rent, to funeral arrangements.

The fieldnote below was written after a patient navigator training session focused on laughter yoga, which featured a nurse who had started introducing laughter yoga in the affiliated academic medical centre's integrative medicine centre.

Fieldnote, 7 February 2013

I smiled as I sat next to Milly, the navigation program director. I was excited, but she definitely didn't seem to be. I asked how she was and she replied, with a wry smile, 'this is one of Marjorie's sessions'.

The hospital's patient navigators sat around the big conference table, and some of the affiliated community health clinic staff and non-profit staff sat in chairs against the wall. It was a pretty professional setting, a conference room with a large table, and windows heavily draped with dark fabric. Lena from the Chinese support group was here, as was Marisol, from the Filipino Senior Center. There were several care navigators from another nonprofit, and one of the facilitators from Amore, the Spanish-speaking support group. People were talking softly to each other or looking at the piece of paper in front of them, a sort of agenda for the meeting. Marjorie had set up a small table near the entrance with water and some healthy snacks that she had picked up from Costco. Several people filled plates while Marjorie welcomed the speaker and made sure she had everything she needed.

Kathy, the speaker, introduced herself as a nurse who had found laughing yoga to be beneficial for her patients. She had taken a course and become a certified instructor. The practice was being taken up in different parts of the healthcare system, and she noted that there were sessions taking place in the academic hospital infusion centres. Milly's eyes cut across toward me, and then to Lisa, the Chinese bilingual patient navigator. Her look was skeptical and a little dubious. Kathy then introduced the work of the day. We would break into small groups and laugh together. There would be no need for jokes or humor, just physically laugh. We would start in groups of two and then move to larger groups. Then we would come back together to talk about how we felt. I looked around the room and watched as uncomfortable looks were shared and people started to pair up. Then Kathy told us to start. It was a slow beginning. I was paired with Olivia, the Spanish-speaking patient navigator. We giggled uncomfortably and just kept kind of doing that, making each other laugh by giving each other looks indicating how uncomfortable and strange this was. And we kept each other laughing.

Toward the close of the session, Kathy asked everyone to share their thoughts on their experience, and how they might integrate this into their own work. Olivia said she had been uncomfortable but ended up having fun. Marisol said it was nice to smile so much with her colleagues. Others mentioned feeling light, happy. When asked about integrating this into their work, no one had much to say. 'I don't know', 'I'm not sure how I would', 'I'm not sure it would be appropriate', were comments thrown out. Milly said very clearly,

'I can't imagine going into a room with someone who has just been diagnosed with breast cancer and starting to laugh. I just think it would be disrespectful.'

Reflections on the session popped up in conversations that occurred over the subsequent weeks. Milly commented, 'can you imagine, walking into a room and going [demonstrating a big belly laugh with an over-exaggerated smile] with our patients?' and Lisa remembered how strange it was to laugh with no reason. Director of the Amore Support Program, a breast cancer survivor herself, shared that she thought prompted laughter in infusion centres was a horrible idea. She compared it to her own experience of putting her head into the freezer when she was undergoing chemotherapy because she was told that keeping her head cold would help her retain her hair, keep it from falling out. Every time she opens a freezer, 15 years later, her body remembers that experience. She is transported back to the coldness. She said she would hate for her patients, who often have little to laugh about in any circumstances, in addition to suffering they experience navigating cancer care in the safety-net system, to re-experience chemo every time they laughed.

Supporting 'survivors'

The leadership of the breast clinic changed in 2015 and the new Director of Medical Oncology expressed a strong interest in cancer survivorship and in working directly with the patient navigation programme. She had become familiar with the programme during her training and one of her goals as the new director was to develop and expand the programme. She viewed the navigators as essential to patient care and felt the potential of the programme had barely been tapped. Her enthusiasm empowered Milly, Patient Navigation Program Director, to seek funds to pilot a group medical visit model for breast cancer survivors. Milly was well aware that the academic medical centre had had a well-developed survivorship clinic in the past that employed group visits and she thought the model would work well with their patients. She received a small grant to pilot the model with English-speaking breast cancer patients who were no longer in active treatment (for example, they had completed chemotherapy and radiation) over the course of six months. The programme recruited three cohorts of six patients to participate in five two-hour group sessions. At the beginning of the first session, the nurse practitioner spoke with each participant individually and walked them through a written summary of the treatment they had received in breast clinic. She also took their weight and measured their blood pressure. Jen, a navigator bilingual in English and Spanish, facilitated the sessions and each week a guest presented on a different health topic, including sexual health education, long-term side effects, healthcare maintenance and emotional health. Milly prepared food for each session, and participants regularly commented on what they liked – and did not – about the ingredients, preparation and presentation of the offerings.

The opportunity posed by the group medical visits was particularly exciting because the sessions took place in the navigation programme offices and the billing structure instituted by the hospital to support the sessions in essence instantiated the programme as a 'navigation clinic'. In the process of setting up the group medical visits, the patient navigation programme had achieved the level of legitimacy and institutional integration they had sought for many years.

Milly recruited a friend who happened to be a sex educator to present on sexuality for the group. The fieldnote below details what occurred during one of her sessions, which turned into quite a raucous affair.

Fieldnote, 7 February 2019

It was the third session of the survivorship group medical visits. Everyone was getting settled – Mindy on the hard green couch, shifting her hips in an attempt to get comfortable. Elsa had just rolled into the room in her wheelchair with her Chihuahua walking beside. She laid out the cloth pad the dog liked to rest on and poured water into his bowl as everyone oohed and ahhed at the puppy. Thelma smiled shyly beside me and asked how I was. She and I had connected on the challenges of parenting teenagers. Her daughter was continually worried about her and had helped her that week with some alternative treatments discussed in the group the week before to help bring Thelma's hair back. She could tell her hairline had receded as it was coming back in after chemo and she kept it covered with hair wraps. Nobue showed everyone that her hair was finally growing back but said with a frown that it is seventy percent white. Morgan, Nurse Practitioner, said that some women experience a change in the texture of their hair after chemo.

The energy was anticipatory; you could feel excitement in the air. Gisela smiled widely at everyone, asking how they were from her chair next to Elsa. Soon the patient navigator facilitator, Jen, entered with her supervisor Milly. Milly worked with her phone to get some music playing through a small speaker and laughed as she did a few dance moves, trying to get Gisela to join her on the floor. Once everyone settled, Jen introduced the speaker and topic for the day – Linda was here to talk about sex. The corners around Thelma's lips tightened and she looked over at Evelyn, an older African American woman sitting across from her. Evelyn gave her a little smile. Linda began by framing the discussion as something that is sometimes tough to talk about, and said that she wants people to feel free 'without shame' to ask questions, 'without judging or blaming yourself. Blame, shame and fear work against you.' Instead, she suggested that we all approach the discussion with optimism and a sense of possibility. She went on to say that 'You may have noticed, because of what you have gone through, changes in your relationship with desire. Medication may be playing a role.' She went on to highlight the physical effects of induced menopause. She pointed to a drawing she had taped to the wall, which depicted female biology in a way strikingly similar to an avocado. Elsa's comment on the likeness set off a few giggles. Linda pointed to the pleasure areas and spoke about the importance of moisture in feeling pleasure. She then stepped back from the biology to talk more generally about intimacy and how it can change with major life changes, different ways of feeling intimacy, and different places on the body – such as around the ears – that can be pleasure centres.

Jen asked, 'do people do things for themselves?' Evelyn said she buys sunflowers because they remind her of her husband. She also mentioned relaxing, writing in a journal, 'having memories that bring a smile to your face. Because I am a widow.' Others mentioned music. Celestyn, 'a good movie'. Linda said, after a long pause, 'I'm here to tell you, you deserve to be happy and to do things for yourself.' Gisela said she sings karaoke in her house with her husband. She likes to sing Celia Cruz. Evelyn rubbed her fingers, leading Linda to comment that a loss of sensation in breast tissue might happen, so you can explore your body to find new pleasure zones. 'It's an opportunity to develop a new relationship with your body. At the end of the day, it's up to you to decide . . . You also need to tell your partner what feels good.' The mood in the room softened as everyone shared, and looked around at others, gauging responses. Linda talked about how each one of us can give ourselves pleasure by just spending a little more time putting lotion on after a shower – rather than slathering it on quickly, take a minute and caress yourself. Everyone smiled.

Linda then turned to vaginal atrophy, and Morgan stepped in, noting that 'everyone's breast cancer is different so not everyone has had hormone blockers, which can exacerbate vaginal atrophy and dryness. Be careful about lubricants. You may have heard that coconut oil is good because it is natural, but it can disrupt your body's Ph and cause a yeast infection. Replense has been studied and has been shown to be effective and safe for introducing moisture into the vagina.' Jen jumped in to say, 'if you are interested in Replense we can get some for you to take home'.

Morgan and Linda start prompting each other, with Morgan noting 'it's not just about sex, there can be burning with urination daily'. Linda noted, 'lubrication is primarily for sexual activity. Not just penetration; it's also for your vulva. There are silicon based and water based lubricants. Silicon based is longer lasting and you use less.' She leaned down to pull out vaginal dilators from her bag and everyone started laughing. She suggested 'these are useful to stretch the tissues that lose their elasticity due to menopause'.

She shared three varieties, each of a different material and each in increasing size, from narrow to wide. The shapes passed from hand to hand around the room, and I watched as women felt the shapes, and touched the surface against palms and cheeks. Linda then turned back to the avocado drawing, gave a short anatomy lesson, and talked about pleasures points. She passed around vibrators shaped to stimulate the different points and repeated her key message of the need to stay relaxed. As she demonstrated the different speeds, she said that there is a connection between the brain and the body. 'Just see if you can have a little more pleasure in your life.'

One vibrator, called the mighty bullet, could be attached to an expander or dildo to turn it into a vibrator. It was so small, she pointed out, you could take it with you anywhere and give yourself some pleasure on the go. Laughter filled the air as women passed around the vibrators, played with the speeds, and touched them to different parts of their bodies. At the end of the session Jen and Milly gave everyone a 'mighty bullet', packets of lubricant, and packets of Replense. Elsa kept repeating how much she wished someone had told her these things earlier, that if she had known about expanders she could have saved herself a lot of pain. Evelyn said, 'That was good. You're never too old to learn something.'

At the beginning of the next session the following week, Elsa looked around the room as she settled in her Chihuahua and asked, with a mischievous look on her face, if everyone had moisturized before coming to the session, eliciting bouts of laughter.

In interviews after the sessions, in which women were asked to reflect on their experiences, they repeatedly commented on their surprise at how much they enjoyed the sexuality session, saying how much fun it was, how the laughing made them all feel so relaxed and how they had actually learned something new. Elsa was adamant about the importance of the session, repeating how much pain she could have avoided had she known about expanders and the other products shared in the session. Several women shared that having Jen and Milly there was important; that it made them feel safe to talk about such a sensitive topic.

Back in the clinic . . .

The kinds of interactions patient navigators have with patients and providers in continuing education training, over the phone and in group medical visits, inform the roles they play in the clinic. At the beginning of each clinic day, patient navigators review their list of patients and plan their movement between rooms by identifying those patients they can just check in on and those who require either linguistic or emotional support. They prioritise patients who may struggle with asking questions of providers, or understanding recommended next steps or those at transition points. These transitions include the receipt of pathology results, movement between stages of treatment (for example, from chemotherapy and radiation to surveillance or aromatase inhibitors) and 'graduation' from breast clinic to surveillance in primary care. The following fieldnote, an expansion of the interaction with which I opened this chapter, details the communication that occurred as Emilia received the news that her surgery was successful – the pathology report showed clean margins – and what her next steps would be. Of note is the manner in which laugher and joking was balanced with information sharing and care delivery and the active involvement of each person in the room in the conversation.

Fieldnote, 15 October 2019

Morgan described Emilia's next steps following her surgery as moving on to the 'last piece'. As she stated, 'It's not really treating your cancer anymore. It's preventing it from coming back. Now we can give you a simple pill with little to no side effects that you can take for five years. What questions do you have?' Emilia responded, 'just about the side effects'. She laughed as she said, 'I don't want to be weirder than I already am.' Her daughter chuckled with her. Morgan responded with a smile and laugh and explained that aromatase inhibitors suppress estrogen, that even after menopause adrenal glands continue to produce a small amount of estrogen. The aromatase inhibitors interfere with the glands making estrogen. Emilia followed with 'But I won't be run down?' Morgan reassured her that she shouldn't be, that that isn't one of the common side effects. 'Women who are further from their change experience fewer side effects because the body is already adapted. The side effects are mainly hot flashes and joint pain.' Emilia's daughter asked if the pill Morgan was recommending was 'the one with the most success rates'. Morgan answered yes; that most of the studies were based on Anastrozole and that was the one they would start with. Next the daughter asked about herbal supplements.

After discussing osteoporosis and the importance of supplemental calcium and Vitamin D, Emilia asked if Anastrozole was expensive 'in case my insurance lapses'. She was considering leaving her current job because of the stress. She had stayed thus far because of the insurance coverage but was in the process of thinking through whether it was worth it or not, and she was afraid she might need to go on Medicaid. Morgan said she didn't know, but could look it up. She turned to the computer and found that it would cost '$177.99 a month out of pocket. But it would be less on Medicare.' After asking about a pretest for bone density the daughter teased Morgan that they had stumped her with the insurance question, 'Like "got cha!"' Everyone laughed loudly, laughter that continued as Morgan suggested she start the breast exam. Emilia joked, 'These have been around, what's one more?'

After the exam Emilia's daughter asked, 'How big is the pill?' Morgan responded that it was 'Medium. Not as big as calcium.' She then looked it up on the computer and showed them a picture of the pills. They both commented, 'Oh, that's not bad.' This led to a medication check. As Morgan looked at the computer Emilia's daughter pulled out a list. Morgan turned to her and said that she thought that what was on the computer was out of date. When she looked at what the daughter handed her, she and Jen started laughing loudly. They had expected a long list, but it only contained one thing – a cholesterol pill. There was almost nothing on it. They repeated several times how funny that was.

Toward the end of the visit Morgan talked through preventive recommendations. She recommended moderate exercise and seemed impressed by Emilia's description of her weightlifting and yoga practice. Laugher erupted again when Morgan mentioned moderation in alcohol consumption. She leaned forward, smiling, and touched Emilia's knee as she said having a glass of wine was okay, but not to drink too much. Emilia looked skeptical. 'Who doesn't drink the whole bottle of wine? I've never understood how people can just drink a little. It's open, you should drink it.' Morgan laughed in response, and Jen giggled from her perch on the file cabinet. Morgan recommended that Emilia just cut back a little bit. Jen agreed with Emilia, saying that she drinks bubbly wine and feels like once it's open, it needs to be drunk. Has less calories too. Emilia looked around as everyone laughed, saying that on holidays, people always give out those decorative wine stoppers. She never understood that. 'Who uses them?'

They left the visit smiling, with a plan to come back in six months. At that follow up visit we laughed again about the wine, and Emilia told Jen that she had actually cut back a bit.

As everyone laughed and contributed to the conversation, Jen asserted a shared experience with Emilia as she described her own appreciation of wine, particularly bubbly wine. They were aligned in their enjoyment; there was no judgement but rather recognition. The next visit reasserted this connection as did the fact that Emilia had heard the recommendation and had 'eased up' on her wine consumption. This sharing was not 'a devolution of one selfhood into another' (Wiltshire 2000: 409, cited in Burke 2014: 30), but rather a softening of the boundaries, a form of relational connection and knowing that supported the clinical goals of the visit.

This form of intersubjective connection differs significantly from many characterisations of the 'biomedical gaze'. Foucault depicted the limitations of this gaze when he noted that, 'in relation to that which he is suffering from, the patient is only an external fact; the medical reading must take him into account only to place him in parentheses' (Foucault 2003: 8). In the clinical exchange between Jen, Emilia, Morgan and Emilia's daughter, Jen extracted Emilia from any parentheses. Rather than being produced by the medical gaze as a breast cancer patient, this discussion encompassed the whole of Emilia, as a fit, funny, wine-drinking woman who has lived in the neighbourhood for over 30 years and watched it change. The conversation turned into a co-creation of value – of knowledge, experience and practice.

Discussion

Intersubjectivity refers to the ways we come into being through the mutual recognition of another (Burke 2014). The examples explored herein highlight the different contexts in which laughter emerges in the work of patient navigation and the role laughter plays in the kind of intersubjective connection patient navigators create with their patients. After the laughter training, patient navigators expressed concern about integrating laughter yoga as taught – without jokes, as a forced physical experience – into their interactions with patients. Comments in the weeks following the training included concerns about appropriateness, respect and the possibility of doing harm rather than healing. These comments stemmed from navigators' recognition of the need for laughter to arise organically, not to be imposed into already challenging contexts. They also reflect the navigators' recognition that in the institutional setting of the safety net the healing value of laughter is sometimes less about its individual physical effects and more about its utility in the face of institutional constraints, lack of resources and bureaucratic barriers that can inhibit the smooth and timely provision of care.

In the survivorship group medical visits, laughter erupted as discussion of sensitive and painful topics such as loss and changes in sexuality unfolded alongside tactile interactions with sex toys. The coy looks women shared as they stroked the expanders and played with the speeds of the vibrators were acknowledging and light. In the clinic, Jen's alignment with Emilia around their enjoyment of wine is another example of this recognition.

> [Intersubjectivity] maintains that the individual grows in and through the relationship to other subjects. Most important, this perspective observes that the other whole the self meets is also a self, a subject in his or her own right. It assumes that we are able and need to recognize that other subject as different and yet alike. (Benjamin 1988: 19–20)

The role of laughter in the intersubjective work of patient navigation, in the relational work that underlies navigators' ability to meet patients' clinical and social needs, aligns with – and differs from – findings from a recent ethnographic study of humour and laugher among incurable patients in cancer centre. This research suggests an elemental connection between humour and subjectivity. Patients reported that humour could 'reinforce or intensify relational bonds' (Buiting et al. 2020: 2428). In addition, humour was found to be useful when broaching difficult topics. Researchers conflate humour with laughter in this analysis, which is distinct from the way Kataria and his followers conceptualise the healing role of laughter. In laughter yoga, the potential alienating aspects of jokes – due to their personal appeal – can get in the way of the physical benefits of laughter. In Buiting and colleagues' research with terminal cancer patients, laughter was considered 'lighter' than humour. Patients and providers in the cancer centre identified 'laughter as humanizing, a reminder of their essential selves' (Buiting et al. 2020: 2430).

The ways laughter emerges in the work of patient navigation in this US safety-net hospital highlight its importance for both the patients and navigators. It is an elemental but rarely commented upon piece of the improvisational work of care provision in low-resource settings (Livingston 2012). While there is growing recognition of the value of patient navigation in cancer care, the relational tools necessary to do it well in fragmented healthcare systems have yet to be clearly defined. Patient navigators at Urban Hospital rely on laughter in many ways – not the laughter therapy practised in the academic medical centre infusion centres, nor that espoused by Madan Kataria's followers – but laughter as they defined it.

Acknowledgements

This work would not have been possible without the friendship and support of Barbara Cicerelli, whose compassion and creativity know no bounds. I would also like to thank the cancer patient navigators and patients who allowed me to listen and sit in on clinic visits, meetings and support sessions. Lastly, I would like to thank the oncology clinic leadership whose support and guidance enabled this research.

References

Benjamin, Jessica. 1988. *The Bonds of Love: Feminism and the problem of domination*. London: Virago.
Berk, Lee S., Stanley A. Tan, William F. Fry, Jerry W. Lee, Richard W. Hubbard, John E. Lewis and William C. Eby. 1989. 'Neuroendocrine and stress hormone changes during mirthful laughter', *The American Journal of Medical Sciences* 298(6): 390–396.

Bourdieu, Pierre. 1977. *Outline of a Theory of Practice*. Cambridge, UK: Cambridge University Press.
Buiting, Hilde M., Remco de Bree, Linda Brom, Jennifer W. Mack and Michiel W. M. van den Brekel. 2020. 'Humour and laughing in patients with prolonged incurable cancer: An ethnographic study in a comprehensive cancer centre', *Quality of Life Research* 29: 2425–2434. https://doi.org/10.1007/s11136-020-02490-w.
Burke, Lucy. 2014. 'Oneself as another: Intersubjectivity and ethics in Alzheimer's illness narratives', *Narrative Works* 4(2): 28–47. https://doi.org/10.7202/1062098ar.
Burke, Nancy J. 2019. 'Stuck in the middle: Clinical trials and patient navigation in the safety-net'. In *Negotiating Structural Vulnerability and Cancer Control: Contemporary challenges for applied anthropology*, edited by Julie Armin, Nancy J. Burke and Laura Eichelberger, 141–166. Albuquerque: University of New Mexico Press.
Burke, Nancy J., Tessa Napoles, Fern Orenstein, Sasha Merrit and Judith Luce. 2015. 'Assessing the impact of post-surgery areola repigmentation and 3-dimensional nipple tattoo procedures on body image and quality of life among medically underserved breast cancer survivors'. San Antonio Breast Cancer Symposium, TX, 5–7 December.
Centers for Medicare and Medicaid Services. n.d. 'In-person assistance in the health insurance marketplaces'. Accessed 14 August 2020. https://www.cms.gov/CCIIO/Programs-and-Initiatives/Health-Insurance-Marketplaces/assistance.
Chebli, Perla, Jocelyne Lemus, Corazón Avila, Kryztal Peña, Bertha Mariscal, Sue Merlos, Judith Guitelman and Yamilé Molina. 2020. 'Multilevel determinants of financial toxicity in breast cancer care: Perspectives of healthcare professionals and Latina survivors', *Supportive Care in Cancer* 28(7): 3179–3188. http://dx.doi.org/10.1007/s00520-019-05119-y.
Clegg, Limin X., Marsha E. Reichman, Barry A. Miller, Benjamin F. Hankey, Gopal K. Singh, Yi Dan Lin, Marc T. Goodman et al. 2009. 'Impact of socioeconomic status on cancer incidence and stage at diagnosis: Selected findings from the surveillance, epidemiology, and end results: National Longitudinal Mortality Study', *Cancer Causes & Control* 20: 417–435. https://doi.org/10.1007/s10552-008-9256-0.
Cousins, Norman. 1976. 'Anatomy of an illness (as perceived by the patient)', *New England Journal of Medicine* 295(26): 1458–1463. https://doi.org/10.1056/NEJM197612232952605.
Cousins, Norman. 1979. *Anatomy of an Illness as Perceived by the Patient: Reflections on healing and regeneration*. New York: W. W. Norton & Company.
Dixit, Niha, Hope Rugo and Nancy J. Burke. 2021. 'Navigating a path to equity in cancer care', *ASCO (American Society of Clinical Oncology) Educational Book* 41: 3–10.
Dudley, Donald J., Joan Drake, Jennifer Quinlan, Alan Holden, Pam Saegert, Anand Karnad and Amelie Ramirez. 2012. 'Beneficial effects of a combined navigator/promotora approach for Hispanic women diagnosed with breast abnormalities', *Cancer Epidemiology Biomarkers & Prevention* 21(10): 1639–1644. https://doi.org/10.1158/1055-9965.EPI-12-0538.
Foucault, Michel. 2003. *Birth of the Clinic: An archaeology of medical perception*. London: Routledge Classics.
Freeman, Harold P. 2006. 'Patient navigation: A community based strategy to reduce cancer disparities', *Journal of Urban Health: Bulletin of the New York Academy of Medicine* 83(2): 139–141. https://doi.org/10.1007/s11524-006-9030-0.
Freeman, Harold P. 2013. 'The history, principles, and future of patient navigation: Commentary', *Seminars in Oncology Nursing* 29(2): 72–75. https://doi.org/10.1016/j.soncn.2013.02.002.
Freund, Karen M., Tracy A. Battaglia, Elizabeth Calhoun, Donald J. Dudley, Kevin Fiscella, Electra Paskett, Peter C. Raich and Richard G. Roetzheim. 2008. 'National Cancer Institute Patient Navigation Research Program: Methods, protocol, and measures', *Cancer* 113(12): 3391–3399. https://doi.org/10.1002/cncr.23960.
Gabitova, G. and Nancy J. Burke. 2014. 'Improving healthcare empowerment through breast cancer patient navigation: A mixed methods evaluation in a safety-net setting', *BMC Health Services Research* 14(407). https://doi.org/10.1186/1472-6963-14-407.
Griggs, Jennifer J., Sarah T. Hawley, John J. Graff, Ann S. Hamilton, Reshma Jagsi, Nancy K. Janz, Mahasin S. Mujahid et al. 2012. 'Factors associated with receipt of breast cancer adjuvant chemotherapy in a diverse population-based sample', *Journal of Clinical Oncology* 30(25): 3058–3064. https://doi.org/10.1200/JCO.2012.41.9564.
Holmes, Dennis Ricky, Jacquelyn Major, Doris Efosi Lyonga, Rebecca Simone Alleyne and Sheilah Marie Clayton. 2012. 'Increasing minority patient participation in cancer clinical trials using

oncology nurse navigation', *American Journal of Surgery* 203(4): 415–422. https://doi.org/10.1016/j.amjsurg.2011.02.005.

Khatchadourian, Raffi. 2010. 'The laughing guru'. *The New Yorker*, 30 August. https://www.newyorker.com/magazine/2010/08/30/the-laughing-guru.

Krok-Schoen, Jessica L., Jill M. Oliveri and Electra D. Paskett. 2016. 'Cancer care delivery and women's health: The role of patient navigation', *Frontiers in Oncology* 6(2): 1–10. https://doi.org/10.3389/fonc.2016.00002.

Livingston, Julie. 2012. *Improvising Medicine: An African oncology ward in an emerging cancer epidemic*. Durham, NC: Duke University Press.

Morishima, Toshitaka, Isao Miyashiro, Norimitsu Inoue, Mitsuko Kitasaka, Takashi Akazawa, Akemi Higeno, Atsushi Idota et al. 2019. 'Effects of laughter therapy on quality of life in patients with cancer: An open-label, randomized controlled trial', *PLoS ONE* 14(6): e0219065. https://doi.org/10.1371/journal.pone.0219065.

Natale-Pereira, Ana, Kimberly R. Enard, Lucinda Nevarez and Lovell A. Jones. 2011. 'The role of patient navigators in eliminating health disparities', *Cancer* 117(S15): 3543–3552. https://doi.org/10.1002/cncr.26264.

Neuhoff, Charles C. and Charles Schaefer. 2002. 'Effects of laughing, smiling, and howling on mood', *Psychological Reports* 91: 1079–1080.

Oluwole, Soji F., Ayoola O. Ali, Albert Adu, Brenda P. Blane, Barbara Barlow, Ruben Oropeza and Harold P. Freeman. 2003. 'Impact of a cancer screening program on breast cancer stage at diagnosis in a medically underserved urban community', *Journal of the American College of Surgeons* 196(2): 180–188. https://doi.org/10.1016/S1072-7515(02)01765-9.

Paskett, Electra D., J. Phil Harrop and Kristen J. Wells. 2011. 'Patient navigation: An update on the state of the science', *CA: A Cancer Journal for Clinicians* 61(4): 237–249. https://doi.org/10.3322/caac.20111.

Pulte, Dianne, Lina Jansen and Hermann Brenner. 2018. 'Disparities in colon cancer survival by insurance type: A population-based analysis', *Diseases of the Colon & Rectum* 61(5): 538–546. https://doi.org/10.1097/DCR.0000000000001068.

Riva, Erika de la, Nadia Hajjar, Laura S. Tom, Sara Phillips, XinQi Dong and Melissa A. Simon. 2016. 'Providers' views on a community-wide patient navigation program: Implications for dissemination and future implementation', *Health Promotion Practice* 17(3): 382–390. https://doi.org/10.1177/1524839916628865.

Robinson-White, Stephanie, Brenna Conroy, Kathleen H. Slavish and Margaret Rosenzweig. 2010. 'Patient navigation in breast cancer: A systematic review'. *Cancer Nursing* 33(2): 127–140. https://doi.org/10.1097/NCC.0b013e3181c40401.

Rodday, Angie Mae, Susan K. Parsons, Frederick Snyder, Melissa A. Simon, Adana A. M. Llanos, Victoria Warren-Mears, Donald Dudley et al. 2015. 'Impact of patient navigation in eliminating economic disparities in cancer care', *Cancer* 121(22): 4025–4034. https://doi.org/10.1002/cncr.29612.

Simard, Edgar P., Stacey Fedewa, Jiemen Ma, Rebecca Siegel and Ahmedin Jemal. 2012. 'Widening socioeconomic disparities in cervical cancer mortality among women in 26 states, 1993–2007', *Cancer* 118(20): 5110–5116. https://doi.org/10.1002/cncr.27606.

Tannenbaum, Stacey L., Tulay Koru-Sengul, Feng Miao and Margaret M. Byrne. 2013. 'Disparities in survival after female breast cancer diagnosis: A population-based study', *Cancer Causes & Control* 24: 1705–1715. https://doi.org/10.1007/s10552-013-0246-5.

Thuret, Rodolphe, Maxine Sun, Lars Budaus, Firas Abdollah, Daniel Liberman, Shahrokh F. Shariat, François Iborra et al. 2013. 'A population-based analysis of the effect of marital status on overall and cancer-specific mortality in patients with squamous cell carcinoma of the penis', *Cancer Causes & Control* 24: 71–79. https://doi.org/10.1007/s10552-012-0091-y.

US Congress. 2005. Patient Navigator Outreach and Chronic Disease Prevention Act of 2005. 29 June. https://www.congress.gov/bill/109th-congress/house-bill/1812.

Vargas, Roberto B., Gery W. Ryan, Catherine A. Jackson, Rian Rodriguez and Harold P. Freeman. 2008. 'Characteristics of the original patient navigation programs to reduce disparities in the diagnosis and treatment of breast cancer', *Cancer* 113(2): 426–433. https://doi.org/10.1002/cncr.23547.

Walsh, James J. 1928. *Laughter and Health*. New York: D. Appleton and Company: New York.

Ward, Elizabeth, Ahmedin Jemal, Vilma Cokkinides, Gopal K. Singh, Cheryll Cardinez, Asma Ghafoor and Michael Thun. 2004. 'Cancer disparities by race/ethnicity and socioeconomic status', *CA: A Cancer Journal for Clinicians* 54(2): 78–93. https://doi.org/10.3322/canjclin.54.2.78.

Whiltshire, John. 2000. 'Biography, pathography, and the recovery of meaning', *Cambridge Quarterly* 24(4): 409–422.

Whitman, Steven, Jennifer Orsi and Marc Hurlbert. 2012. 'The racial disparity in breast cancer mortality in the 25 largest cities in the United States', *Cancer Epidemiology* 36(2): e147–51. https://doi.org/10.1016/j.canep.2011.10.012.

5
Morality tales of reproductive cancer screening camps in South India

Cecilia Coale Van Hollen

One early morning in July 2015, I was sitting in an open-air waiting area of the outpatient clinic at the Tamil Nadu Government Cancer Hospital in Kancheepuram.[1] I looked up to see a series of posters on the wall. Most were straightforward public health announcements about the dangers of smoking and the importance of breast self-examination and regular cervical cancer screening. But one caught my eye. At the centre was a large picture of a Hindu couple during their marriage ceremony, dressed in traditional wedding garb, with bountiful jasmine garlands around their necks. Below this couple, in red font, the poster said (in Tamil): There is no protection like moral sex (*ozhukkamana udaluravu oppatra padukappu*) (see Figure 5.1). The only indication on this poster that it was even about cancer was the name of the hospital at the top and the small international cancer symbol of the crab in the bottom right corner. There was no mention of what kind of cancer this referred to. What was clear was that cancer is associated with immoral sexuality. Since this poster hung directly across from the gynaecological oncologist's office of this public government hospital that caters primarily to low-income patients, it was also clear that this message was intended for lower-class and lower-caste women. The idealised Tamil bride depicted in the poster symbolised cancer prevention for women. As I was to discover, such moralising messages were a mainstay of public health programmes to prevent cancer and to promote screening for reproductive cancers in Tamil Nadu, South India.

India carries a disproportionate percentage of the world's cancer mortality burden. This is particularly so for breast and cervical cancers,

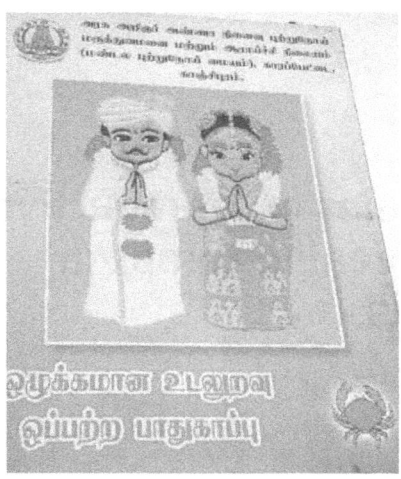

Figure 5.1 Government cancer poster. © Department of Health and Family Welfare, State of Tamil Nadu, India.

the leading forms of cancer among women in India. The vast majority of Indian women do not have access to Pap smears or mammograms for early detection of cervical and breast cancer.[2] The disparity in access to early cancer screening and treatment between low- and middle-income countries such as India, on the one hand, and high-income countries on the other, is particularly glaring for these two cancers, given the remarkable progress made in treatment outcomes if they are detected at an early stage (Farmer et al. 2010; Mallath et al. 2014). One result of this disparity is that more women die from both cervical and breast cancer in India than anywhere else in the world (Davies 2013; Raina 2013). Thirteen per cent of all deaths from breast cancer worldwide occur in India and 25 per cent of all women who die from cervical cancer in the world are Indian.[3]

During the first decades of the twenty-first century, international and local government and non-government organisations (NGOs) stepped up efforts to promote and provide screening and early treatment for cervical and breast cancer in low-income communities in India. With support from the World Bank, the South Indian state of Tamil Nadu was the first state in India to incorporate these screenings into its public primary health programme. Whereas high-income countries use Pap smears and mammograms, many of the recent government and NGO interventions in India rely heavily on low-cost, low-tech methods of visual screening for cervical cancer – VIA and VILI[4] – that were developed in

India, and for breast cancer, clinical breast exams and instructions for breast self-examination.

Although all cancers are stigmatised to some degree in India because they are often viewed as fatal, cervical and breast cancers carry an added, unique kind of stigma because they affect parts of women's bodies that are associated with sexuality – a taboo and highly censored topic. With better access to early detection and treatment – and thus, better health outcomes – cervical and breast cancer could become less stigmatised in India, thereby further encouraging women to make use of cancer screening.

Based on ethnographic research in Tamil Nadu during the summers of 2015 and 2016, in this chapter I analyse the messages conveyed through visual and oral presentations at public health 'camps' designed to educate primarily lower-class women about cervical and breast cancer and to encourage them to undergo screening for these cancers. I argue that in the process of conveying information about the importance of regular cancer screening, these messages also convey highly normative middle-class, upper-caste ideas about gender, morality and modernity and neoliberal assumptions of individual responsibility. In doing so, these programmes may inadvertently further the stigma of these two forms of cancer among women in South India. These educational interventions also seem to serve as a conduit to simultaneously promote other public health and social development campaigns without clearly demonstrating how recommendations for or against various practices are specifically associated with cancer risk. Furthermore, while these campaigns promote individual behaviour changes to prevent cancer, they do not address broader social transformations needed for individual women to be able to change their practices to follow the recommended guidelines.

A critical analysis

Inspired by Foucault's (1978) concept of biopower, feminist critical medical anthropologists have shown that biomedical and public health science and practice can serve to reify patriarchal values and hierarchies even if such power may be resisted. They have also demonstrated that gender inequalities are interwoven with other social relations of power such as class, race, ethnicity, nationality and colonial and neocolonial relationships within biomedical and public health projects (Martin 1987; Ram and Jolly 1998).

Similarly, historians of medicine in India have documented ways that public health measures were used to serve biopolitical projects in colonial India in part by disseminating middle-class Victorian values about gender roles, marriage, reproduction and sexuality (Levine 1994; Whitehead 1995). Scholars of postcolonial India have shown how this tendency continued through government and NGO public health programmes that have been part and parcel of developmentalist and nationalist projects to craft modern Indian citizens. Postcolonial programmes to improve women's health have served to promote idealised, homogenising middle-class norms for culturally appropriate modern reproductive and sexual behaviour while denigrating practices that do not conform to such ideals (Ramberg 2014; Van Hollen 2003).

Sontag's (1978) seminal work revealed how metaphors of cancer in American and European literature and public culture blamed victims of breast cancer for being overly repressed while shoring up historically specific configurations of capitalism that encouraged conspicuous consumption. Douglas (1992) further argued that the discourse of risk in the science of epidemiology supplanted a discourse of sin while masking a persistent assumption of moral blame and individual responsibility. The work of these two authors inspired critical ethnographic research on discourses of cancer causality and risk. Anthropologists found that moralising discourses of cancer blame the victims of cancer and deflect attention away from other political–economic and environmental factors contributing to cancer incidence and mortalities (Jain 2013). Some anthropologists have shown that discourses of cancer causality often blame cancer victims for not following appropriate gender scripts (Hunt 1998; Martínez 2018). My work examines such discourses of cancer causality, gender and individual responsibility that circulate within public health educational programmes in the South Indian context.

I draw inspiration from these above-mentioned studies in feminist critical medical anthropology, critical public health in colonial and postcolonial India and the discourse of cancer causality and risk. I show that while educational campaigns at cancer screening camps in Tamil Nadu provide an important public health service to low-income communities, they also act as a conduit for the promotion of modern middle-class and upper-caste norms for Tamil women. These programmes frame cervical and breast cancer as resulting from individual lifestyle 'choices' relating to marriage, sexuality and reproductive behaviours and practices associated with sanitation, diet and exercise that echo long-standing colonial and postcolonial international and national development agendas in India. They do so in ways that condemn these practices and equate them with either uneducated backward traditionalism attributed to the lower class or overly Westernised modernity attributed to the upper class. Embedded in these messages is the promotion of parallel social and public health campaigns that discourage child marriage and chewing betel *paan* and promote family planning, latrine use, menstrual hygiene and breastfeeding. Yet there is a lack of clear information about how these issues are directly related to cervical and breast cancer risk.

Public health planners in India conceptualise cervical cancer as overwhelmingly affecting rural, lower-class, under-educated women. Cervical cancer is constructed as a disease that results from practices of 'backward', uneducated women who get married too young, have too many children, have multiple sexual partners, have too many abortions and do not eat nutritious, fresh foods. In contrast, public health planners conceive of breast cancer as primarily affecting affluent, educated, urban, upper-class women. Breast cancer is viewed as a disease resulting from an overly modern Westernised lifestyle for women who marry too late, have too few children, do not breastfeed, eat too much fatty food and do not get enough exercise. In both instances, underlying messages emphasise that inappropriate behaviours of women from different class backgrounds may put them at risk for cancer. The juxtaposition of these two critiques makes the promotion of idealised middle-class normative behaviour for Indian Tamil women strikingly apparent.

Reproductive cancer screening camps

My research assistants and I observed six cervical and breast cancer educational screening camps run by three organisations.[5] The term 'camp' is used in India to refer to temporary health services that are brought directly into communities on a given day to promote public health education and to provide medical services. Typically these camps take place in underserved rural and urban sites and are facilitated by government or non-government organisations. Although the forcible sterilisation camps of Indira Gandhi's Emergency period in the 1970s were widely condemned, generally members of lower-income communities have a favourable impression of public health camps in India and see them as convenient alternatives to visits to government hospitals for preventative health screening and minor ailments. Of the cancer camps that we observed, four were organised by the Cancer Institute – two in a village and two in a suburb of the state capital city, Chennai. The Cancer Institute is one of the best-known NGOs for cancer care in India. One of the camps we attended was in a clinic at the Rural Women's Social Education Centre (RUWSEC). RUWSEC is a small NGO run by and for lower-caste (*dalit*) women, which advocates for gender equity and sexual and reproductive health rights. The final educational camp was observed in a village near Kancheepuram, to the south-west of Chennai, and was run by an NGO called the Noble Foundation, working in tandem with the Government Cancer Hospital. This government hospital, formally known as the Government Arignar Anna Memorial Cancer Hospital, is the only public tertiary specialty cancer hospital in the state, with a population of over 70 million.

RUWSEC used its community health workers to recruit women whom they knew from villages where they worked to attend their camps. These RUWSEC health workers themselves lived in the villages from which they recruited women for these cancer screening camps and they had been involved in these cervical and breast cancer screening and testing programmes for several years before my research. Over time, they had managed to convince women in their communities of the value of these programmes and women and men generally agreed that it was beneficial for the whole family for women to undergo cancer screening. The other two organisations used a combination of recruitment methods. These included door-to-door recruitment in the vicinity of the camp, during which the organisers of the camps would go to individual homes in nearby villages to inform women that they were holding a free health camp and encourage them to attend. The Cancer Institute also approached groups of women at work sites for the government's Mahatma Gandhi National Rural Employment Guarantee Act (MGNREGA) where they were gathered in the hopes of getting daily manual labour jobs. Those who were not chosen for MGNREGA work on a given day were encouraged to attend the free health camp instead. Several women who were recruited through door-to-door methods or at MGNREGA work sites were under the impression that they were coming to a general health camp, similar to other health camps with which they were familiar. They only learned that these were screening camps for cancer once the meetings were already underway. Two of the Cancer Institute camps were organised at the request of women who belonged to women's micro-finance self-help organisations that are prevalent among lower-income communities in India.

The Noble camp and the two rural Cancer Institute camps were held in government elementary school buildings; the other two Cancer Institute camps took place on the flat rooftop of the home of a self-help group member, under the welcome shade of a huge colourfully embroidered canopy. Women attending these camps typically received light snacks and drinks; the self-help group that organised the rooftop camp provided a full vegetarian South India *thali* meal served on banana leaves.

At each camp, groups of approximately 20 women between the ages of 20 and 70, but mostly middle-aged, sat on the floor listening to presentations by primarily female public health social workers and general practitioner doctors.[6] The aim of the presenters was to assuage women's fears about cancer by telling them that unlike the depiction of cancer in movies, they should not assume they will die immediately if they have cancer. Rather, with early detection through screening, cervical and breast cancers can be stopped in their tracks. They encouraged women to undergo clinical screening immediately after the educational programme, to spread this information in their communities and to get checked every year free of cost at the state government's Primary Health Centres in their localities or at the Cancer Institute or a RUWSEC clinic.

The presenters at these camps began by asking women if they knew what cancer was, if they had heard of cervical and breast cancer, if they knew what caused these cancers and what the symptoms were. These initial enquiries were met with silence or a few murmurs by some women indicating that they had heard of these cancers or they had not heard of them, that they had recently heard on television that they should begin screening at age 30 or 25, that they did not know what the symptoms were and that smoking and chewing tobacco or betel *paan* caused cancer. Many of the younger women in these groups publicly displayed their embarrassment and discomfort about talking about issues concerning women's reproductive and sexual practices with shy smiles, giggles and downcast eyes. In some cases this may have been due to a genuine discomfort but it was also a way of publicly performing gendered norms of modesty. When it was clear that most of the women in attendance were not inclined to say anything publicly, the leaders would move on to give a presentation on all of these issues, with very little interaction between the presenters and the women in attendance for the remainder of the session, apart from one exceptional anecdote described in the discussion of breast cancer causes and prevention. This does not, however, mean that women accepted wholesale the moralising messages about cancer causality that are the focus of this chapter. In fact, my broader ethnographic research revealed that lower-class and lower-caste Tamil women typically held substantially different views about the causes they viewed as increasing cancer incidence in their communities (Van Hollen, Krishnan and Rathnam 2019).

In post-screening interviews, women explained that they were reticent to speak up in these camps in part because they felt too shy (*koocham*) to talk publicly about women's reproductive and sexual practices discussed at these camps, whether it was in front of strangers or among members of their self-help groups, co-workers from their work sites, neighbours or even relatives from their families. Furthermore, they explained that the people presenting at these camps were important, educated people (*periyavanga*, 'big people') who expect respect and listening silently is a sign of respect. Many felt that this respect was deserved and they valued the information provided by the more educated public health workers. At the same time, they questioned what good could come from questioning or challenging such 'big people' at these camps.

Listening to Sundari

Each NGO running these camps had its own presentation style and materials, using oral, video and paper-based media. Yet the content of the messages and the degree to which they promoted normative ideas about appropriate behaviour for women in Tamil Nadu was strikingly consistent. The social workers and doctors who facilitated the Cancer Institute awareness programmes handed out two pamphlets – a green one for cervical cancer and a pink one for breast cancer – and they used these pamphlets to guide them through their presentations. These pamphlets primarily contained cartoon-style pictures along with some words in Tamil. A fictional character named Sundari (literally 'the beautiful one') was on the cover of each pamphlet and appeared on each page (see Figure 5.2).

By Tamil standards, Sundari has a fair complexion, indicating probable upper-caste identity. She is wearing a clean and neatly tied sari that covers her ankles, indicating respectable middle-class status. Her *pottu* (*bindi*) on her forehead indicates her Hindu identity. Her long hair, braided with jasmine flowers, indicates her femininity but controlled sexuality. Her *tali* (marriage necklace) indicates her status as a married woman. Like the picture of the bride on the poster in the Kancheepuram clinic described above, Sundari embodies an idealised Tamil woman. And she is here to educate. The cover of each pamphlet says: 'Let's listen to what Sundari has to say!' I will let Sundari be our guide and will bring in similar points made in the RUWSEC and Noble camps to show how these cancer screening camps reproduce normative gendered values while providing an important public health service. Echoing the format of these camps, I begin with an analysis of the longer set of educational messages about cervical cancer, followed by a shorter discussion on messages about breast cancer; I then consider the cervical and breast cancer messages combined.

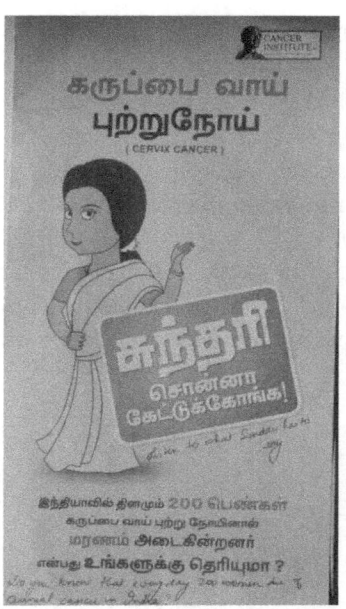

Figure 5.2 Cervical cancer pamphlet cover. © Cancer Institute (WIA)

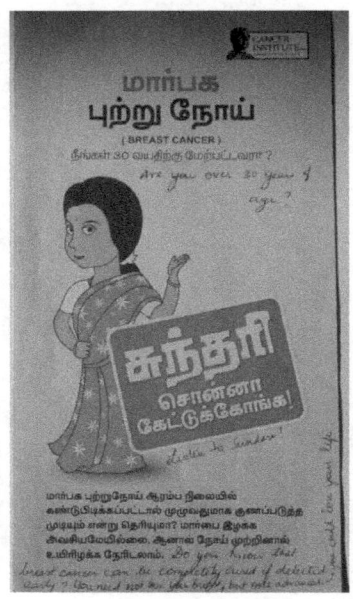

Figure 5.3 Breast cancer pamphlet cover. © Cancer Institute (WIA)

Cervical cancer: causes and prevention

The public health workers open the green cervical cancer pamphlet and begin by giving lessons about behaviours that could lead to cervical cancer and which must be avoided to reduce risk. There are six pictures to teach us about practices that should be shunned (see Figures 5.4 and 5.5).

First, we see that you should avoid getting married at a young age. There is a picture of an older husband and a child bride. The husband has darker complexion, suggesting lower-caste and lower-class identity. It is a

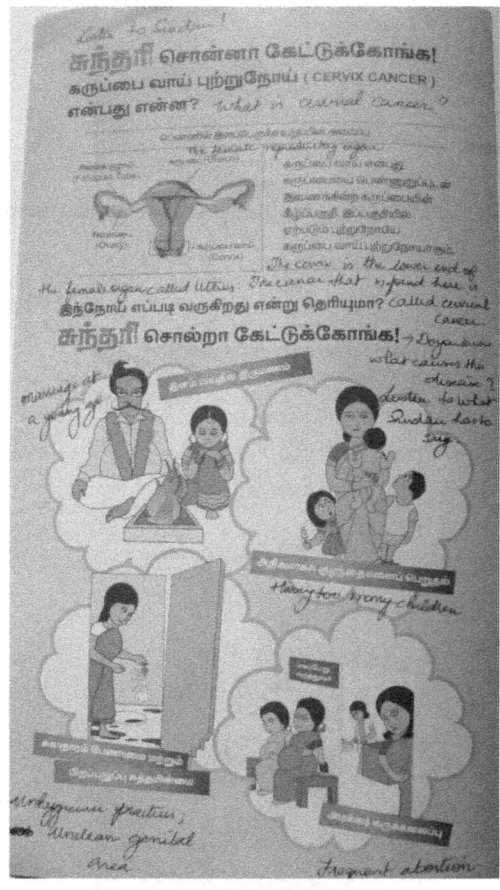

Figure 5.4 Cervical cancer pamphlet page on causes of cancer. © Cancer Institute (WIA).

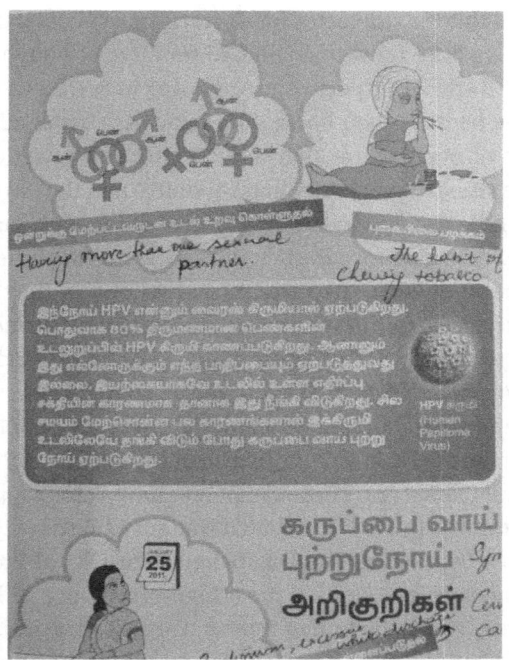

Figure 5.5 Cervical cancer pamphlet page on causes of cancer. © Cancer Institute (WIA).

Hindu marriage, as represented by the fire for the worship to Lord Agni and by the clothing and accessories. It represents what is considered a 'backward' form of marriage that is not acceptable to a modern, educated Hindu woman like Sundari, our teacher. Marriages between child brides and older husbands were historically considered acceptable for upper-caste Tamil Brahmin communities. Such marriages were condemned by colonial administrators, Indian nationalist social reformers and women's rights advocates. As a result, marriages with child brides have become 'an anachronism inconsistent with a modern, middle-class way of life' in Tamil Nadu and most other states in India (Fuller and Narasimhan 2008: 740). Today, marriages with brides who are not legal adults occur primarily among lower-class, lower-caste communities in Tamil Nadu and recent campaigns against these practices target that demographic.

Early marriage was also the first thing mentioned by the leader of the RUWSEC educational programme as a causal factor for cervical cancer. She explained that early marriage exposes women to sex at an earlier age and this is a risk factor for cancer. She explained that the ideal age for marriage is 21 for women and 25 for men, although legally they can marry at 18 and 21 respectively. According to her, 21 was an optimal age for women because their bodies and minds are better adapted to the requirements of marriage at that age. Their bodies would be able to withstand the stress of pregnancy and childbirth and they would be more mature to handle the new relationships that come with marriage. She said they would be able to 'adjust' better in the house of their husbands and in-laws because when they are 21, they will know they have to 'live by making sacrifices' (*vittukkoduththu vaazhanum*). The *average* age of marriage for women in Tamil Nadu in 2014 was 21.2,[7] indicating that many in fact married before that age; others married later.

Transnational and Indian women's rights groups have been waging campaigns against child marriage – particularly against child brides – in India since the colonial era. These campaigns have been stepped up in the twenty-first century. In 2016 the United Nations Children's Fund and the United Nations Population Fund launched their Global Programme to End Child Marriage in 12 'of the most high-prevalence or high-burden countries' in the world, including India.[8] It seems that these campaigns are reflected in cervical cancer prevention campaigns. The problem is that there was virtually no discussion about why early marriage per se could put women at risk for cervical cancer. Here we see that because talking about sex is taboo, marriage comes to stand in for Tamil women's initiation into sexual activity. The implication is that Tamil women do not engage in premarital sex. This assumption is not always borne out in reality, particularly as trends have been moving towards women marrying at later ages for several decades (Nag 1995). Furthermore, the suggestion that delayed sexual activity resulting from delayed marriage will reduce the risk of cervical cancer does not help women to understand the links between cervical cancer and the risk of contracting the human papillomavirus (HPV) through unprotected sex with multiple partners or via unprotected sex with their spouses who have multiple partners. This point is raised as a separate issue in these awareness camps.

According to the American Cancer Society, there is an increased risk of cervical cancer if a woman's first full-term pregnancy is before the age of 17. There is no conclusive understanding of why this is so.[9] To the extent that marriage is used to stand in for the beginning of women's reproductive lives and first full-term birth, these messages may help prevent cervical cancer. However, unspoken assumptions about the relationship between cervical cancer, marriage, reproduction and sex obscure more than they clarify about the biology of cervical cancer. These messages reinforce modern social movements against child marriage, establish an appropriate age for women to marry and reassert the cultural value of self-sacrifice for Tamil women as wives and daughters-in-law.

In the next picture of the Cancer Institute cervical cancer flyer, we see that women should avoid having too many children; this was also mentioned by the leader of the RUWSEC screening camp. The picture in the pamphlet to convey this message shows a mother with three children; the mother looks very sad. For over half a century, the governments of India and Tamil Nadu and countless transnational NGOs and international governments have been telling Indian women that the 'small family', with one or two children and no more, is a happy family and that they should undergo sterilisation after having their second child. These family planning programmes have targeted lower-class communities and represented lower-class people as incapable of controlling their sexual and reproductive practices without such interventions. As if to underscore the assumption that marriage at the age of 21 and female sterilisation after two children should be the norm, the woman leading the RUWSEC programme explained that 'women could begin cancer screening at the age of 25, after they have married and had two children and have done the *kudumba kattupadu* (family planning) operation (i.e. female sterilisation)'.

The American Cancer Society website mentioned says there is evidence that having three or more children is linked to increased risk of cervical cancer, but that the reasons for this are unclear. In the screening camps, messages about having too many children followed well-worn paths of pre-existing population control programmes without providing insights into possible causal connections between multiparous births and cervical cancer. The long-standing official policy in Tamil Nadu that set targets to incentivise public health workers and medical practitioners to encourage lower-class women to use birth control ended in 1995, following widespread condemnation of the abusive nature of such targets (Dhanraj 1991). Yet healthcare providers and public health workers continued to pressure women to undergo sterilisation because they believed this was in the best interest of women and of the nation (Van Hollen 2003). It seems that this impulse within the public health sector to urge lower-class women to have fewer children continues to circulate through these cervical cancer prevention campaigns.

The next picture in the pamphlet says that women must avoid unhygienic practices and unclean genitals; they must use a latrine with running water and keep the latrine and their bodies clean. The woman in the picture is frowning as she steps in what might be human faeces or might be menstrual blood. In this picture, the woman is in a separate bathroom with a toilet and a running tap. Most people from poor rural communities in Tamil Nadu (and throughout India) do not have their own latrines; poor urban people living in subsidised public housing have access to pit latrines but live with chronic water shortages; rural women use the fields to defecate and running water is scarce. This is likely the situation for many of the lower-class rural women attending these camps. The woman leading the RUWSEC camp also stated that poor hygiene could lead to cancer. She said that the female organs (*penn kuri*) have openings so if women are not hygienic during urination, defecation or menstruation, this could lead to repeated infections of the female reproductive tract that could cause cancer. She said that this is why women should wash after urination as well as defecation, and use sanitary methods and maintain good hygiene during their menstrual period.

These cancer prevention campaigns seem to find common cause with state, national and transnational organisations' campaigns for sanitation in India. There is a long history of public health sanitation programmes dating back to the colonial era, which represent lower-class and lower-caste Indian women as dirty and in need of social and moral reform through good hygiene (Whitehead 1995). Muthulakshmi Reddy, a social reformer and founder of the Cancer Institute, was involved in charity programmes to provide latrines to lower-class women in the early twentieth century (Basu 1986). Such sanitation programmes have been reinvigorated through Prime Minster Modi's Swachh Bharat Abhiyan (Clean India Mission) to encourage communities to build and use communal free-standing latrines to achieve an 'Open Defecation-Free India'.[10] Menstrual hygiene campaigns in India to prevent reproductive tract infections are also proliferating (Garg, Goyal and Gupta 2012). Although both of these public health campaigns have merits, neither can succeed through education about lifestyle changes without addressing the fundamental social, political and economic problems of lack of access to latrines and water for washing (Coffey and Spears 2017). Without actively engaging in such structural transformations, these cervical cancer educational camps may inadvertently blame poor women for getting cervical cancer because they have neglected to keep themselves clean. This may reinforce stereotypes about lower-class and -caste women as dirty and backwards and reassert the superiority of middle-class, upper-caste women as represented by Sundari. It also misrepresents the cause of cervical cancer.

The fourth picture in the Cancer Institute cervical cancer pamphlet is of women at an abortion clinic. It states recurrent induced abortions may cause cervical cancer, a point that was also raised in the RUWSEC screening camp. In this picture, the woman who has just had an abortion and the doctor who has performed it both look very glum and a woman who is in line to get an abortion is giving a suspicious sideways glance. Medically induced abortions have been legal in India since 1971 and have been subsidised by international organisations and government and non-government organisations involved in India's family planning programme. Although abortion is considered a *mahāpātaka* (great sin) in the *dharmaśāstras* (ancient Sanskrit Hindu texts), morally charged political debates about abortion found elsewhere have been relatively absent in India due to the acceptance that abortion has a role in India's population control campaigns. Despite its legality, abortion is a taboo subject that women cannot always openly discuss within their families. Therefore, women sometimes resort to unsafe abortions to maintain secrecy of an unintended pregnancy, resulting in serious health problems (Visaria and Ramachandran 2007). Yet research in Tamil Nadu demonstrated that, among the younger generation, women felt that having a large family and being pregnant at an advanced age was even more shameful than having an abortion (Anandhi 2007).

Within this context, it is surprising that the cervical cancer prevention messages present abortion as a risk factor for cervical cancer when the findings from epidemiological studies to determine the causal link between induced abortions and cervical cancer is inconclusive. When I enquired about this with the Cancer Institute doctor in charge of these educational programmes, she said that they were using a 1990 study by L. I. Remennick for their preventative messages about abortion. In that study, Remennick (1990) lays out a strong case that such a link is 'biologically highly plausible' (259) and calls for more robust epidemiological research, but also concedes that an 'initial attitude of researchers towards abortion usually determines the way they interpret results, since outcome risk measures are often of moderate value and/or borderline statistical significance' (263). There is evidence that transnational Christian discourses that view abortion as a sin are on the rise in Tamil Nadu with the growing popularity of the Pentecostal Church (Van Hollen 2013). This trend may be seeping into public health messages about cervical cancer.

At the top of the next page of the pamphlet, there is an abstract representation of international symbols of men (♂) and women (♀) in two clusters of interlocking groups (see Figure 5.5). The first is of one woman interlocked with two men and the second of one man interlocked with two women. Beneath this is an explanation that having more than one sexual partner can cause cervical cancer. This supports a powerful cultural norm in India that sexual relations should be monogamous and between a husband and wife. The woman leading the RUWSEC screening camp also warned that having multiple sexual partners was a risk factor for cancer. As she put it: 'For every man, one woman (*oruvannukku oruththi*) is the best way to live. That is in accordance with our Indian culture (*kalacharam*).' But she also recommended that women should get their husbands to wear condoms to be safe from cancer. The organisers of these camps make a point to say that cancer *itself* is not contagious. They distinguish cancer from the (usually) sexually transmitted and intensely stigmatised HIV/AIDS disease that was a focal point of public health campaigns in the state a decade earlier. Nevertheless, such presentations run the risk of leaving women with the impression that cancer itself is a sexually transmitted disease (without full understanding of the role of the sexually transmitted HPV in cancer), that the best prevention is monogamy (without a clear explanation about protected versus unprotected sex) and that if a woman gets cervical cancer she and/or her husband must not be upholding Indian cultural standards of morality.

The last picture about causal factors is of an old white-haired woman chewing the stimulant betel *paan* (a combination of betel leaf, areca nut and lime). Instead of sitting cross-legged, as a demure Tamil woman is expected to do, the woman in this picture is uncouth, sitting with her legs stretched out, her ankles inappropriately exposed, spitting out the red juice that is secreted from chewing *paan* and leaving a red puddle on the floor. Since the British colonial era, the government has tried to prevent people from spitting betel *paan* juice. There is renewed attention to this under Modi's Swachh Bharat campaign, using the legal system to punish those found spitting in public places. The campaign against spitting *paan* juice is couched within a middle-class discourse of civility aimed against members of lower-class communities who are more likely to use *paan* today.

While smoking tobacco, chewing tobacco and *paan* are widely used among lower-income men in India, women from this socio-economic sector rarely smoke but may use smokeless products. This tends to be the case more so among rural rather than urban women and older rather than younger women (Gajalakshmi, Whitlock and Peto 2012). Chewing tobacco and *paan* increase the risk of oral and throat cancers and this is an important health message to convey to the public. However, whereas smoking tobacco has been linked to increased risk of cervical cancer, research on smokeless tobacco and *paan* causing cervical cancer has been inconclusive. Furthermore, the visual contrast in the pamphlets between the proper middle-class comportment of Sundari versus the improper demeanour of the woman spitting *paan* juice may further stigmatise cervical cancer as an affliction associated with the uncivilised lifestyle choices of members of lower-class, lower-caste communities, without addressing the social context that leads people to engage in these practices.

Below this picture, the text on the pamphlet explains that cervical cancer is often caused by HPV. It states that although HPV can be found in the bodies of approximately 80 per cent of married women, it does not harm most women due to natural immunities. But, it warns, due to the reasons portrayed in the above-mentioned pictures, the body's natural immunity may be weakened, rendering women with HPV vulnerable to getting cervical cancer.

On the last page of this pamphlet is a statement recommending the HPV vaccine for girls between 9 and 13 to prevent cervical cancer. Although the Government of India has considered including the HPV vaccine in the national immunisation programme, it has faced stiff resistance from some activist groups due to concerns about potential harmful effects of the vaccine and to negligence in informed consent procedures by multinational pharmaceutical companies in clinical trials for these vaccines among tribal communities (Sarojini, Anjali and Ashalata 2010). Others have questioned the validity of epidemiological data used to recommend universal HPV vaccination in India (Mattheij, Pollock and Brhlikova 2012). The vaccine is available in private Indian clinics but the cost is prohibitive for lower-income individuals. Neither the Cancer Institute nor RUWSEC emphasised the vaccine in their educational camps in part due to concerns that once vaccinated women might not undergo screening, even though the HPV vaccine does not prevent all cervical cancer. The Noble Foundation, however, showed two videos promoting both the HPV vaccine and Pap smears. The first video states that girls between 9 and 19 should get the HPV vaccine and all women should get regular Pap smears. It does so by appealing to men's sense of duty to protect the women in their lives. The film states that while women give birth and take care of the family, it is men's duty to take care of women. If men want to be good husbands, brothers or fathers, they should protect girls and women by taking them for HPV vaccines and Pap smears. Patriarchal norms that women are expected to take care of the family while men should be the protectors of women are clearly reinforced through this cancer prevention campaign. Although there were no men recruited for this camp, the programme was broadcast to the whole village through booming loudspeakers installed outside for all to hear.

Breast cancer: causes and prevention

In the pink pamphlet that the Cancer Institute presenters handed out at the camps, Sundari recommends regular breast self-exams and annual clinical breast exams (see Figure 5.3). There are also a series of 'dos and don'ts' to prevent breast cancer. The first is the directive to breastfeed to prevent cancer. The public health educators recommend that mothers breastfeed for at least one full year and suggest those who do not breastfeed are at an elevated risk for breast cancer. In the process, they tap into another public health campaign to promote breastfeeding for infant health. This other campaign represents modern upper-class urban lifestyles and multinational milk-formula companies as posing a danger to infants and to what are purported to be traditional and highly valued cultural ideals of Tamil womanhood (Van Hollen 2003, 2013). Public health workers present these messages as if individual women have the power to simply change this lifestyle behaviour, without addressing the broader socio-economic constraints that might make it virtually impossible for some working women to breastfeed, even if they wanted to.

The public health educators at these camps also say that delaying the birth of the first child can increase the risk of breast cancer. Therefore, they stress that it is important not to get married at too advanced an age in order to avoid breast cancer. A doctor at one of the camps stated explicitly, 'People who haven't married and haven't had children are more likely to have breast cancer.' Once again, we can see an emphasis placed on *marriage* in relation to cancer risk, so promoting normative gender practices for women. As noted, women are encouraged to get married and have children in their twenties.

Middle- and upper-class women are increasingly getting married at later ages than was the case one or two generations ago. Some of those who can afford to are pursuing higher education and career opportunities before marriage and have a greater say in the marriage agreement because their consent is now expected (Fuller and Narasimhan 2008). This can create intergenerational conflicts in which parents may castigate their daughters for defying traditional cultural norms and accuse them of being corrupted by Western values if they want to defer marriage while daughters criticise their parents as old-fashioned. When educational programmes about cancer prevention present 'late marriage' as a risk factor for breast cancer without providing more nuanced information linking the age at first childbirth and breast cancer risk, they may end up reproducing normative cultural ideas about women and marriage held by older generations. This could contribute to stigmatising women who get breast cancer if they are then blamed for bringing the disease upon themselves by 'selfishly' choosing to delay marriage to pursue their education or career.

The connection between marriage and cancer implied in the cervical cancer prevention messages differs from that implied in the breast cancer prevention messages due to differing demographic assumptions about the relationship between socio-economic class and these two cancers. Cervical cancer is presented by public health planners as a problem of uneducated, rural, poor women who have too many children at too young an age. Breast cancer, in contrast, is presented as a problem of overly modern, wealthier, educated, urban, upper-class women who marry too late and who may end up having difficulty conceiving children when they do marry. Yet these messages are combined in NGO awareness camps that provide both cervical and breast cancer screening simultaneously to primarily lower-class groups of women.

The breast cancer pamphlet also tells women to avoid eating fatty foods. From the picture of a cut of red meat, it seems that we should particularly avoid eating meat, implying that a vegetarian diet is best. This echoes early colonial-era claims in British medical journals that cancer did not affect Indians because of their vegetarian practices – an argument that is specious not only because Indians did suffer from cancer during the colonial era, but also because the vast majority of Indians are not vegetarian (Banerjee 2020). In South India, where vegetarianism is more prevalent than in many other parts of India, it is associated with higher-caste groups, particularly with Brahmins.

This pamphlet further instructs women to get regular exercise to prevent breast cancer. The exercise of choice depicted in the pamphlet is yoga. Although many people around the world have the impression that yoga has been widely practised throughout India for centuries, and continues to be practised, in reality it has only recently become trendy in India and is generally a middle- to upper-class and upper-caste phenomenon. Prime Minister Modi and his Bharatiya Janata Party, whose primary political base consists of middle-class, upper-caste Hindus, have actively promoted yoga as a national symbol of pride in Indian 'traditions'. The public health messages about breast cancer causality and prevention tap into anxieties about the negative impact of Westernised, modern, urban, gluttonous and sedentary lifestyles. The recommended antidote appears to be to engage in what are considered to be good 'traditional' middle-class, upper-caste Hindu Indian cultural practices such as vegetarianism and yoga. Women who get breast cancer may thus be blamed for not being good traditional Indian citizens by not taking care of themselves through such practices.

The only time that I saw a woman openly challenge the recommendations of the presenters at these educational camps was in response to the suggestion that women should be getting more exercise by practising yoga or going to the gym. Upon hearing this, a wiry woman in her fifties abruptly stood up from the floor. Her anger was evident by the intensity with which she looked the public health worker in the eye. 'How can you say that we need to exercise more when we have spent our whole lives working all day long in the fields?' she asked in an accusatory tone. The doctor replied that women should at least spend time walking very fast each day so that they would sweat and that it would only count as exercise if they sweat. In response, the woman said that all they ever do is work hard and sweat all day long and that *that* is what was killing people in her village. She walked out of the room, bristling. The public health educator continued to explain the health benefits of regular yoga practice and no one else uttered a word.

Intervening interventions

Although different messages about prevention for cervical cancer and breast cancer reflect discreet class-specific moral assumptions, these awareness programmes address both of these cancers together (and the clinical screenings for cervical and breast cancer take place at the same time). The result is that women attending these camps, typically from lower socio-economic groups, are presented with the totality of all of these messages. Combined, the key information provided about cancer causality and prevention at each of these camps can be summarised by nine messages conveyed over 30 minutes to the groups of women gathered:

1. Get married at the right age: not too young and not too old. The ideal age for a woman to marry is 21.
2. Have monogamous sex within marriage only.
3. Have children but do not have 'too many': no more than two. Get sterilised after two.
4. Breastfeed for at least one year.
5. Do not have 'too many' abortions and use condoms.
6. Wash your body with clean running water in a latrine when menstruating, defecating and urinating.

7. Eat a healthy diet (avoid fatty foods, such as meat).
8. Avoid betel *paan* (and tobacco).
9. Exercise regularly (especially yoga).

One aim of this edited volume, *Cancer and the Politics of Care*, is to interrogate the concept of the *intervention* in global public health programmes for cancer. When we consider this list of the combined messages regarding reproductive cancer prevention for women in South India, it is clear that the educational programmes at these camps facilitate multiple kinds of interventions simultaneously. The stated goal of these programmes is to encourage behaviour change as a public health measure to prevent cancer; such educational interventions are an important component of any public health agenda. However, when we review the list of these combined messages, it is apparent that such educational programmes also facilitate sociocultural interventions by prescribing behaviours deemed essential for an idealised middle-class Tamil woman. They thus intervene to (re)produce gender norms in the society and seek to mould women according to a narrow set of feminine ideals. Furthermore, these public health programmes for reproductive cancer prevention are implicitly aligned with and promote several other social and public health interventions. This is so even when the link between cervical and breast cancer causality and these other interventions is not always clearly articulated, not well understood within the scientific community and, in some cases, not agreed upon within the scientific community.

None of this would be a surprise for feminist critical medical anthropologists, critical scholars of public health in India or critical social scientists interested in discourses of cancer causality and risk. Such scholars argue that biomedical and public health knowledge and practice is inherently and inevitably embedded within sociocultural contexts. We cannot escape this. Nevertheless, we can use this analytical lens to shine a light on how public health interventions intervene and to consider the effects of these multiple simultaneous interventions. This is not only an important exercise for feminists or others concerned with issues of social equity. It is also crucial for public health policymakers since at times the implicit interventions may negatively impact the uptake of the explicit public health intervention. They also risk further stigmatising cancer patients despite public health goals to destigmatise cancer.

My ethnographic interviews with reproductive cancer patients and survivors demonstrate that they all grapple with the stigma associated with assumptions that they have brought these cancers upon themselves by marrying too early or too late, by not breastfeeding properly, by being sexually promiscuous, by having too many or too few children, by being dirty, by chewing *paan* or by being ignorant or irresponsible. Women frequently told me that family members, neighbours and medical-care practitioners would make comments suggesting that they had cancer because of such transgressions. Even if no one said this directly, women worried deeply that people thought this. Sometimes they would resist such accusations. Other times, they were overwhelmed by feelings of guilt and blamed themselves. They tried to keep their cancers secret to avoid ostracism and to mitigate the impact that moral accusations might have on the prestige of their families.

I did not carefully examine the extent to which such moralising discourses of these educational programmes might inadvertently discourage women from undergoing cancer screening due to fears of social stigma that might result from a cancer diagnosis. This is an important question for future researchers. The organisers of the RUWSEC screening camps told me that when they began these projects, women from the lowest-caste *dalit* communities were initially reluctant to undergo screening because they saw it as one more example of a legacy in which those in power consider them to be inherently dirty. Furthermore, lower-class and lower-caste Indian women are often wary of public health interventions on their reproductive bodies since they have historically been the targets of family planning interventions carried out without consent. Because the RUWSEC health educators were themselves *dalit* women, they were able to overcome this initial resistance in the villages where they worked.

The moralising discourse conveyed through these educational programmes could inadvertently deter women from undergoing cancer screening if the women fear that a cancer diagnosis might threaten their moral and social standing in their communities. For example, stating that cervical cancer can result from sex with multiple partners without thoroughly explaining the prevalence of HPV throughout the whole population, as well as the relationship between HPV, cervical cancer and factors that compromise the immune system, could deter women from getting screened for fear that they could be accused of promiscuity. Stating that abortions cause cervical cancer, without careful explanation of scientific debates surrounding this, could deter women from cancer screening if they fear that others will suspect them of having had multiple abortions. Attributing cervical cancer to having 'too many' children could deter women from going to public hospitals for cancer screenings if they think they will be blamed by healthcare practitioners for not undergoing female sterilisation after their second child. Women who have not been able to follow recommendations for long-term breastfeeding may hesitate to get screened for breast cancer if they think that healthcare workers and their family and friends will blame them for being bad mothers. My ethnographic research with cervical and breast cancer patients reveals that these forms of moralising blame are not hypothetical. Women reported being accused of all of these things following their cancer diagnosis and suffered psychologically from the stigma of such blame. It is, therefore, not a stretch to suggest that such moralising discourses surrounding cervical and breast cancer could potentially have harmful consequences for women's health and well-being.

Conclusion

The public health messages about cervical and breast cancer causality conveyed in these educational camps focus on getting women to engage in particular practices and to avoid other practices. These programmes seem to presume that lower-class, lower-caste women can be empowered to live healthier lives through education about healthy lifestyle choices, while doing little to address underlying local and global political, economic and sociocultural structural inequalities contributing to their ill health. Educational outreach about healthy practices has an important role to play in health promotion. Yet when educational messages attribute cancer risk to individual behaviour choices without challenging broader social and economic factors contributing to cancer aetiology and morbidity, their public health impact will be limited.

I have demonstrated that these public health education programmes about cervical and breast cancer causality and prevention reproduce and promote normative ideas about appropriate middle-class, upper-caste moral conduct for Tamil women. With better access to early detection and treatment and thus better survival rates made possible through screening, cervical and breast cancer should become less stigmatised in India, thereby further encouraging people to make use of cancer screening. However, the moral assumptions embedded in the discourses of causality conveyed in the educational portion of the screening camps may have the unintended consequence of furthering the stigma of cervical and breast cancer. Lower-class and lower-caste women who are the targets of these educational programmes worry that other people will hold them responsible for not living up to such middle-class norms for Tamil women when they are diagnosed with these reproductive cancers. Ironically, this could deter women from undergoing screening, thereby complicating efforts to provide these women with much-needed screening, early detection and early treatment.

Acknowledgements

Funding for this research was provided by the American Institute of Indian Studies, the Woodrow Wilson International Center for Scholars, Syracuse University and Yale-NUS College. I am also grateful to the following institutions in India for support and affiliations for this project: Rural Women's Social Education Centre, Cancer Institute (WIA), Government Arignar Anna Memorial Cancer Hospital and the Research Institute and Indian Institute of Technology-Madras. And I would like to thank the editors of this volume, Linda Bennett, Lenore Manderson and Belinda Spagnoletti, for their insightful editorial feedback on this chapter. This research received ethics approval from the Syracuse University IRB.

Notes

1. A version of this chapter has been published in my book, *Cancer and the Kali Yuga: Gender, inequality and health in South India* (Van Hollen 2022).
2. Although this is a commonly reported statement, statistics on rates of Pap smear or mammogram use among women in India are not readily available. A 2019 study states that '[less than] 1/3 women between 30–49 years in India reported ever having received *any* kind of cervical cancer screening' (https://www.cdc.gov/mmwr/volumes/68/wr/mm6801a4. htm#:~:text=Among%20women%20in%20India%20aged,partners%2C%20wealth% 2C%20and%20marriage. Accessed 11 August 2020). Another study suggests that rates of breast cancer screening among women in India are lower than rates of cervical cancer screening (https://www.ncbi.nlm.nih.gov/pmc/articles/PMC4711217/. Accessed 11 August 2020).
3. See Mallath et al. (2014: e206); FICCI-FLO (Federation of Indian Chambers of Commerce). 2017. 'Call for action: Expanding cancer care for women in India', 21 September. https://www. ficciflo.com/wp-content/uploads/2017/09/Expanding-cancer-care-for-women-in-India.pdf. Accessed 16 September 2022.
4. Visual inspection with acetic acid; visual inspection with Lugol's iodine.
5. Shweta Krishnan and Shibani Rathnam.
6. The Cancer Institute and RUWSEC camps were all run by women. The Noble camp had male and female presenters.
7. See https://www.thenewsminute.com/article/three-charts-brides-kerala-and-tn-have-gotten-younger-nine-years-44797#:~:text=While%20women%20in%20Kerala%20were,to% 2021.2%20years%20in%202014. Accessed 8 December 2020.
8. See https://www.unicef.org/protection/unfpa-unicef-global-programme-end-child-marriage. Accessed 29 January 2021.
9. See https://www.cancer.org/cancer/cervical-cancer/causes-risks-prevention/risk-factors. html. Accessed 9 January 2018.
10. See https://swachhbharat.mygov.in/sb-challenges. Accessed 3 March 2017.

References

Anandhi, S. 2007. 'Women, work, and abortion practices in Kancheepuram District, Tamil Nadu'. In *Abortion in India*, edited by Leela Visaria and Vimala Ramachandran, 62–99. New Delhi: Routledge.
Banerjee, Dwaipayan. 2020. *Enduring Cancer: Life, death, and diagnosis in Delhi*. Durham, NC: Duke University Press.
Basu, Aparna. 1986. 'Introduction'. In *The Pathfinder: Dr. Muthulakshmi Reddi*. Delhi: All India Women's Conference.
Coffey, Diane and Dean Spears. 2017. *Where India Goes: Abandoned toilets, stunted development and the costs of caste*. New Delhi: HarperCollins Publishers India.
Davies, Will. 2013. 'India has most cervical cancer deaths'. *The Wall Street Journal*, 10 May. Accessed 17 September 2013. http://blogs.wsj.com/indiarealtime/2013/05/10/india-has-highest-number-of-cervical-cancer-deaths/.
Dhanraj, Deepa, dir. 1991. *Something Like a War*. Women Make Movies.
Douglas, Mary. 1992. *Risk and Blame: Essays in cultural theory*. New York: Routledge.
Farmer, Paul, Julio Frenk, Felicia M. Knaul, Lawrence N. Shulman, George Allyn, Lance Armstrong, Rifat Atun et al. 2010. 'Expansion of cancer care and control in countries of low and middle income: A call to action', *Lancet* 376 (9747): 1186–1193. https://doi.org/10.1016/S0140-6736(10)61152-X.
Foucault, Michel. 1978. *The History of Sexuality*. New York: Vintage Books.
Fuller, C. J. and Haripriya Narasimhan. 2008. 'Companionate marriage in India: The changing marriage system in a middle-class Brahman subcaste', *Journal of the Royal Anthropological Institute* 14(4): 736–754.
Gajalakshmi, Vendhan, Gary Whitlock and Richard Peto. 2012. 'Social inequalities, tobacco chewing, and cancer mortality in south India: A case-control analysis of 2,580 cancer deaths among non-smoking non-drinkers', *Cancer Causes & Control* 23(S1): 91–98.
Garg, Rajesh, Shoba Goyal and Sanjeev Gupta. 2012. 'India moves towards menstrual hygiene: Subsidized sanitary napkins for rural adolescent girls – issues and challenges', *Maternal and Child Health Journal* 16(4): 767–774.
Hunt, Linda M. 1998. 'Moral reasoning and the meaning of cancer: Causal explanations of oncologists and patients in southern Mexico', *Medical Anthropology Quarterly* 12(3): 298–318.
Jain, S. Lochlann. 2013. *Malignant: How cancer becomes us*. Berkeley: University of California Press.
Levine, Philippa. 1994. 'Venereal disease, prostitution, and the politics of empire: The case of British India', *Journal of the History of Sexuality* 4(4): 579–602.
Mallath, Mohandas K., David G. Taylor, Rajendra A. Badwe, Goura K. Rath, V. Shanta, C. S. Pramesh, Raghunadharao Digumarti et al. 2014. 'The growing burden of cancer in India: Epidemiology and social context', *The Lancet Oncology* 15(6): e205–212. http://dx.doi.org/10.1016/S1470-2045(14)70115-9.
Martin, Emily. 1987. *The Woman in the Body: A cultural analysis of reproduction*. Boston, MA: Beacon Press.
Martínez, Rebecca G. 2018. *Marked Women: The cultural politics of cervical cancer in Venezuela*. Palo Alto, CA: Stanford University Press.
Mattheij, I., A. M. Pollock and P. Brhlikova. 2012. 'Do cervical cancer data justify HPV vaccination in India? Epidemiological data sources and comprehensiveness', *Journal of the Royal Society of Medicine* 105(6): 250–262. https://doi.org/10.1258/jrsm.2012.110343.
Nag, M. 1995. 'Sexual behaviour in India with risk of HIV/AIDS transmission', *Health Transition Review* 5: 293–305.
Raina, Pamposh. 2013. 'India ranks no. 1 in cervical cancer deaths'. *India Ink: The New York Times*, 10 May. Accessed 17 September 2013. http://india.blogs.nytimes.com/2013/05/10/india-ranks-number-one-in-cervical-cancer-deaths/?_php=true&_type=blogs&_r=0.
Ram, Kalpana and Margaret Jolly. 1998. *Maternities and Modernities: Colonial and postcolonial experiences in Asia and the Pacific*. Cambridge, UK: Cambridge University Press.
Ramberg, Lucinda. 2014. *Given to the Goddess: South Indian Devadasis and the sexuality of religion*. Durham, NC: Duke University Press.
Remennick, Larissa I. 1990. 'Induced abortion as cancer risk factor: A review of epidemiological evidence', *Journal of Epidemiology & Community Health* 44(4): 259–264.

Sarojini, N., S. Anjali and S. Ashalata. 2010. 'Findings from a visit to Bhadrachalam: HPV vaccine "demonstration project" site in Andhra Pradesh'. Delhi, India: SAMA Resource Group for Women and Health.

Sontag, Susan. 1978. *Illness as Metaphor*. New York: Random House.

Van Hollen, Cecilia. 2003. *Birth on the Threshold: Childbirth and modernity in South India*. Berkeley: University of California Press.

Van Hollen, Cecilia. 2013. *Birth in the Age of AIDS: Women, reproduction, and HIV/AIDS in India*. Palo Alto, CA: Stanford University Press.

Van Hollen, Cecilia. 2022. *Cancer and the Kali Yuga: Gender, inequality and health in South India*. Berkeley: University of California Press.

Van Hollen, Cecilia, Shweta Krishnan and Shibani Rathnam. 2019. '"It's partly in our hands; It's partly in the hands of the goddess": Cancer patients' quest for well-being in India', *Purushartha: Sciences sociales en Asie du Sud* 36: 179–206.

Visaria, Leela and Vimala Ramachandran. 2007. *Abortion in India: Ground realities*. New York: Routledge.

Whitehead, Judy. 1995. 'Bodies clean and unclean: Prostitution, sanitary legislation, and respectable femininity in colonial north India', *Gender & History* 7(1): 41–63. https://doi.org/10.1111/j.1468-0424.1995.tb00013.x.

6
Intersections of stigma, morality and care: Indonesian women's negotiations of cervical cancer

Linda Rae Bennett and Hanum Atikasari

Our first encounter with cervical cancer stigma in Indonesia was during a preliminary field trip in 2018 when we visited stakeholders engaged in cancer prevention and care. As we sat in a circle at a community-based cancer organisation (cancer CBO), drinking sweet tea and sharing snacks, we began the process of getting to know one another and our involvement in cancer advocacy and research. For many women, this involved telling their own cancer stories. Bunga, a middle-class woman in her mid-fifties, had recently completed treatment for Stage IIB-cervical cancer,[1] and had subsequently joined the cancer CBO as a volunteer. She had chosen not to disclose her diagnosis to her children or extended family and relied solely on her husband for support. Her reasons for this choice provide keen insight into why and how some women evade or contain stigma through selective disclosure:

> If I told my children that I had cervical cancer it was likely they would blame their father. They are well educated, they would go to the internet and see it there, the risk factor [having multiple sexual partners]. I needed my family to stay close, if they blamed their father it would be harder for everyone. It's better to handle it alone, just with my husband. We could do that because my children are outside, not at home. But it's not like that for everyone. Until now they don't know I had this type of cancer, just that I had reproductive health problems.

Bunga's reasoning around selective disclosure included her desire to protect herself, her husband and her whole family from the potential harm of a stigmatising diagnosis derived from popular associations between cervical cancer, promiscuity and blame. Bunga's story, and those of others who sat around the table that day, confirmed that in Indonesia cervical cancer stigma is pervasive and contagious, that is, knowledge of a diagnosis can confer stigma by association to women's partners and children. What also struck us from this initial encounter was that cervical cancer stigma had serious implications for the care available to women affected by cancer and the care they provided for others while living with cancer.

Our discussion in this chapter positions women affected by cancer as subjective agents in navigating stigma, acknowledging that they make decisions to mediate stigma and its associated suffering; they are not merely victims of stigma. This involves exploring what women affected by cancer did about stigma, how they lived with it and managed its impacts. We discuss women's selective disclosure of their diagnosis, their re-articulation of causation narratives, their establishment of safe relationships and social environments free from stigma and their reclassification of cancer. This approach enables us to explore how women's negotiations of stigma are necessarily shaped by the local moral contexts of their lives, while at the same time embodying the potential for challenging existing norms (Parker and Aggleton 2003).

Erving Goffman's original conceptualisations of 'enacted stigma' – acts of discrimination against individuals with a stigmatising condition – and 'felt stigma' – referring to a person's embarrassment or shame associated with a stigmatising condition — are relevant for our description of Indonesian women's experiences (Goffman 1963). However, our analysis within the specific cultural and moral complexes of contemporary Indonesian society focuses on the workings and impacts of 'moral stigma' (Yang et al. 2007). Moral stigma is highly salient precisely because a diagnosis of cervical cancer threatens to rupture the moral subjectivity of Indonesian women, while questioning the moral integrity also of those closest to them, their partners and children. The moral stigma attached to cervical cancer is rooted in the widespread belief that it is caused by sexual promiscuity and those affected by this form of cancer are held responsible due to their moral/sexual deviance. Our deployment of the concept of moral stigma refers both to the highly moralised nature of cervical cancer stigma and its propensity to disrupt the moral status of others close to women affected by this cancer.

The moral stigma projected at women affected by cervical cancer can be differentiated from the fear surrounding other prominent cancers in Indonesia, such as breast and lung cancer. While cancers in general are feared in the popular imaginary, both because they often lead to death and because their treatment is understood to be brutal (Sunarsih et al. 2018), other cancers do not immediately attract moral condemnation because they are not associated with immorality and promiscuity;[2] only HIV and other sexually transmissible diseases share this level of moral stigma (Newland et al. 2021; Waluyo et al. 2015; Waluyo, Nurachmah and Rosakawati 2006). The discrepancy in stigma between cervical cancer and other cancers drives inequalities between different cancers, in terms of the degree of care afforded to women and their associated social suffering. In this sense, we add to a growing understanding of the unequal treatment of different cancers and those who live with them.

Our conceptualisation of 'care' is an inclusive one. We follow prior anthropological concern for considering care in its specific cultural and historical context in order for it to be adequately understood (Kleinman and van der Geest 2009; Martin, Myers and Viseu 2015). In conceptualising practices of care we characterise its different forms as innately relational, occurring between individuals, families, cancer CBOs and survivor groups, as well as between cancer patients and those who offer care within the health system. We apply this relational lens also in our analysis of how cancer is experienced, building on Livingston's (2012: 6) assertion that 'cancer is something that happens between people'. Our emphasis is less about physical acts of care that occur when women undergo treatment in a hospital environment (compare Chapter 8 by Varaleki, this volume) and more about care as a social process occurring across multiple social fields: emotional and psychological care, informational support, practical support to access treatment and to live with cancer and specific acts of care involved in evading or managing the stigma. We extend earlier thinking on care (Bennett 2015; Kleinman and van der Geest 2009; Mol 2008; Mol, Moser and Pols 2010) by unpicking how the moral stigma deriving from cervical cancer shapes who is considered worthy of care. We also reveal how women's strategies for mediating moral stigma shape the extent and nature of care available to them, as well as the care they offer others whilst living with cancer.

Living with cervical cancer in Indonesia

> Ali texted while her daughter and husband were out looking for a laundry, so we could chat privately. They only have two sets of clothes each and two bed sheets. The sheets have to be washed daily

because Ali has both bladder and bowel incontinence, as well as an open wound from the radiotherapy burns on her right thigh and hip. I called her on WhatsApp, and her tone is so different when she is not trying to contain her suffering in front of her family. The pain in her voice was palpable. She needed to cry, but not in front of her daughter.

She was worried about finances again. Her husband hasn't worked since they arrived in Yogyakarta for her treatment, and she feels embarrassed to keep asking the extended family for support. Ali feels grateful they qualified for a room in the *rumah singgah* [free cancer patient hostel], as all their savings were spent on the journey to Java. It's a single room with one mattress on the floor. She stressed that others have not been so lucky and have to pay for accommodation because the *rumah singgah* is always full.

They have enough cash to eat just once a day and she can't afford the protein formula recommended by her oncologist. She is worried about her constant weight loss; she is now 40kgs. Ali confided she can't stand or walk unsupported and now feels she will need a wheelchair to get to the hospital for treatment. She asked her oncologist when she could expect to walk again; apparently he avoided the question. She hoped I'd have an answer, but sadly I don't.

Ali is frustrated with the pace of her treatment; so far it has taken twice as long as she was told it would. This might be partly due to COVID-19 putting pressure on staffing, but also because her constant haemorrhaging is causing the need for intermittent blood transfusions. The treatment can only continue when her haemoglobin levels are high enough. She has had five transfusions so far this month, one bag each time due to limited blood supply (another COVID-19 consequence). Our chat ended with her request that I pray for her treatment to be successful, and my promise to do so and to follow up with the CBO to see if they can provide a wheelchair free of charge. (Bennett's field diary entry – 10 November 2020)

This diary extract provides a glimpse into the multiple hardships Indonesian women face in navigating cervical cancer. Indonesia has a population of 270 million people, living across 34 provinces and 6,000 islands, resulting in highly varied access to healthcare between different geographical regions and classes. Medical infrastructure for cancer diagnosis and care is inadequate to cover demand, with only 16 of the nation's 34 provinces able to provide nuclear medicine, including the radiotherapy and brachytherapy required to treat cervical cancer at inoperable stages (Octavianus and Gondhowiardjo 2022). The distribution of cancer treatment centres is also highly uneven, heavily concentrated in large cities on the islands of Java and Bali. Women living rurally and beyond these central islands must undertake substantial travel to access diagnosis and care, so delaying diagnosis. Survival among Indonesian women diagnosed with cervical cancer is very low, with the most recent research indicating a five-year cervical cancer survival rate for patients receiving care at the nation referral hospital of just 34 per cent, primarily as a result of later stage diagnosis (Nuranna and Fahrudin 2019). In 2020, GLOBOCAN estimated that in Indonesia more than 50 women died from cervical cancer each day, underlining the imperative of understanding how the women live with and die from this disease (Globocan 2020).

The scheduling and duration of treatment is suboptimal for most women who must access care through the national health insurance scheme. Diagnosis is frequently delayed due to the low availability of staging technologies such as MRI machines and CT scans. Diagnosis can take up to a month, followed by a minimum waiting time of one month from diagnosis to treatment. Women in this study reported frequent interruptions to treatment, related to their own health and the availability of staff to provide the highly specialised care required. Health service and treatment delays at multiple points impact on survival rates and many women expressed concern that these delays might jeopardise their chances of survival.

As noted, one factor contributing to the high mortality rate is late diagnosis. This in turn is the result of the low availability and uptake of cervical cancer screening, despite a national screening programme with the stated goal of providing free screening via either visual inspection with acetic acid or a Pap smear for up to 70 per cent of women aged between 35 and 45. Recent estimates suggest that only 12 per cent of eligible women between 30 and 50 years of age have ever taken up screening (Ministry of Health Republic of Indonesia 2020). Rates of repeat screening are not monitored, but are likely to be even lower. Multiple barriers to screening occur on the demand side because of women's lack of confidence in the efficacy of screening, fear of a positive screening result, low knowledge of cervical cancer and screening, shame associated with undergoing pelvic exams and time and transportation constraints (Robbers et al. 2021). Supply-side barriers include a lack of skilled screening providers, limited health promotion on cervical cancer, resource constraints on equipment and medical supplies and lack of training and supervision of health workers tasked with screening (Robbers et al. 2021).

Ali's experiences, above, illuminate that for most women it is not merely a struggle to reach diagnosis, but also an ongoing struggle to manage the continuing physical suffering associated with cancer and treatment side effects. The costs associated with accessing treatment, such as travel and accommodation, can be enormous and often qualify as catastrophic health spending, particularly for women who do not live close to treatment centres (half of Indonesia's population still lives rurally). Poverty and cramped living conditions can also compromise women's ability to maintain adequate nutrition and hygiene whilst undergoing treatment, further compromising their physical resilience. Even elite women who initially enter the cancer care system as private patients, in the hope of quicker diagnosis, often switch to the public system for treatment because even with private health insurance the cost of treatment as private patients is extremely high. The financial hardship women and their families experience when seeking treatment adds to women's psychological distress and, for some, manifests in guilt. This guilt often relates to the accumulation of family debt, or opportunities that may have been forgone by other family members in order to meet the costs of treatment, for example financing higher education for women's children or grandchildren. Cancer CBOs and other charity organisations provide financial and practical support to many women seeking treatment, but their resources are limited and inadequate in the face of the rising incidence of cervical cancer.

In this context of combined physical, economic and psychological suffering, women must also negotiate the social suffering associated with stigma. As we explore later in the chapter, stigma is not only directed at women affected by cancer, but also at their loved ones, and hence the social suffering associated with stigma can be transferred to others. This creates a layer of care responsibilities for women, complicating their need for care themselves.

Methodological approach

In this chapter we draw on ethnographic case studies of 31 Indonesian women ever diagnosed with cervical cancer, with fieldwork occurring over 20 months from March 2019 to January 2021. We applied a novel methodology for constructing cancer biographies that we refer to as 'biographies of vulnerability and resilience' (BOVR). This approach was designed to place women's experiences of living with cervical cancer within the wider context of their personal histories and to avoid reducing their identities and health to their experiences of cancer. To achieve this, we constructed biographies through the collection and synthesis of life histories and illness narratives with women affected by cancer, in-depth interviews with a support person nominated by these women and participant observation of women's daily lives and their engagement with cancer CBOs and the health system. The BOVR framework applied a grounded theory approach, whereby we explored women's experiences as holistically as possible (Strauss and Corbin 1994) and allowed lines of enquiry to be iteratively guided by women's meanings of their experiences and the issues they identified as most significant. Our focus on stigma was not predesignated, but emerged organically as a pervasive concern of women, influencing how they experienced and navigated cervical cancer from diagnosis onwards.

During preliminary stakeholder engagements in 2018, stigma was raised as a potential obstacle. While members of cancer CBOs were highly supportive of the research, they warned that many cervical cancer survivors were reluctant to speak openly or publicly about their disease due to its associated shame. Without cancer CBO networks, patient support groups and compassionate oncologists it would have been impossible to find women with a diagnosis because of their relative 'invisibility' as cancer survivors. Nevertheless, when we established the trust required to invite women into the research via cancer-based networks, many were keen to participate and did not shy away from discussing the impacts of cervical cancer stigma and other forms of social suffering on themselves and their loved ones.

Face-to-face interviews and participant observation occurred between April 2019 and March 2020; in response to the COVID-19 pandemic, thereafter, we shifted to phone and video interviews. Women initiated ongoing contact with the research team via mobile phone and social media to update us on their cancer trajectories and share insights that occurred after formal interviews. We also maintained contact to provide support to women, fact check and for data triangulation. Communication with these women has continued and is ongoing at the time of writing. Bennett and Atikasari both engaged with women through participant observation, via WhatsApp chats and conducted interviews with them in Indonesian or Javanese, according to their preferences. We also interviewed cancer advocates and cancer CBO volunteers (N=16) and health professionals involved in screening, diagnosis and care (N=50). We primarily draw on women's experiences in this chapter and use pseudonyms throughout to protect their anonymity.

The research was initially centred in Yogyakarta and Jakarta, the two Indonesian cities with the greatest number of cancer treatment centres. The conversion to phone and video interviews had the effect of widening the geographical breadth of the study. Our final self-selected sample included 31 women ever-diagnosed with cervical cancer: 14 were aged 34–50, correlating loosely with reproductive age, with the remaining 17 aged 51–63, all of whom reported being post-menopausal. The majority of women recruited were Muslim (N=24); the remaining seven were Catholic or Protestant. Participants resided in 12 of Indonesia's 34 provinces, but all had sought cancer treatment in either Jakarta or Yogyakarta. Nearly half (N=14) had undertaken costly and time-consuming travel across provincial borders to reach care. We did not seek to recruit women who were in treatment or receiving palliative care due to our concerns regarding their vulnerability and need for privacy; however, some women initiated ongoing dialogue with us as their cancer progressed, which provided some insight into their experiences of later stage cancer and palliative care.[3] At the time of writing three of the 31 women who shared their experiences with us had passed away as a result of cervical cancer.

Lower cervical cancer survival rates among disadvantaged women are driven by differences in access to and engagement with health services (compare Chapter 3 by Luxardo and Bennett, this volume), as reflected in the skewing of our sample towards women able to afford diagnosis. Women most disadvantaged and alienated from the Indonesian health system were excluded because we had no way of identifying them, which we acknowledge as a serious limitation. All but one of the women who contributed to this study had been married, 24 were still married and six were widowed or divorced. All but two were mothers: 16 women had one or two children and 13 women had three or more children. Educational attainment among women in our sample was high compared with national standards, reflecting the enhanced capacity of women with higher formal education and higher incomes to achieve diagnosis. All women were literate and had some secondary education, and the majority had regular access to mobile phones and the internet. Four women chose not to discuss their income, and for the remaining 27 we assessed their socio-economic status according to the quintiles used by the Indonesian Bureau of Statistics.[4] Accordingly, 13 women were classified as being 'upper class', three as 'middle class', six as 'aspiring middle class', four as 'vulnerable' and one as 'poor'. Poor, vulnerable and aspiring middle-class women all required financial support additional to their regular household incomes to navigate treatment. However, wealth and elevated class status provided women with no protection from the stigma associated with cervical cancer.

Women's navigation of stigma

Selective disclosure

We began this article with Bunga's strategy of selective disclosure. This was commonly adopted to limit the impact of stigma and blame. Women typically practised two forms of selective disclosure – they were selective about 'who' they disclosed to and were selective about 'what' they disclosed. Some women practised both forms of selective disclosure and for many this also required their loved ones to maintain a certain degree of discretion or secrecy, primarily to avoid the moral judgement of others. Rita, a 47-year-old cancer advocate, explained: 'When you acknowledge a person has cervical cancer it can be like instantly judging them, making a moral judgement about someone.' Thus, the choice not to disclose is a tactic to evade the moral judgement of others and the stigma flowing from that judgement.

A common form of selective disclosure women practised was to refrain from naming their specific type of cancer within their immediate social circles of friends, neighbours and workmates. Cervical cancer treatment requires significant time – including recovery from surgery and extended periods of combined radiation/chemotherapy, has visible bodily effects – such as hair and weight loss – and is often ongoing. As a result, it is extremely difficult for women to hide their illness. By acknowledging that they have an unspecified cancer, women are able to explain their changing appearance and absence from everyday routines including work, while containing potential malicious gossip. For instance, Nelly, a public servant aged 45, had undergone two treatment regimens at different stages of her cancer, requiring long absences from work. She fully disclosed her diagnosis to her boss in order to access sick leave and trusted her boss, who was a person with 'experience herself in dealing with cancer, because her mother had died of cervical cancer'. However, Nelly and her boss agreed to keep the nature of her cancer concealed from her other colleagues to reduce the likelihood of judgemental responses and gossip.

Some women limited disclosure to their immediate family members and some disclosed only to their primary support person or carer, as was the case for Bunga at the beginning of this chapter. Women's explanations for these tight circles of disclosure typically involved concern over limiting stigma directed towards both themselves and family members. Many women wanted to avoid being blamed for the disease, or their husbands being blamed, because sexual promiscuity is so widely interpreted not as a risk factor but as causing cervical cancer. Women worried that negative moral judgements about their own sexuality would lead to referred stigma to their male partners and their daughters (see Indrah's story in the subsection 'Reclassifying cancer'). This was confirmed by the stigmatising discourses that some women experienced at or immediately following diagnosis. Rohana (aged 51), who had relocated from an outer island to Java to achieve diagnosis and undergo treatment, described her experience of enacted stigma at diagnosis:

> At that time [at diagnosis] the doctor asked a lot of questions . . . he asked if my husband was a driver [transport worker]. I said 'no'. If that was relevant then I would have told him, or asked about it. There was no need to ask that question.
>
> Other friends [peers with cervical cancer] also shared that the doctor asked about their husbands' occupation. No one likes this question. It's like saying that the husband is behaving badly with other women.

When initial encounters with diagnosing clinicians involved moral judgement of women's husbands, and themselves by association, women responded by seeking to minimise further judgement through the careful management of disclosure.

Women who disclosed their diagnosis only to their key support person tended to be particularly reliant on that support person. Key support people were often positioned as the sole supporters available to facilitate access to treatment, to assist women in coping with the physical hardships of living with cancer and to act as women's only confidants. As a result, key support people struggled at times to cope with highly intensified care responsibilities and were unable to seek support themselves without betraying confidences. This was particularly apparent when daughters acted as the sole support person for their mothers. Another obvious effect was to limit the scope of support available to women from others in their families and social networks.

Re-articulating causality

Rather than limiting disclosure, some women responded to their diagnosis by seeking to disrupt the association between cervical cancer and sexual transgression, offering alternative explanations of causality and so deflecting stigma. Citra was a happily married middle-class woman in her mid-forties who had recently been diagnosed with Stage IIA cancer when we met her. In her interview she sought to reconcile her sexual subjectivity and life experiences with information she had accessed via the internet. She had read that 'having multiple sexual partners' was the highest risk factor for the disease and felt angry and confronted by this information. Citra asserted that she had only one sexual partner throughout her life and believed that her husband had been faithful. She openly rejected the popular (stigmatising) assumption that women who develop cervical cancer had multiple sexual partners. Instead, she explained her cervical cancer as caused by an intrauterine contraceptive device (IUD) which she had previously used.

In her informal cancer support group, Citra informed the other women that she had contracted human papillomavirus (HPV) from using an IUD. She attempted to dissociate from the implications of promiscuity and to protect her marital bond, via the counter-narrative of being happily married, rejecting the assumption of extra-marital sex and speaking of a 'good' husband who offered her significant support. Four other women in the study asserted that their use of modern family planning methods, not promiscuous behaviour, had caused their cancer. Linking cancer aetiology to family planning can be interpreted as an effective normalising narrative, given that married women's use of modern contraception is ardently promoted by the Indonesian government. Hormonal contraceptive use by married couples is not stigmatised in any way (although condom use is) and is strongly associated with idealised notions of women as responsible for disciplining their bodies for the good of their family and the nation (Bennett 2005; Spagnoletti et al. 2019). This is in direct contrast to the stigmatising narrative of the sexually promiscuous undisciplined woman who has brought cervical cancer upon herself.

When women interpreted cervical cancer causality through such normalising narratives, they maintained dominant constructions of 'good' and 'bad' women and chose not to emphasise biomedically 'accurate' explanations of disease aetiology. While a number of oncologists we interviewed asserted that women patients 'did not, or could not' comprehend the cause of their cancer, women may also actively choose to construct cancer causality in ways that deflect stigma and a degraded social identity (Goffman 1963) and maintain a valued moral subjectivity. This strategy of re-articulating causality makes sense according to the local moral worlds of women, but it becomes problematic when we consider its implications for the possibilities of cervical cancer prevention and care. An unintended effect of the circulation of misinformation about the causes of cervical cancer among women is the othering of cervical cancer risk. Women who do not perceive themselves at risk because they have only one sexual partner and believe their husbands do not have other partners, or do not use modern contraceptives, are less likely to engage in screening, placing them at greater actual risk of developing the disease.

> We can ask our women friends [cancer peers] whatever we want [about the cancer experience], we don't have to be embarrassed like with doctors and nurses, because we are the same ... I'm not going to ask a doctor about how to handle my relationship with my husband, they [doctors and nurses] already think we swap [sexual] partners. It's safer just to talk to our friends [cancer peers] who won't judge us.

Setty, who is quoted above, explicitly mentioned the safety of these peer relationships, grounded in the understanding that women who have experienced the same cancer will not judge others.

For many women, maintaining a safe social space for socialising and support extended beyond their treatment and was managed digitally via closed WhatsApp groups. While these spaces are limited to virtual interaction, they provide crucial social outlets, free of stigma and where disclosure is not an issue. For women who have travelled extensively to access care, virtual social groups enable them to maintain contact with distant peers who they cannot meet in person (Manderson et al. in press). These digital relationships are also important for women who are socially isolated following their cancer diagnosis, as was common for women who chose not to disclose their cancer widely.

Cancer CBOs also provided safe physical spaces for women to meet without the threat of moral stigma. They also provided meaningful opportunities for women to volunteer to support other women, practically and psychologically. Rohaini, head of one of Indonesia's oldest cancer CBOs with 40 years of advocacy experience, often remarked that there was nothing more powerful in supporting a woman to take up treatment than the 'testimony and support of another woman survivor'. In illness narratives, we also observed how women's sense of solidarity with and support from other survivors positively influenced their decisions around pursuing and completing treatment. Small boarding houses run by cervical cancer survivors were often preferred over free generic cancer patient hostels by women who could afford them, because they were experienced as environments free from judgement and moral stigma.

The term solidarity is an appropriate description of the social strategies women developed to manage the impacts of stigma and meet their specific support needs. Moral stigma had great propensity to spoil women's public identities, in the sense that Goffman (1963) used this term, and disrupt their prior social relationships. However, solidarity formed in the context of non-judgemental relationships with other survivors acted to restore their social identities and moral subjectivities. We suggest that the function of solidarity between women affected by cervical cancer adds to prior conceptions of biosociality (Gibbon and Novas 2007), as it is driven by not merely a shared experience of a disease, but also by the shared project of creating safe relationships and alternative spaces free from the norms of mainstream morality.

Reclassifying cancer

The association between promiscuity, immorality and cervical cancer was more acutely felt by some women than others and the intensity of felt stigma for different women was commonly linked with marital status. Ethnographers of Indonesia have documented a pervasive stereotype, across multiple ethnic groups, that constructs widows and divorcees as promiscuous and sexually available (Mahy, Winarnita and Herriman 2016; Parker, Riyani and Nolan 2016). The convergence of stigma associated with being a divorcee diagnosed with cervical cancer was felt deeply by Indrah, who was a sole parent of three children, aged 8, 12 and 16 when we met her. Indrah had faced multiple hardships, and living with cancer in her forties was an additional struggle compounding the already difficult circumstances of her life (Manderson and Warren 2016). Indrah had married young and endured three unsuccessful marriages, of which two were marked by infidelity. When we met her, she was unemployed, impoverished and responsible for caring for her children without financial support from their fathers or her extended family.

Members of our research team regularly texted and spoke with Indrah by phone to provide moral support and help alleviate her social isolation. Every call began with Indrah apologising for her intrusion and reminding the caller that she was not a *perempuan nakal* (badly behaved woman) or a *perempuan kacau* (promiscuous woman). Indrah struggled daily with the experiences of intersectional stigma flowing from her status as a serial divorcee, a single woman and a woman diagnosed with cervical cancer (Turan et al. 2019). This intersectional stigma had a profound impact on Indrah's mental well-being and sense of self-worth. She experienced severe depression, disclosed suicidal ideation and constantly sought to reassure people of her good character. During each interaction with the research team, Indrah also expressed concern for her children. This included fears over their stigmatisation via association and her regret that she could not adequately provide for their material needs. She went to great lengths to guard her teenage daughter's sexual reputation, which she feared was at risk from moral stigma, by ensuring that her daughter was never alone with any adult or adolescent male.

After attending a follow-up appointment to assess her cancer status, Indrah contacted a member of our team and explained that her oncologist had informed her that the cancer had progressed beyond her cervix, into her pelvic cavity and uterus, consistent with a Stage IIIB diagnosis. While reflecting on this new information, Indrah expressed significant relief because she felt able to reclassify her cancer as *kanker kandungan* (literally, womb or uterine cancer). *Kanker kandungan* is often used to refer to gynaecological cancers associated with reproduction rather than sex (for example, ovarian, uterine and endometrial cancers) and so are not automatically stigmatised. Indrah understood that her cancer had progressed to the point where additional treatment could prolong her life but would not cure her. Yet she expressed considerable relief that she would not die of the deeply stigmatised cervical cancer. Indrah's deflection of stigma by embracing her 'new diagnosis' of *kanker kandugan* allowed her to shore up her moral subjectivity and reclaim a more legitimate social identity, which she hoped would result in less associated stigma for her children.

As our research progressed, other women also moved into the later stages of cancer and we witnessed their reclassification of cancer once it had spread. This was accompanied by a shift in their representation of the illness in dialogue with us, family and friends. For instance, Ali, aged 53, shared her thoughts after receiving the news that her cancer had progressed to Stage IV:

> The cancer is now in my bones and lungs, it won't be long now. I know soon I'll see my father in heaven . . . At least I'm finished with the cervical cancer . . . the treatment for that cancer was so traumatic . . . I can't handle that again . . . before I go, I can tell my family and close friends that I have bone and lung cancer. It's much better for the family [to know about lung and bone cancer], better for them not to remember that I had cervical cancer.

Neither Ali nor Indrah rejected the dominant moral paradigm that associates cervical cancer with promiscuity. They aimed to reclaim a positive moral subjectivity for themselves, and by association their loved ones, through the reclassification of their cancer. These experiences highlight how women's management of stigma so often extends to care for their loved ones and can extend to a commitment to minimise the social suffering of others even beyond their own life span.

Discussion: moral stigma and capacities for care

Containment has been established as a salient concept in prior ethnographies of cancer and aptly applied to describe people's efforts to contain the impacts of cancer on the lives of themselves and others (Andersen et al. 2010; see also Chapter 9 by Greco, this volume). In the context of moral stigma, we have described how women's containment of stigma through selective disclosure is effective in limiting the social suffering associated with their disease. These containment practices can be understood as both forms of self-care and care for others vulnerable to moral stigma via association with women affected by cervical cancer. Care for others often focused on women protecting their daughters and their male partners from moral stigma; for some women this form of care extended to their wider kin group. Women's prioritisation of care for others remained paramount across different stages of their cancer trajectories up until the end of women's lives, as Indrah's and Ali's accounts illustrate.

Indonesian women's choices to enact care by limiting the potential impacts of moral stigma make sense in their local moral worlds. Similar strategies of limited disclosure have been observed by women living with cervical cancer in other societies where promiscuity and sexual immorality are linked closely with cervical cancer. For instance, ethnographic work on women's experiences of cervical cancer by Hunt (1998) in Mexico, Gregg (2003, 2011) in Brazil and Martínez (2018) in Venezuela have all illuminated the extraordinary impact of dominant sexual moralities on cultural understandings of cervical cancer. What have not been explored to date are the inherent contradictions between practices of care that limit disclosure or reclassify cancer and the costs of those practices in limiting women's possibilities for care.

The care available to women affected by cervical cancer is shaped by their own strategies for mediating stigma. Women can only request and receive care, related to their cancer, from those to whom they have disclosed. In the biographies we collected, we observed that narrow circles of disclosure tended to limit the scope of care available to women. Conversely, wider fields of disclosure tended to generate greater capacities for care among women's extended families, religious communities and other social networks. We also witnessed unintended impacts of selective disclosure on those who were the sole carers of women affected by cancer. Key support people who were women's only confidants tended to experience extremely high care burdens, which in turn constrained their capacities for care. The requirement of secrecy around their care roles also prevented them from seeking out or receiving support themselves. Our interviews with key support people confirmed that for some it was extremely difficult to be the sole carer for a woman negotiating cervical cancer and that carers benefited greatly when they could draw on wider circles of support from cancer CBOs, peer volunteers and extended family. Our contention is that the varied strategies performed by women, with the purpose of avoiding or limiting moral stigma, had the unintended effect of constricting the capacities for care available to them.

Capacities for care are simultaneously shaped by an individual's sense of entitlement to care and society's moral judgements about who is deserving of care. The prominent association between sexual promiscuity and blame for cervical cancer acts to devalue women's social identities and in turn their social legitimacy as cancer patients. This phenomenon of victim blaming has been widely observed by other researchers of cervical cancer (Dyer 2010; Gregg 2003; Martínez 2018; see also Chapter 3 by Luxardo and Bennett, this volume). In our research, victim blaming limited capacities for care among women who had internalised a high degree of intersectional stigma and so struggled to ask for and receive care. This was the case for Indrah and two other women of lower socio-economic background, all of whom had been married multiple times and had been divorced or widowed. Perhaps one of the most harmful impacts of moral stigma we encountered was when it undermined women's self-worth to the extent that they no longer believed they were deserving of care.

Women's rejection of dominant causation narratives and their re-articulation of causation without reference to sexual behaviour – as occurred for Citra and others – negated women's blame for their cancer and established their sense of entitlement to care as respectable moral subjects. This expanded the capacities for care for a number of women because it enabled them to confidently assert their right to care. However, the negation of blame through re-articulating causality did not challenge the notion that immoral women are undeserving of care. It allowed some women to re-establish their moral worth, but ultimately it failed to challenge the idea that women's right to care was subject to sexual reputation. In her ethnography with Brazilian women living with cervical cancer, Gregg (2003) describes how women tended to hold themselves accountable for their cancer as a consequence of their failure to conform with dominant moral constructions of female sexuality. Some but not all women in our study also struggled to challenge the normative association with sexual immorality and cervical cancer. In the longer term, widespread social legitimation of care for women affected by cancer will necessarily require the de-stigmatisation of the disease.

Contexts in which Indonesian women are consistently working to expand capacities for care include cervical cancer advocacy, both physical and virtual, including cancer CBOs and the social support networks of cervical cancer survivors themselves. As noted, one of the fundamental reasons why these spaces and relationships are so successful at enhancing capacities for care is because they are stigma free. Acceptance and belonging negate stigma and shared experiences of navigating cervical cancer validate women's identities. Becoming a peer volunteer supporting other women diagnosed with cervical cancer is validating for women who volunteer as well as for those they support. Through the processes of guiding recently diagnosed women through treatment options and supporting them to access treatment, cervical cancer survivors greatly enhance the capacities for care available to other women. In doing so, most volunteers share their own stories – understood locally as giving testimony – and these testimonies have the power to disrupt the silence and stigma surrounding cervical cancer in Indonesia. We propose that sharing testimony and other forms of solidarity practised by women in our research constitute important practices of care in themselves and, over time, have the potential to erode social barriers to care that are driven by stigma.

Conclusion

Morality, stigma and capacities for care exist in dynamic relationship with one another and are vital in shaping the choices and experiences of Indonesian women living with cervical cancer. Our exploration of women's strategies for navigating moral stigma such as selective disclosure, re-articulating causality, reclassifying cancer and seeking solidarity, establish that these choices can be read as both forms of self-care and care for others who are targets for stigma by association. In the local moral worlds of Indonesian women, cervical cancer stigma creates the necessity for care practices directed at the containment and evasion of social suffering. While strategies of solidarity can enhance the care available to some women, those who choose limited circles of disclosure subsequently experience constrained capacities for care.

For a disease that is both preventable via HPV vaccination prior to sexual debut and highly treatable if detected in its earlier stages it is also crucial that prevention be prioritised. For adult women to take up regular screening, and to facilitate the HPV vaccination of their daughters, they require an accurate understanding of risk in relation to HPV and cervical cancer. Moral stigma, and women's readings of causality, deflect risk perception away from women and girls who wish to be constructed as morally upright. Thus, cancer care along the full trajectory from prevention to treatment requires that moral stigma be eroded and eventually extinguished. This requires the promotion of narratives of causality that are not morally loaded, are free from blame and are expressed in non-judgemental terms across society-wide platforms including within the health system. If cervical cancer stigma is not actively rejected it will continue to erode the care available to women affected by the disease, perpetuating inequalities between different forms of cancer in the Indonesian context.

Our conceptualisation of care in the context of cervical cancer has revealed how care is performed by women affected by the disease, rejecting notions of care as a unidirectional process and cancer patients as passive recipients of care. It has added to the growing understanding of cancers as innately relational and as necessarily navigated between and through complex human relationships. Where capacities for care have been diminished through women's containment practices, hierarchies of care can be observed in which moral subjectivity and social acceptability are placed above women's needs for other forms of support, which could be accessed via wider circles of disclosure. We have emphasised women's choices in relation to how they have navigated moral stigma, deliberately avoiding narratives that position women as passive victims in the face of stigma; women clearly did not view themselves in such terms. However, women's choices and the capacities for care available to them are constricted by persisting cultural norms that vilify sex outside of marriage (particularly for women) and link individuals' rights to care with their perceived moral worth. Moral stigma ultimately acts as an antithesis to realising the full possibilities of care that should be available to Indonesian women living with cervical cancer.

Acknowledgements

We thank the Australian Research Council for funding this research under the Discovery Projects Scheme, and the co-investigators on this project: Professor Barbara McPake, Professor Lenore Manderson and Professor Siswanto Wilopo. Contributions of the authors to this chapter are summarised as study design by Linda Rae Bennett, ethnographic fieldwork conducted by Bennett in 2018 and 2019 and by Hanum Atikasari in 2020, data coding and extraction by Atikasari with supervision from Bennett, data analysis and theoretical framework by Bennett, first draft of chapter produced by Bennett with subsequent drafts and theoretical input by Atikasari and Bennett. We also wish to thank the transcribers who worked on our interviews and the administrative staff at the Centre for Reproductive Health at Gadjah Mada University. Finally, our thanks are extended to all the women whose stories feature in this chapter for sharing their time and experiences with us.

Notes

1. In this chapter we use the conventional biomedical classifications for cervical cancer staging, which include pre-cancer, followed by Stages I through to IV, with Stage IV being the palliative care stage.
2. In parts of South Asia qualitative research has confirmed that women living with breast cancer often experience significant stigma and discrimination, both from their families and wider society (Nyblade et al. 2017). However, in the Indonesian context those diagnosed with breast cancer typically receive a high degree of compassion and discourses around breast cancer treatment and survival are highly visible in public, indicating the ease with which people discuss breast cancer compared to the silence around cervical cancer.
3. We initially chose not to recruit women receiving palliative care because this was the first ethnographic work to be conducted on cervical cancer in Indonesia. We aimed to establish an appropriate level of cultural sensitivity around communicating about cancer before engaging with women at the end of their lives, but as noted some women contacted us as their cancer progressed and wanted to share their experiences of late stage cancer. The gap in the initial study (on palliative care) is now the focus of Hanum Atikasari's current PhD project, which builds on the relationships and expertise she developed as a research assistant during the initial research.
4. These quintiles are: poor – with a monthly income of 1 million rupiah or less, vulnerable – with a monthly income of 1 to 3 million rupiah, aspiring middle class – with a monthly income of 3.1 to 5 million rupiah, middle class – with an income of 5.1 to 8 million rupiah and upper class – with a monthly income of over 8.1 million rupiah.

References

Andersen, Rikke Sand, Bjarke Paarup, Peter Vedsted, Flemming Bro and Jens Soendergaard. 2010. '"Containment" as an analytical framework for understanding patient delay: A qualitative study of cancer patients' symptom interpretation processes', *Social Science & Medicine* 71(2): 378–385. https://doi.org/10.1016/j.socscimed.2010.03.044.

Bennett, Linda Rae. 2005. *Women, Islam and Modernity: Single women, sexuality and reproductive health in contemporary Indonesia*. London and New York: Routledge Curzon.

Bennett, Linda Rae. 2015. 'Sexual morality and the silencing of sexual health within Indonesian infertility care'. In *Sex and Sexualities in Contemporary Indonesia: Sexual politics, diversity, representations and health*, edited by Linda Rae Bennett and Sharyn Graham Davies, 148–166. London and New York: Routledge.

Dyer, Karen E. 2010. 'From cancer to sexually transmitted infection: Explorations of social stigma among cervical cancer survivors', *Human Organization* 69(4): 321–330. https://doi.org/10.17730/humo.69.4.a750670h0784521j

Gibbon, Sahra and Carlos Novas. 2007. 'Introduction: Biosocialities, genetics and the social sciences'. In *Biosocialities, Genetics and the Social Sciences*, edited by Sahra Gibbon and Carlos Novas, 11–28. London: Routledge.

GLOBOCAN. 2020. 'Indonesia fact sheet 2020'. Accessed 17 August 2022. https://gco.iarc.fr/today/data/factsheets/populations/360-indonesia-fact-sheets.pdf.

Goffman, Erving. 1963. *Stigma: Notes on the management of a spoiled identity*. New York: Prentice Hall.

Gregg, Jessica L. 2003. *Virtually Virgins: Sexual strategies and cervical cancer in Recife, Brazil*. Stanford, CA: Stanford University Press.

Gregg, Jessica L. 2011. 'An unanticipated source of hope: Stigma and cervical cancer in Brazil', *Medical Anthropology Quarterly* 25(1): 70–84. https://doi.org/10.1111/j.1548-1387.2010.01137.x.

Hunt, Linda M. 1998. 'Moral reasoning and the meaning of cancer: Causal explanations of oncologists and patients in southern Mexico', *Medical Anthropology Quarterly* 12(3): 298–318. https://doi.org/10.1525/maq.1998.12.3.298.

Kleinman, Arthur and Sjaak van der Geest. 2009. '"Care" in health care: Remaking the moral world of medicine', *Medische Anthropologie* 21(1): 159–168. https://hdl.handle.net/11245/1.314817.

Livingston, Julie. 2012. *Improvising Medicine: An African oncology ward in an emerging cancer epidemic*. Durham, NC: Duke University Press.

Mahy, Petra, Monika Swasti Winarnita and Nicholas Herriman. 2016. 'Presumptions of promiscuity: Reflections on being a widow or divorcee from three Indonesia communities', *Indonesia and the Malay World* 44(128): 47–67. https://doi.org/10.1080/13639811.2015.1100872.

Manderson, Lenore and Narelle Warren. 2016. '"Just one thing after another": Recursive cascades and chronic conditions', *Medical Anthropology Quarterly* 30(4): 479–497. https://doi.org/10.1111/maq.12277.

Manderson, Lenore, Belinda Rina Marie Spagnoletti, Linda Rae Bennett and Siswanto Wilopo. In press. 'Digital communication and cervical cancer in Indonesia: Expanding access while exacerbating digital divides', *Psycho-Oncology*.

Martin, Aryn, Natasha Myers and Ana Viseu. 2015. 'The politics of care in technoscience', *Social Studies of Science* 45(5): 625–641. https://doi.org/10.1177/0306312715602073.

Martínez, Rebecca G. 2018. *Marked Women: The cultural politics of cervical cancer in Venezuela*. Stanford, CA: Stanford University Press.

Ministry of Health Republic of Indonesia. 2020. *National Health Profile Report – 2019*. Jakarta: Ministry of Health Republic of Indonesia.

Mol, Annemarie. 2008. *The Logic of Care: Health and the problem of patient choice*. London: Routledge.

Mol, Annemarie, Ingunn Moser and Jeannette Pols. 2010. *Care in Practice: On tinkering in clinics, homes and farms*. Bielefeld, Germany: Transcript Verlag.

Newland, Jamee, Dwi Lestari, Mashoeroel Noor Poedjanadi and Angela Kelly-Hanku. 2021. 'Co-locating art and health: Engaging civil society to create an enabling environment to respond to HIV in Indonesia', *Sexual Health* 18(1): 84–94. https://doi.org/10.1071/SH20125.

Nuranna, Laila and Aziz Fahrudin. 2019. 'Survival rate of cervical cancer in national referral hospital in 2012-2014', *Indonesian Journal of Internal Medicine* 51(2): 145–150.

Nyblade, Laura, Melissa Stockton, Sandra Travasso and Suneeta Krishnan. 2017. 'A qualitative exploration of cervical and breast cancer stigma in Karnataka, India', *BMC Women's Health* 17(1): 1–15. https://doi.org/10.1186/s12905-017-0407-x.

Octavianus, Steven and Soehartati Gondhowiardjo. 2022. 'Radiation therapy in Indonesia: Estimating demand as part of a national cancer control strategy', *Applied Radio Oncology* 11(1): 35–42.

Parker, Lyn, Irma Riyani and Brooke Nolan. 2016. 'The stigmatisation of widows and divorcees (*janda*) in Indonesia, and the possibilities for agency', *Indonesia and the Malay World* 44(128): 27–46. https://doi.org/10.1080/13639811.2016.1111677.

Parker, Richard and Peter Aggleton. 2003. 'HIV and AIDS-related stigma and discrimination: A conceptual framework and implications for action', *Social Science & Medicine* 57(1): 13–24. https://doi.org/10.1016/S0277-9536(02)00304-0.

Robbers, Gianna Maxi Leila, Linda Rae Bennett, Belinda Rina Marie Spagnoletti and Siswanto Agus Wilopo. 2021. 'Facilitators and barriers for the delivery and uptake of cervical cancer screening in Indonesia: A scoping review', *Global Health Action* 14(1). https://doi.org/10.1080/165497 16.2021.1979280.

Spagnoletti, Belinda Rina Marie, Linda Rae Bennett, Michelle Kermode and Siswanto Agus Wilopo. 2019. '"The final decision is with the patient": Reproductive modernity and preferences for non-hormonal and non-biomedical contraceptives among postpartum middle class women in Yogyakarta, Indonesia', *Asian Population Studies* 15(1): 105–125. https://doi.org/10.1080/ 17441730.2019.1578532.

Strauss, Anselm and Juliet Corbin. 1994. 'Grounded theory methodology: An overview'. In *Handbook of Qualitative Research*, edited by Norman K. Denzin and Yvonna S. Lincoln, 273–285. Thousand Oaks, CA: SAGE.

Sunarsih, Irene Marcellina, Yayi Suryo Prabandari, Teguh Aryandono and Soenarto Sastrowijoto. 2018. 'Exploring possible causes for delays seeking medical treatment among Indonesian women with breast cancer', *Asian Journal of Pharmaceutical and Clinical Research* 11(6): 284–288. https://doi.org/10.22159/ajpcr.2018.v11i6.25211.

Turan, Janet M., Melissa A. Elafros, Carmen H. Logie, Swagata Banik, Bulent Turan, Kaylee B. Crockett, Bernice Pescosolido and Sarah M. Murray. 2019. 'Challenges and opportunities in examining and addressing intersectional stigma and health', *BMC Medicine* 17(1): 1–15. https://doi.org/10.1186/s12916-018-1246-9.

Waluyo, Agung, Elly Nurachmah and Rosakawati Rosakawati. 2006. 'Perceptions of HIV/AIDS patients and their families about HIV/AIDS and community stigma against HIV/AIDS patients'. *Jurnal Keperawatan Indonesia* 10(2): 61–69. https://doi.org/10.7454/jki.v10i2.175.

Waluyo, Agung, Gabriel J. Culbert, Judith Levy and Kathleen F. Norr. 2015. 'Understanding HIV-related stigma among Indonesian nurses', *Journal of the Association of Nurses in AIDS Care* 26(1): 69–80. https://doi.org/10.1016/j.jana.2014.03.001.

Yang, Lawrence Hsin, Arthur Kleinman, Bruce G. Link, Jo C. Phelan, Sing Lee and Byron Good. 2007. 'Culture and stigma: Adding moral experience to stigma theory', *Social Science & Medicine* 64(7): 1524–1535. https://doi.org/10.1016/j.socscimed.2006.11.013.

7
Untimely liver cancer and the temporalities of care in rural Senegal

Noémi Tousignant

The timing of liver cancer in Senegal – which manifests mostly in young and middle-aged adults and which usually progresses rapidly from symptoms to diagnosis then death – places a heavy burden of both emotion and responsibility on health workers. Doctors and nurses told me about being deeply affected by the intensity of their patients' suffering and of feeling powerless to act on the course of their disease. Yet, in their accounts of care, what they emphasised as most troubling was the youth of their patients, their own certainty that death was imminent and inevitable and how quickly patients then died. In other words, they pointed to the *untimeliness* of liver cancer deaths as a central challenge in providing care.

In this chapter, I explore how Senegalese health workers – in particular nurses who run rural health posts – treat this untimeliness as a problem both *for* and *of* care. Cancer's untimeliness constricts possibilities for action, threatening to unsettle care's moral and material capacities (Cook and Trundle 2020). Yet an untimely death, nurses and other caregivers insist, also calls for care. It exists in a moment in which care matters intensely, not just for patients' comfort but also for the social and material relations that are affected by their suffering and dying. Care for the dying cannot *transform* the untimeliness of their disease and death; it cannot prevent, delay, prolong or even hasten rhythms of damage. Yet care can, to some extent, *form* the temporal outline and qualities of a brief end-of-life and its aftermath. In this chapter, I approach the temporal limits and possibilities of care, as described by rural health workers, as a window into the situatedness of liver cancer in Senegal. I ask how the untimeliness of cancer and care are mediated and made 'different' (McMullin 2016) by local social and ecological histories, biomedical knowledge, health infrastructures and practices and so on. At the same time, I reflect from this case study on the temporalities of care and how they depart from and are enmeshed with (rather than defined in opposition to; see Mol 2008) other modes of engaging with cancer, particularly those of biomedical knowledge-production and control. Following Maria Puig de la Bellacasa (2015: 692), a feminist attention to care can 'draw attention to the significance of practices and experiences made invisible or marginalized by dominant, "successful", forms of technoscientific mobilization'.

Cancer time

In many settings, cancer is surrounded by an intense, heavily resourced (and highly profitable; see Jain 2013) 'biotechnical embrace' (Del Vecchio Good, cited in McMullin 2016: 252). An enduring faith in 'the paradigm of early detection' (Löwy 2010: 356) has oriented the building of diagnostic and therapeutic systems, yoking cancer to a 'regime of hope' (Löwy 2011). These systems thus create and are driven by an 'imagined time of biomedicine' that, in Camilo Sanz's (2017: 192) apt term, *synchronises* the 'rhythms' of time-sensitive interventions with cancer's (imagined) progression through stages of treatability. This idealised synchrony, in which intervention is rendered effective by its timeliness, is often at odds with actual trajectories through healthcare, even for those with privileged access. It sets up deviations from this ideal, such as belated diagnosis, as a personal failure, while drawing attention away from other, more uncertain temporalities of causation and fatality (Jain 2013). For a global majority, however, minimal or partial access to biomedical resources make synchronised cancer care an implausible or even unimaginable fantasy. In such settings, diagnostic and treatment delays are the norm, arising from systemic failures in the provision and accessibility of healthcare (Banerjee 2020; Livingston 2012; Sanz 2017). 'Dissonance' thus arises with a 'discourse of hope' that depends on the conditions of prompt intervention (McMullin 2016: 253).

Attention to temporality can thus illuminate the situated materialisations of cancer and its care, especially as shaped by economic and techno-infrastructural inequalities. Sanz (2017: 190) describes how cancer care for low-income patients in Colombia is thrown 'out-of-sync' by insurance companies' deferral of treatment. Following neoliberal reforms, the insurance industry was entrusted with upholding a legal provision of universal access. Yet, in practice, the time taken to process and verify claims – cadenced by business imperatives – means that cancer patients often only receive treatment when their condition has progressed beyond such treatments' therapeutic effectiveness. Similarly blaming delayed care on failed healthcare systems, and thus shifting the 'burden of responsibility' away from 'already vulnerable patients', Banerjee (2020: 23) further locates cancer in Delhi within the longer temporal arc of sufferers' trajectories. Rather than a rupture, the diagnosis of cancer builds onto prior vulnerabilities that include economic precarity, fragile social relations and the 'infrastructural . . . failure and violence' of healthcare and other public systems (Banerjee 2020: 4).

In Senegal, liver cancer generally presents in clinical settings as an *acutely* fatal condition. This is, to some extent, a product of gaps in the availability and affordability of public healthcare. Yet liver cancer differs in important ways from cancers of other organs – such as breast, cervix or prostate – that have well-scripted ideal tempo-technological trajectories in contexts with well-resourced medical systems. Liver cell (or hepatocellular) carcinoma, the dominant form of primary liver cancer worldwide, is one of the most preventable but least curable cancers. This is partly due to its aetiology – chronic viral infections (with hepatitis B and C) are the main risk factors – and these are amenable to immunising and antiviral technologies. It is also due to its symptomatology, with tumours often remaining 'silent' until they have advanced beyond treatability. Yet liver cancer's biomedical possibilities and ideals are also shaped by its geographical distribution, with 85 per cent of recorded cases occurring in low- to middle-income countries, mainly of eastern Asia and sub-Saharan Africa (Yang et al. 2019).

This distinctive spatial pattern drove aetiological research in the mid-twentieth century, in the hope that geography might offer causal clues and that cracking this specific mystery might illuminate more general mechanisms of cancer causation (Mueller 2019). By the early 1980s, hepatitis B was identified as the main risk factor and a vaccine was on the market, making liver cancer the first 'vaccine-preventable' cancer. For the next decades, hepatitis B vaccination – which fitted well into the dominant framing and resourcing of global health – became the overriding focus of calls to address liver cancer in the resource-poor settings where it was most prevalent. This fixation on vaccination drew attention away from the study and control of other (co-)factors of liver cancer. Treatment and care for those who have or, due to chronic hepatitis B, are at risk for liver cancer have also remained largely absent from global policy discourse – although this has started to change in the past decade. Yet although vaccination was held up as the only feasible liver cancer strategy in settings such as Africa (Muraskin 1995), it remained unimplemented due to the high cost of vaccines; while their price dropped, it was seen as 'too expensive' for purchase by African countries or the donors supporting their immunisation programmes until the early 2000s.

The imagined temporality from which rapidly fatal liver cancer is 'out of sync' is not only a clinical one of prompt detection and treatment. Globally, and even in some well-resourced settings such as in Europe, most cases of liver cancer are diagnosed too late for curative treatment and prognosis is poor (Yang et al. 2019). Nina Lykke (2019) suggests that a lack of therapeutic options stems from liver cancer's biomedical neglect as a cancer of the global south. Certainly, the likelihood of being diagnosed early enough for expensive surgical interventions (transplantation, resection or ablation) or other palliative treatments that can prolong survival time, and the likelihood of being able to obtain such interventions, is amplified by access to either private wealth or public welfare. The highest rates of early diagnosis and the longest median survival times have been found in Taiwan and Japan (60 months for the latter), countries with a rare combination of high incidence and sufficient resources to implement comprehensive screening programmes (Yang et al. 2019). While median survival time after diagnosis is only 24 months in Europe, it is lowest – only 10 weeks in one multi-country study (Yang et al. 2017) – in sub-Saharan African countries, where very high rates of incidence combine with severely under-resourced health systems and where nearly all patients with liver cancer present 'very late' (Ladep et al. 2014: 787). Moreover, age of onset of late-stage liver cancer has been found to be lower in Africa, particularly in West Africa and for hepatitis B-associated cancers, than in other parts of the world (Yang et al. 2019).

In Senegal, I was told, rare individuals diagnosed early enough for treatment are advised by doctors to seek care, in order of preference, in Europe or North Africa; options that are clearly out of reach for most Senegalese, particularly those from rural areas. In the vast majority of cases that are diagnosed close to death, the clinical temporality of end-of-life care is not out of sync with curative or life-prolonging care, which is a rare occurrence across the globe, and is particularly difficult to imagine under the current conditions of Senegalese healthcare. Rather, it is in tension with the *preventive temporality* that has dominated global discourse and policy, largely to the exclusion of care – including antiviral treatment of hepatitis B as a form of 'secondary prevention' (Ladep et al. 2014: 783). Calls for prevention are anchored in a well-defined *aetiological temporality* (a chronic process starting in early life) and in anticipatory futures when significant amounts of liver cancer will have been averted by vaccination (compare Muraskin 1995) or by 'test-and-treat' strategies to slow or halt the damage wrought by hepatitis B infections. The clinical temporality of end-of-life care fills the gaps of missing or deferred prevention, as the next-generation impact of universal hepatitis B vaccination (introduced in Senegal in 2004) is still awaited and many teens and adults (10–20 per cent) are already infected.[1] They are also likely heavily exposed to aflatoxin, the metabolite of a crop fungus that is both a liver carcinogen on its own and interacts synergistically with hepatitis infection (Yang et al. 2019).

Ethnography and the time of care

Liver cancer's rapid and fatal progression in Senegal presents both practical and ethical challenges to direct ethnographic observation. As I will describe, this is compounded by widespread concealment of diagnosis and prognosis. I therefore opted to conduct interviews with health workers and some family members who had, in the past, cared for individuals who had since died of liver cancer. Although I also spoke to specialists working in urban tertiary care, here I draw mostly on a set of 15 semi-structured interviews with primary care nurses in a south-central rural district of Nioro bordering Gambia and about an hour's drive – at its closest edge, on the main road – to the regional capital of Kaolack. Nioro has comparatively good agricultural conditions and is a major producer of peanuts and corn; it has one of the highest average household incomes among Senegal's rural districts (Faye et al. 2019). Still, poverty levels are high across Senegal's agricultural heartland, estimated at around 80 per cent, using one definition of the poverty line, with more than 60 per cent of households in Nioro District (Faye et al. 2019). Nioro, home to larger-scale farmers and traders, is also marked by particularly high levels of inequality between households (Faye et al. 2019). In early 2019, I spent four non-consecutive weeks in Nioro District, accompanied by Aissatou Diouf, an experienced research assistant. We toured a non-random sample of *postes de santé* (village-level clinics), which are headed by mainly male state-certified nurses called *infirmier chef de poste* (ICP, Head of Clinic Nurse), working alongside female midwives, who are responsible for prenatal care. These clinics form the primary level of Senegal's 'pyramidal' healthcare system. We also visited the secondary level *centre de santé* (a small hospital with inpatient facilities and a laboratory) in Nioro town (the district centre), which is the only district facility staffed by doctors, and private clinics run by retired state nurses. In addition, I interviewed several professionals at the regional hospital in Kaolack, a large tertiary care institution with specialised services. We conducted most interviews with professionals in French (the language in which they are trained and receive official instructions) but encouraged nurses and midwives to switch to Wolof – spoken by most Senegalese, either as a mother tongue or, in multi-ethnic cities or zones such as Nioro, as a lingua franca – when describing interactions with their patients.

Nurses play a vital role in Senegal's 'health pyramid', with ICPs providing first-line services to about two-thirds of the population (Seck 2010). Health in Senegal, as in many sub-Saharan settings, is marked by stark urban–rural disparities. These are, in part, a legacy of French colonial health policies, which sought to reach the vast rural spaces of its two African federations mainly through mobile disease control campaigns, supported by a few centralised and specialised institutions of medical research, care and training (compare Bado 1996). Dakar, the capital of French West Africa and then of the Republic of Senegal, was and remains relatively well equipped, with public (including teaching) hospitals as well as a thriving network of private clinics, practices and medical laboratories. There have been sustained efforts to increase primary healthcare capacity in rural areas since the 1980s, through investments in immunisation programmes, decentralised management and cost-recovery policies in the 1990s and, since circa 2000, the roll-out of donor and state-funded programmes to improve maternal and infant health as well as to diagnose and treat malaria, HIV and tuberculosis (compare Faye et al. 2013; Foley 2010). While decentralisation has brought resources, such as new facilities, staff and tools including rapid tests and drugs, to rural areas, it has also shifted significant technical, monitoring and financial responsibility to ICPs, midwives and non-professional community health workers (Foley 2010; Hane 2017; Tichenor 2016).

In 2019, when I conducted fieldwork, Nioro District was served by 51 posts (including ex-ICP-run private clinics; see République du Sénégal 2020b). At the overarching regional level (comprising three health districts), each post covered a theoretical average of a circa 4 km radius (close to the national average of about 5 km) and a population of about 6,300, with a nurse-to-population ratio of 1:4083. The latter is in marked contrast with this region's doctor-to-population ratio of 1:31,223, whereas Dakar has much closer ratios of 1:1716 for nurses and 1:3962 for doctors. In addition, the vast majority of Senegal's specialist doctors, including oncologists and internists, work in Dakar's clinics and hospitals.[2] A handful of facilities in Dakar provide specific curative or palliative treatment for liver cancer, such as surgical ablation or chemoembolisation, to those lucky enough to be diagnosed early and who can afford both the procedure and the significant additional cost, as one specialist pointed out, of hospitalisation time. Imaging services for liver cancer diagnosis are available in Kaolack, but the hospital there, and the health centre in Nioro town, can only provide symptomatic treatment of pain, although they do not have opiates or strong opioids. These can also treat oedema and ascites (fluid in the abdomen), which not all ICP are able or willing to do.

Most patients diagnosed with liver cancer are therefore sent home, with any professional end-of-life care likely provided by the nearest ICP. Nurses' interview-elicited accounts of this care gave me only a small and partial window into their practices and the relations in which these are embedded. For example, my interviewees likely described themselves as doing the best they could – eliding errors, failures, missteps and so on – under conditions that severely challenge 'good care'. Josiane Tantchou (2018) has described how the material – spatial, technical and remunerative – conditions of many African clinical settings generate acute dilemmas for nurses about how and for whom to care. Here, ICPs pointed to material constraints on their capacity to care well, notably in access to pain medication, but especially to temporal factors, which they generally described themselves as managing successfully. That said, they did not idealise the power of their care to bring about a 'good death' or to maintain or restore harmonious relations among kin. Even though I could not observe what nurses, while caring, *performed* as good' through 'a matter of practical tinkering' (Mol, Pols and Moser 2010: 12, 13), I got a sense, through nurses' descriptions, of what they think good care can do *within*, and *to*, the constraints posed by liver cancer's untimely deaths.

The limits of my ethnographic engagement with dying and care also arise from the scope of my broader project. In it, I investigate how liver cancer's location in West Africa has, over time, transformed with the epistemological and technological capacities of global biomedicine. Doing this entails lengthy archival and oral historical research on biomedical interventions into West African liver cancer, starting in the mid-twentieth century when, prior to Senegal's political independence from France in 1960, late colonial French clinicians began collecting case notes and tissues samples from their dying and dead patients in a Dakar hospital to elucidate the mystery of this peculiarly 'African' cancer. I also trace how, in the 1970s, Senegal became a hub for research on hepatitis B virus as a cause of liver cancer. Senegal, and then Gambia, were selected as sites for some of the earliest and most ambitious trials of hepatitis B vaccine, which were initially meant to prove the viral causation of cancer (rather than as a pilot public health intervention). I further explore the deferral of protection from known and suspected liver carcinogens, particularly through delays in the provision of hepatitis B vaccine, as well as in the history of aflatoxin research and regulation, which is deeply entangled in the politics of Senegal's peanut export economy (a colonial legacy and still a key sector).

My broader project thus approaches Senegal as a site of recurring cancer and death in relation to past histories of Senegalese participation in biomedical progress – through the bodies of the exposed, dying and dead, as well as the practice and expertise of care providers – and of techno-scientific anticipation and of deferred protection. Combining ethnography with history allows me to locate end-of-life care, first as the outcome of past failures to convert Senegalese participation in biomedical research into timely protection. Secondly, I consider how some experts anticipate a delayed, awaited future when more Senegalese have been protected by hepatitis B vaccination (given to most born after the early 2000s) and, perhaps, by slowly expanding access to antiviral therapy (see Tousignant 2021) and access to the recently introduced aflatoxin control technology. This timeframe opens possibilities for broader accounts of how inequalities in liver cancer prevention and care have been generated, maintained and justified by and through techno-scientific progress.

This longer historical view informs how and why I attend to care, but the nurses I spoke to did not directly refer to this historical context when describing their practices or the continued need for end-of-life care. In the core section of this chapter, I stick to the times and tempos of care which the nurses made ethnographically present: the brief intervals between a specific person's care-seeking and death and the regular repetition of these events in their clinical experience. This illuminates care as a mode of (inter)action that, following recent commentators, calls for an engagement – by both carers and their ethnographers – with the specificities of present situations. 'The art of care', concludes Annemarie Mol (2008: 28) from observing its banal, tentative enactments, 'is to act without seeking to control.' In the same vein, Mol, Pols and Moser (2010: 10) write that care 'involves living with the erratic'. Critical scholars have cautioned that care, and appeals to its essential goodness, often maintains existing relations of power, reproducing harmful effects and paternalistic justifications (for example, Duclos and Sánchez Criado 2020; Murphy 2015). Yet there has been renewed energy to recuperate the critical potential of care both as a theoretical orientation towards 'non-dominative' modes of being together (Woodly et al. 2021) and as an empirical attentiveness to often neglected non-productivist practices (Puig de la Bellacasa 2015). For example, Vincent Duclos and Tomas Sánchez Criado invite us to move away from care as 'repair', as an 'abstract project' or 'epic narrative', and instead to attend, following Mol and others, to care as 'an art of the singular' and a 'speculative ethics' (Duclos and Sánchez Criado 2020: 8–10). Noting an etymological resonance between 'to carry' and 'to care', Emily Yates-Doerr (2020: 235) writes that 'caring thus conceived implies a commitment to attending to problems as they materialise and transform'. While none of these authors seek to cut moments of care off from past and future – on the contrary, they invite attention to continuities, potentiality and anticipation – they describe caring as a response to *present* suffering and damage that does not escape into techno-science-driven fantasies of future control, progress and resolution. Puig de la Bellacasa (2015) explicitly attends to care as a mode of 'making time' that is in tension with fast and futuristic late capitalist temporalities. Here, I explore how, in their accounts, nurses make time for and with end-of-life care against impossible interventionist temporalities of preventing or delaying death.

Nurses in Senegal describe how they must attend to an immediate present in which a person with liver cancer is *already* dying. They suspend their desire to postpone or avert death to instead work in, and on, the brief time when their care is essential, even as it offers little. When describing this care, nurses rarely referred to why and when specific cases of liver cancer might have started, to pasts when hepatitis B vaccine was not available in Senegal or to futures when cancer cases might wane due to current vaccination. While nurses complained that patients and their families came to them 'late', usually after consulting non-biomedical healers, they did not evoke ideal clinical scenarios of early detection and possible treatment; they know that such scenarios are implausible under current conditions of diagnostic and therapeutic availability. In other words, they recounted care in the present tense without switching into the past- and future-oriented aetiological and preventive temporalities that dominate research and policy discourse on liver cancer, particularly as it affects Africans.

This does not mean that nurses are unable to act or see beyond the immediate present or locate cancer diagnoses within longer personal, family and community histories (compare Banerjee 2020). They experience liver cancer as a regular occurrence; most nurses spoke of seeing one to two cases per year on average, up to three or four, and they told me of families and villages that experience repeated deaths. They thus interweave times of care with the endemicity of liver cancer in this region. Some nurses also spoke of a recent increase in hepatitis B testing in the district, particularly as part of prenatal care, and the 2016 introduction of an at-birth dose of vaccine; these events both affected their own practice and that of the midwives with whom they work. This opens up new opportunities to give preventive advice, through which some nurses are tentatively stretching the clinical temporality of liver cancer towards anticipatory modes of risk management. I return, briefly, to these extended temporalities of liver cancer care in the concluding section. First, however, I examine how nurses spoke of the challenges of caring within the constraints of an untimely end-of-life.

Caring for the untimely

When articulating what they find hard about caring for people with liver cancer, many nurses first evoke their patients' young age. 'What disturbed me the most', says Nurse Ndiaye,[3] 'is that the majority is under 40.' Similarly, Nurse Seck states: 'It's striking, so striking. Because normally the cases we've had, they're young, eh, 20–25 years old, and, they're finished . . . they're dead . . . it's hard, really hard.' Some nurses expanded on the meaning of age in relation to life stage and family relations: 'It's mostly youth . . . a kid in his prime, who was recently married, or just had his first [child's] baptism' (Nurse Dieng). Most also complained about delays in seeking care, explaining that clinics were the patients' 'last recourse' after consulting traditional healers. 'Usually, we see these cases at the last moment, the terminal phase, that's the last moment . . . it's when . . . it's finished!' Only one nurse suggested, vaguely, that more might be done 'when it's diagnosed very early maybe . . .'; the rest did not dream aloud about the possibility of early detection and of curative or life-extending treatment elsewhere, agreeing with Nurse Ndao: 'no one [can do anything], even if it's in France, in the United States, they won't be able to treat. It's already attacked, it's finished.' What they seem to find hard is initiating care so close to death. As Nurse Diatta explained: 'They are typical cases, I had three like that, who came in a terminal phase. And then . . . ouf! There's nothing to do. You don't refer. You do nothing. Just counsel the family.'

As this last statement illustrates, the untimeliness of cancer and care – the youth of victims, the nearness of death – merge with nurses' feelings of powerlessness as healers, as well as with the heavy emotional weight and responsibility of knowing the patient's prognosis. Nurse Niang explains he finds it hard because 'you're [also] thinking about their family. For example, a youth . . . at that moment [they] have a young family, it's not easy to tell people, that . . . it's finished.' I often ask if they can remember a particular striking case. Many, like Nurse Gaye, say that, because they are usually young men, *every* case is striking. He continues: 'Aaaah! You know you can't do anything . . . it's hard for us, as care providers, for the family . . . Oof! You know that that one, I can't do anything for him.'

Despite such common statements, all nurses describe doing *something* for cancer patients. In most cases, the first thing they say they do is refer to the regional hospital. This is usually only to confirm what they already know, as Nurse Boye – who has retired from public service to move into private practice – puts it: 'in most cases I don't need an ultrasound. It's only for confirmation.' Other nurses confidently list telltale signs and symptoms. Several admit that, when patients 'lack means' or their death seems imminent, they do not refer at all. Nurse Gaye, for example, explains 'when I see that that one, if we [refer] him it's just to refer him, I already know he no longer has a chance . . . I refer him but, also explaining to family members, maybe they don't, no longer have to spend their money . . .'. Several health workers cited cases in which patients died before making it to the hospital.

It is unclear what value nurses see in referring. Perhaps they hope for a different or early enough diagnosis; they did not tell me of any such cases, but hospital specialists insist that other, non-fatal conditions present similarly. Or they may find it useful to obtain diagnostic certainty and 'hard' evidence. Nurse Dieng admits that he occasionally does *not* refer, but only when he thinks family members are 'up to it' – that they will be strong and trusting enough to accept that going to the hospital is unnecessary. What *is* clear is that nurses do not expect the act of referring to shift any responsibility for care away from them. From the hospital, most patients, nurses say, are sent home and 'returned' to the village clinic nurse's care with their test results – in a sealed envelope, some nurses specify – and a follow-up appointment for a time (two, three or four months later) when the patient is likely to already be dead. 'In 90% of cases they are sent home', explains Nurse Guissé, 'because they can't do anything more.'

The untimeliness of liver cancer disrupts the prescribed distribution of responsibilities across levels of the health system, in which primary care nurses are meant to manage conditions for which they are given specific tests, drugs and protocols and to refer more complex conditions 'up'. Several nurses mentioned the 'obligation to refer' and some hinted that they felt resentful towards hospitals seeking to free beds and get 'rid' of dying patients, thereby leaving nurses alone with the full responsibility of caring and explaining. When I remarked to Nurse Dieng that the task of delivering information seems to be left to nurses, he retorted: 'And what did you want?' He then explains: 'Us, the ICP we are everything. We are social workers, everything . . . surgeons . . . Frankly, it's chaos over there.' Despite suggesting that the health system places too high a burden on primary care nurses, like others he finds it appropriate for liver cancer patients to die at home and to be 'accompanied' by the most proximate health worker.

The mainstay of what many nurses refer to as 'palliative' care is giving painkilling drugs. A few say they prescribe diuretics for oedema, and one admitted removing excess fluid from the abdomen (ascites), despite this being a medical procedure reserved for doctors. Most, however, focused on patients' pain, which Nurse Ndiaye described as 'unsettling' and disturbing for family members, and Nurse Thiam, simply, as 'very atrocious'. Descriptions of pain elicited, for nurses, expressions of powerlessness and pity. A few nurses said they prescribe only paracetamol and ibuprofen. 'Is that enough?' I ask. 'Is that enough . . .' Nurse Gaye echoed, 'well, it depends on what the patient feels [laughs bitterly].' Many described prescribing tramadol, the strongest analgesic available outside Dakar hospitals, where morphine is unavailable. Some progress to injections or infusions when the pain worsens, a few describing doing home visits at 'the end'. 'Is that enough?' I asked Nurse Niang. 'Even after tramadol injections', he answered, 'the pain returns after a few hours . . . It's so hard. Too, too hard, even. It's a really unbearable pain . . .' Nurse Guissé responded: 'At the beginning it's enough [pause] but at the end, no, no [quiet laugh].' I then asked him whether stronger painkillers would help: 'Oh yeah, it would be better [repeats, trailing off] . . . Sometimes it's so hard! You see them dying and suffering at the same time. [It would be better if] we could help them die peacefully.' Even at the regional hospital, a doctor is angry that they lack 'the means for a proper [end-of-life] accompaniment . . . they suffer enormously . . . atrociously . . . We don't have morphine, we don't have morphine derivatives . . . [we only have] tramadol . . . and . . . it's unbearable, [repeats, more softly], it's unbearable.'

This situation, and particularly the unavailability of strong opiates and opioids, is consistent with the global inequalities in access to effective palliative care and pain relief that has recently drawn greater attention – notably, from a Lancet Commission (Knaul et al. 2018). It also confirms other anthropologists' observations of the centrality of pain in experiences of cancer and care where therapeutic options are limited by scarcity and inaccessibility (Banerjee 2020; Livingston 2012). Yet I would not say that pain treatment is 'often the only form of cancer care [patients] receive' (Banerjee 2020: 11). Nurses speak of managing the prognostic knowledge of their liver cancer patients' imminent and inevitable deaths as central to what they do for these patients and their families. Strategically revealing or concealing this knowledge, they say, powerfully affects the qualities, relations and legacy of an untimely death. By contrast, nurses describe referrals for diagnostic confirmation and pain treatment – the main bodily interventions they initiate – as having a weaker impact on experiences of disease and death. In other words, knowledge management is at the heart of end-of-life care, rather than an accessory to acts of bodily care such as pain relief.

Prognosis as care

Nurses described prognostic knowledge as a potent but dangerous resource. Handling this knowledge properly, they said, requires skill and insight into local relations. Without exception, nurses (as well as rural and urban doctors) insisted that it is imperative to conceal patients' prognosis from them, as well as their diagnosis – since cancer in general and liver cancer in particular, is associated with dire prognoses. Several described the lengths to which they go to hide prognoses. Patients and their kin, some said, are really 'clever' and will get suspicious if you prescribe the same thing twice, or if the prescription is 'small' or too cheap, and therefore disproportionate to the severity of their illness. As Nurse Niang put it: 'if you prescribe a medicine that costs only 1500 francs, they'll come back and say . . . there's a problem! I'm very ill! . . . Why didn't you prescribe me something really expensive? . . . so you try, really, to camouflage things [little laugh].' Similarly, Nurse Seck said he 'tries to change the medicines . . . today we might prescribe paracetamol, tomorrow we prescribe Doliprane . . . then Panadol . . . you see, they are all paracetamol. It's to avoid the patient wondering, hunh? I've already been prescribed this box.' Nurse Diarra recalled: 'I even had a case . . . a doctor told him he had liver cancer. I said no, it's not true, I really calmed him down . . . he had regained confidence . . . After his death, his father came all the way here [from another district], and his mother, to thank me . . . at the beginning . . . he wouldn't leave his room, no longer ate, but after you reassured him, he went out, he ate, really . . .' Other nurses similarly spoke of fostering hope and calmness in their patients to preserve the quality of their end of life. Maintaining hope, and keeping open a therapeutic orientation, also gives meaning to the bodily care they provide. For example, Nurse Niang avoids telling patients that their condition is incurable; instead, he insists that it is stubborn and requires prolonged treatment. Switching from French to Wolof, he illustrates how he explains this: 'The treatment, really, it will last long. You will come [to the clinic], we will give you medicines and check your body, then you will come again . . .'

Anthropologists have approached practices of concealment or partial truth-telling around cancer as situated (see Banerjee 2020: 8; Bennett 1999). Banerjee (2020: 7), focusing especially on how patients and families hide cancer diagnoses rather than doctors withholding these from patients, describes 'concealment as a practice [that] helped sustain possibilities of relations that disclosures might foreclose'. What is kept open in nurses' explanations of why they conceal is not only the patient's hope for recovery but their continued interaction with their material and social surroundings – food, friends, family – as well as the value (at times literally) of the treatment that nurses prescribe and provide. As in the practices observed by Elizabeth Bennett (1999: 402) in north-east Thailand in the mid-1990s, 'softening' the truth of a cancer diagnosis also seeks to protect patients from the further violence of harsh disclosure that threatens patients' psychological integrity.

Conversely, revealing the fatal prognosis to someone in the patients' network is a way of preventing or closing off futile, wasteful and potentially harmful efforts to seek further diagnostic and therapeutic resources. Here too, however, the potential 'harshness' of disclosure must be prevented by carefully selecting the right person to tell. Both the telling and the selection of who to tell, I suggest, are also part of how nurses describe themselves as enacting good care. 'You don't tell [just] anyone', explains Nurse Boye, 'you identify someone solid . . . someone who can bear it . . . as I know this area well, I can identify someone who can keep a secret, a . . . someone also who is able to take it . . . also someone who has influence over the patient's treatment.' Other nurses, especially older ones, similarly refer to their accumulated local expertise as crucial to their capacity to sensitively navigate prognostic disclosure, and therefore to care well. Nurse Diarra described an occasion when his instinct failed him: the father of a teen with liver cancer was 'always praying' and yet he fainted when the nurses told him his son would die and that he should stop wasting money on traditional healers and instead turn his son over to the nurse's palliative care. The nurse was disappointed both by the father's reaction and his own capacity to gauge moral and emotional strength. As this example suggests, many nurses implicitly gender the qualities they seek in disclosure candidates – namely, authority, discretion and fortitude – as masculine. Given that most ICPs are men (all but one in our sample), as are the majority of patients diagnosed with liver cancer (a widely acknowledged epidemiological trend, but also an observation that nurses insisted on), practices of disclosure reinforce a largely male environment of liver cancer care defined as such.[4]

Some of the sought-for qualities, such as discretion, are associated with a need to preserve the affective environment of end-of-life care that concealment from patients and other relatives seeks to create. Others, such as those with authority over the patient's treatment, are sought by nurses so that disclosure will interrupt unnecessary treatment-seeking, whether in urban medical facilities or with traditional healers, both of which they present as a waste of money and, implicitly, of the patient's remaining time. Prognostic revelation can therefore be a means of stopping futile attempts to synchronise illness with biomedical or other forms of therapy – what Sanz (2017), in the Colombian context, calls *vueltas*; a movement that leads nowhere. Nurses are particularly wary of non-biomedical healers who, they warn, might 'take' or 'eat' a family's money, promising cures and asking for exorbitant sums. Moreover, what healers might offer is not just useless but, according to nurses, can be toxic to both livers and social relations. Nurses argued that liver cancer's main sign – a painful, swollen belly and digestive trouble – is usually diagnosed as the result of an ill-intentioned person giving the victim something to eat. According to nurses, healers often prescribe emetic substances, even though these can accelerate death. Accusations arising from healers' diagnoses can also create tensions in families and communities that may last beyond death (see Tousignant 2021).

Besides preventing unnecessary treatment, prognostic revelation can also, some nurses suggest, turn informed family members' attention towards providing company and comfort to dying patients. For example, Nurse Niang explains: 'Three quarters [of patients] come to me in the terminal phase. I take two relatives, to tell them that it's over. What you can do now, is just accompany [the patient]. [In Wolof:] Stay close to them, [switching back to French,] have empathy for them . . . get closer and closer, care for their needs, and all.' Other nurses similarly spoke of using disclosure to encourage relatives to be more attentive to patients' needs, from making special foods to simply spending time by their side. In other words, they use disclosure to foster more caring interactions around patients, shifting the focus away from bodily and biomedical intervention and towards social and emotional support.

Liver cancer's incurability and intractable pain, and nurses' inability to stave off death or fully relieve pain, unsurprisingly figure prominently in nurses' accounts of the challenges of care. Yet these features of the disease are enmeshed with and amplified by its temporal qualities – striking young men at the 'prime of life', bringing them swiftly to suffering and death. Knowing a patient will die soon complicates and disrupts nurses' capacity to provide good care, placing intense pressure on them to protect the quality of a short end of life. They often seek diagnostic certainty through referral, but in some cases decide that time is too short. In any case, they do not generally expect higher-level medical facilities to take up any of the burden of care.[5] Nurses are left with the heavy responsibility of managing pain as well as diagnostic/prognostic knowledge. By prescribing and administering analgesics, nurses seek to act, albeit imperfectly, on the body's brief end of life. Yet their accounts suggest that it is by concealing and revealing their knowledge of death's imminence that they wield the most power over how this brief time is lived and cared for. Managing prognostic knowledge is a way of turning an untimely death over to their care and that of close relatives, among whom they choose allies in protecting this brief time from what they see as useless, expensive and potentially harmful quests for further diagnosis and treatment of the disease. With these meagre means, nurses seek – they say – to cultivate calmness, trust and closeness, an affective environment of good relations that they hope will last beyond death. Liver cancer's untimeliness threatens to render care impotent. Yet untimeliness is also the focus nurses' care, a focus that extends beyond the body's suffering and includes the social and material relations that an untimely death, untimely therapeutic quests and untimely money-spending threaten to disrupt.

Conclusion: extending and inhabiting times of care

While liver cancer's brief end-of-life temporality dominates rural nurses' clinical narrated practice and experience, this moment is not sealed off from other (possible) rhythms. Most obviously, the specific instances of care they describe are situated within their longer experience of working in this area – some hinting at how their knowledge of local social and kinship relations is an asset in managing prognostic knowledge – as well as liver cancer's endemic temporality in the region. The latter manifests as a regular occurrence of cases in their clinical practice (one, two or more every year). Nurses also told me stories of families or communities in which cases are frequent, including among their own relatives and friends. Their familiarity with the disease makes them confident in their capacity to make clinical diagnoses even without imaging and to predict a rapid and inevitable death. While, as I described, they conceal this knowledge from patients and most of their kin, they also admit that residents of the district – whom nurses believe to have a higher liver cancer incidence than other parts of Senegal – are familiar with the disease, its symptoms and its generally fatal outcome. In some cases, they hint, concealment is thus a 'fiction' (Banerjee 2020: 6).

The recent expansion of hepatitis B screening in prenatal care and blood drives, as well as the introduction of at-birth hepatitis B vaccination in 2016, has created new situations when nurses and midwives evoke liver cancer in an anticipatory mode: as a potential event that can be averted by intervening in the present. This was not, I was told, the case with the other doses of hepatitis B vaccine that were introduced in 2004, as part of a combined vaccine, which was not promoted with specific reference to hepatitis and its consequences. When speaking with expectant mothers about at-birth vaccination, or giving advice to those with positive screening tests, midwives and nurses have started integrating aetiological and preventive temporalities of liver cancer into clinical care. As I describe in more detail elsewhere (Tousignant 2021), health workers' experience of frequent positive tests and their understanding of how fatty foods and especially peanut consumption can facilitate infection and accelerate liver damage points to carcinogenic landscapes rather than individual exposures, as the aetiological source of liver cancer; peanuts, a key cash crop in Senegal, are omnipresent in this district's agriculture and diets. That said, nurses and midwives mainly advise patients diagnosed with hepatitis B (mainly mothers screened during prenatal care and young men screened during blood drives) to modify their diets and, in rare cases, to seek further expensive biomedical assessment and antiviral treatment, thereby shifting responsibility onto individuals for cancer prevention.

In various ways, then, Senegalese nurses do situate liver cancer's regular occurrence and future risk, as well as their own clinical judgement and practice, within longer timeframes of local medical, economic, food and social relations. In their accounts of care, nurses hint at some of the longer-term processes that shape experiences of liver cancer, as well as emerging clinical temporalities around hepatitis B prevention, screening and treatment, which would merit further ethnographic study. Significantly, however, when speaking about liver cancer, nurses focus on the short time in which patients are dying, a time in which the care they provide cannot 'do anything' yet is urgently needed. This draws attention to the specificity of care as a mode of intervention that, even if arising within broader temporal relations, cannot evade the present and the pressing calls of the fragile bodies and relations that inhabit it. Most patients are sent home from secondary and tertiary care institutions with a deferred appointment. The responsibility for their end-of-life care falls, by default, on primary care nurses. Speaking of this responsibility, nurses rarely evoke the past and future tenses of missed or anticipated opportunities for early detection and prevention that arise from ideal narratives of cancer control. With few tools at their disposal, including too-weak painkillers and diagnostic referrals that only confirm what they already know, nurses in Senegal are left to practise a form of 'bare' care that focuses intensely on the untimely moment of imminent death. While deploring that they cannot do much in terms of survival or relief, nurses describe this bare care – particularly the careful concealment and disclosure of prognosis – as having potentially powerful effects on the social and material relations of an end of life.

This care labour is largely invisible in global discourse on liver cancer's preventability and incurability. The untimely deaths that elicit this care can be situated in the gaps and failures of global and national public health discourse and action in West Africa. The high regional prevalence of this cancer has, since the 1950s, been a focus of biomedical research. Yet the aetiological knowledge and preventive strategies that arose from this research have only recently begun to alter the epidemiology of liver cancer risk and incidence. Moreover, access to the diagnostic evaluation of treatable liver damage, including early cancer, is severely limited in Senegal, as is access to treatment options that include antiviral drugs, surgery and chemotherapy (Périères et al. 2021). Left to care for patients near death, care nurses must deal with the untimeliness not just of growing tumours and foreshortened lives but of a global biomedicine whose potentially protective effects have long been deferred and delayed.

Acknowledgements

The research for this chapter was generously supported by a Wellcome Trust University Award (209911/Z/17/Z). Its drafting benefited from the close readings and feedback of the volume editors, especially Lenore Manderson and Linda Bennett, and from conversations with members of the Grid Oncology and Maps of Malignancy projects at King's College London.

Ethics statement: The protocol for the research for this chapter was reviewed and approved by the UCL Research Ethics Committee (Office of the Vice-Provost (Research)) and Comité National d'Éthique pour la Recherche en Santé (Senegal, Ministry of Health). Participants provided consent to be interviewed; to protect their confidentiality, their names and any identifying information have not been used in this chapter.

Notes

1. There is a lack of fine-grained data on infection prevalence across geographical, age and epidemiological groups in Senegal. In one of the first extensive serosurveys conducted since the 1970s, Périères and colleagues (2021) found a rate of 12.4 per cent of chronic infection in the 15–34 age group. Screening of blood donations in 2018 found a 10.5 per cent positivity rate among Nioro's 712 donors (République du Sénégal 2020a).
2. According to République du Sénégal (2020a), only 35 per cent of Senegal's general practitioners (254 in total) and 40 per cent of its state nurses (1,795 in total) are located in Dakar, compared with 100 per cent of its cancer specialists (including paediatric and surgical, about 21 in total) and 83 per cent of its specialists in internal medicine and gastroenterology (37 in total).
3. All nurse names are pseudonymous last names (by which ICPs are commonly referred, with the honorific 'doctor'), selected from among common Senegalese names without regard for ethnic associations.
4. Women likely perform many of acts of care in the home but may not be informed of the patients' diagnosis or identify it in biomedical terms. Further ethnographic study is needed to elucidate the gender dynamics of liver cancer care in West Africa (as of hepatitis B; see Tousignant 2021).
5. Doctors in Kaolack and Nioro nevertheless insisted that they do hospitalise and/or provide more complex symptomatic treatment (such as draining ascites) to those who need it.

References

Bado, Jean Paul. 1996. *Médecine coloniale et grandes endémies en Afrique*. Paris: Karthala.

Banerjee, Dwaipayan. 2020. *Enduring Cancer: Life, death, and diagnosis in Delhi*. Durham, NC: Duke University Press.

Bennett, Elizabeth S. 1999. 'Soft truth: Ethics and cancer in northeast Thailand', *Anthropology & Medicine* 6: 395–404.

Cook, J. and C. Trundle. 2020. 'Unsettled care: Temporality, subjectivity, and the uneasy ethics of care', *Anthropology and Humanism* 45: 178–183.

Duclos, Vincent and Tomás Sánchez Criado. 2020. 'Care in trouble: Ecologies of support from below and beyond', *Medical Anthropology Quarterly* 34: 153–173.

Faye, Ndeye Fatou, Moussa Sall, François Affholder and Françoise Gérard. 2019. 'Inégalités de revenu en milieu rural dans le bassin arachidier du Sénégal', Papiers de Recherche AFD No. 115. Accessed 30 December 2021. https://agritrop.cirad.fr/593810/1/In%C3%A9galit%C3%A9s%20de%20revenu%20en%20milieu%20rural%20au%20S%C3%A9n%C3%A9gal.pdf.

Faye, Sylvain Landry, Frédéric Le Marcis, Fatoumata Samb and Mouhamed Badji. 2013. 'Politiques de lutte contre le paludisme en Casamance, Sénégal: une activité de santé publique soumise aux contextes de conflit et de décentralisation', *Global Health Promotion* 20: 59–67.

Foley, Ellen. 2010. *Your Pocket Is What Cures You: The politics of health in Senegal*. New Brunswick, NJ: Rutgers University Press.

Hane, Faoumata. 2017. 'Production des statistiques sanitaires au Sénégal: entre enjeux politiques et jeux d'acteurs', *Santé publique* 29: 879–886.

Jain, S. Lochlann. 2013. *Malignant: How cancer becomes us*. Berkeley: University of California Press.

Knaul, Felicia Marie, Paul E. Farmer, Eric L. Krakauer, Liliana De Lima, Afsan Bhadelia, Xiaoxiao Jiang Kwete, Héctor Arreola-Ornelas et al. 2018. 'Alleviating the access abyss in palliative care and pain relief – an imperative of universal health coverage: The Lancet Commission Report', *The Lancet* 391: 1391–1454.

Ladep, Nimzing G., Olufunmilayo A. Lesi, Pantong Mark, Maud Lemoine, Charles Onyekwere, Mary Afihene, Mary M. E. Crossey and Simon D. Taylor-Robinson. 2014. 'Problem of hepatocellular carcinoma in West Africa', *World Journal of Hepatology* 6: 783–792.

Livingston, Julie. 2012. *Improvising Medicine: An African oncology ward in an emerging cancer epidemic*. Durham, NC: Duke University Press.

Löwy, Ilana. 2010. *Preventive Strikes: Women, precancer, and prophylactic surgery*. Baltimore, MD: Johns Hopkins University Press.

Löwy, Ilana. 2011. '"Because of their praiseworthy modesty, they consult too late": Regime of hope and cancer of the womb, 1800–1910', *Bulletin of the History of Medicine* 85: 356–383.'

Lykke, Nina. 2019. 'Making live and letting die: Cancerous bodies between Anthropocene Necropolitics and Chthulucene Kinship', *Environmental Humanities* 11(1): 108–136.

McMullin, Juliet. 2016. 'Cancer', *Annual Review of Anthropology* 45: 251–266.

Mol, Annemarie. 2008. *The Logic of Care: Health and the problem of patient choice*. London and New York: Routledge.

Mol, Annemarie, Jeannette Pols and Ingunn Moser. 2010. *Care in Practice: On tinkering in clinics, homes and farms*. Bielefield, Germany: Transcript Verlag.

Mueller, Lucas M. 2019. 'Cancer in the tropics: Geographical pathology and the formation of cancer epidemiology', *BioSocieties* 14: 512–528.

Muraskin, William. 1995. *The War against Hepatitis B: A history of the international task force on hepatitis B immunization*. Philadelphia: University of Pennsylvania Press.

Murphy, M. 2015. 'Unsettling care: Troubling transnational itineraries of care in feminist health practices', *Social Studies of Science* 45(5): 717–737.

Périères, Lauren, Aldiouma Diallo, Fabienne Marcellin, Marie Libérée Nishimwe, El Hadji Ba, Marion Coste, Gora Lo et al. 2021. 'Hepatitis B in Senegal: A successful infant vaccination program but urgent need to scale up screening and treatment (ANRS 12356 AmBASS survey)', *Hepatology Communications* 6(5): 1005–1015. https://doi.org/10.1002/hep4.1879.

Puig de la Bellacasa, M. 2015. 'Making time for soil: Technoscientific futurity and the pace of care', *Social Studies of Science*, 45: 691–716.

République du Sénégal. 2020a. 'Annuaire des statistiques sanitaires et sociales 2018'. Ministère de la santé et de l'action sociale. Accessed 30 December 2021. https://www.sante.gouv.sn/sites/default/files/Annuaire%20Satatistiques%20sanitaires%20et%20sociales%202018.pdf.

République du Sénégal. 2020b. 'Rapport annuel de suivi de la carte sanitaire'. Ministère de la santé et de l'action sociale. Accessed 30 December 2021. https//www.sante.gouv.sn/sites/default/files/Carte%20sanitaire%20Senegal%20Rapport%20annuel%20de%202019_1.pdf.

Sanz, Camilo. 2017. 'Out-of-sync cancer care: Health insurance companies, biomedical practices, and clinical time in Colombia', *Medical Anthropology* 36(3): 187–201.

Seck, Awa. 2010. 'Sénégal', *Recherche en soins infirmiers* 1: 90–93.

Tantchou, Josiane C. 2018. 'The materiality of care and nurses' "attitude problem"', *Science, Technology, & Human Values* 43(2): 270–301.

Tichenor, Marlee. 2016. 'The power of data: Global health citizenship and the Senegalese data retention strike'. In *Metrics: What counts in global health*, edited by Vincanne Adams, 105–124. Durham, NC: Duke University Press.

Tousignant, Noemi. 2021. 'Filtering inequality: Screening and knowledge in Senegal's topography of hepatitis B care', *Frontiers in Pharmacology* 11. https://doi.org/10.3389/fphar.2020.561428.

Woodly, D., R. H. Brown, M. Marin, S. Threadcraft, C. P. Harris, J. Syedullah and M. Ticktin. 2021. 'The politics of care', *Contemporary Political Theory* 20 (4): 890–925.

Yang, Ju Dong, Pierre Hainaut, Gregory J. Gores, Amina Amadou, Amelie Plymoth and Lewis R. Roberts. 2019. 'A global view of hepatocellular carcinoma: Trends, risk, prevention and management', *Nature Reviews Gastroenterology & Hepatology* 16: 589–604.

Yang, Ju Dong, Essa A. Mohamed, Ashraf O. Abdel Aziz, Hend I. Shousha, Mohamed B. Hashem, Mohamed M. Nabeel, Ahmed H. Abdelmaksoud et al. 2017. 'Characteristics, management, and outcomes of patients with hepatocellular carcinoma in Africa: A multicountry observational study from the Africa Liver Cancer Consortium', *The Lancet Gastroenterology & Hepatology* 2: 103–111.

Yates-Doerr, Emily. 2020. 'Antihero care: On fieldwork and anthropology', *Anthropology and Humanism* 45: 233–244.

8
Rehumanising illness: practices of care in a cancer ward in Athens, Greece

Falia Varelaki

One morning Panos,[1] a 67-year-old man with lung cancer, was admitted to the third floor ward, which I refer to as Ward A, of the public cancer hospital in Athens. I heard the director of the oncology clinic, Dr Alexandris, talking about him – his 'old friend' from medical school, who had 'had a great career in his life as an ear-nose-throat doctor, but had no family'. When I entered the single room with the doctors on their morning rounds, Panos was sitting alone in his bed, staring out of the window, waiting for his chemotherapy treatment to finish. Just before we left the room, Dr Alexandris carefully took Panos' hand, trying not to press on his IV and cause him pain, and said: 'Please don't worry my old friend. We will take care of you now. You are not alone.'

Hospitals are distinctly medicalised spaces, where 'the bodies of patients are confined, and for a time controlled, with the primary goal of sustaining and prolonging life' (Makrinioti 2008: 18–20). As a place where lives begin and sometimes end, a hospital is a place where you can observe rituals and relationships but, above all, it is a place in which life events and the emotions around them can be experienced with all of the senses. During my fieldwork on Ward A, I observed that it was possible to see, hear, smell, taste and even touch pain, sorrow and death. In this chapter, I discuss such moments as observed during my fieldwork on the ward from 2016 to 2019. In line with Julie Livingston (2012: 6), I interpret cancer as a relationship rather than a disease, 'as something that happens between people'. Experiences of cancer are accompanied with narratives of pain, disfigurement, loneliness and often death, rendering them social experiences. In addition to manifestations of suffering, care also constitutes an important part of such narratives. Practices of care can be evidenced on many layers, in many moments and through different perspectives. Doctors, nurses, patients' family members and friends and patients through their relationships with other patients, perform practices of care in their efforts to heal the pain of both body and soul. Bodily pain with cancer disease and as caused by chemotherapy treatments in muscles and bones, but also bodily and emotional pain, are caused by bodily and identity disfigurement and by the feeling that death is close.

The practices of care on Ward A, as reflected in the exchange between Panos and Dr Alexandris, occurred on a daily basis during my fieldwork. In this chapter, I explore how care unfolds in the daily operations of Ward A and the lives of those within it. I describe the relationships that developed between patients and medical staff in order to identify the meanings, practices and politics of care from the latter's perspectives. Ethnographic analysis illuminates the service gaps that are created within the biomedical healthcare system and the practices of care arise within these gaps. I also explore cancer care as an intervention occurring within the Greek public health system and reflect on the concept of 'care' and its role in social relationships.

The ethnographic material presented in this chapter derives from field research conducted as part of my doctoral studies between October 2016 and March 2019 in Athens, the capital of Greece. I conducted an initial 12 months of fieldwork and several follow-up visits, mainly in a cancer hospital in Athens and, specifically, in one of its two oncology wards and its associated outpatient clinic. Here people with various different types of cancer received treatment. My participation in the daily life of Ward A and its associated outpatient clinic was limited to observations, activities and conversations in which I could engage as a non-medical person. I also spent time in the chemotherapy unit and in staff meetings. During this hospital-based fieldwork, I conducted 19 semi-structured in-depth interviews with 11 doctors, four nurses and four other hospital employees. Their ages were between 23 and 65, 13 were women and 6 were men. Notes from observations and informal conversations supplemented these data.

This chapter brings new insight and understanding to how practices of care are performed and contextualised within the context of cancer politics in Greece. To illustrate this, I outline the concept of care as it is developed through anthropological perspectives and point out some methodological issues of the research. I then provide details of cancer care in Greece and contextualise practices of care within Greece's public healthcare system, focusing on the gaps within which these practices of care arise. I illustrate the improvised aspects of care as they are performed by healthcare professionals and the intimacies that are developed. Finally, I interpret care as a humanising practice. The insights that emerge contribute to efforts to develop a deeper consideration of the politics of care, adding to the collective dialogue on care pursued throughout this book.

The concept of 'care'

According to the prevailing scholarly representation of care, the most common use of the term involves two individuals: a subject who acts and offers care and a subject who receives care as the object of the former's act. This schematic representation signifies the activity of the former and the passivity of the latter. However, since practices of care are structured around relationships of interconnectedness and interdependence, role separation between caregivers and care recipients seems to be faint (Sevenhuijsen 1998) and care as a relationship is not a one-way process. Rather, it operates in the midst of reciprocity, with the continuous and reciprocal flow of care shaping relationships and leading us to further question what care is. In order to find the answer we must seek to define its meanings within specific contexts. We must further ask: How is care contextualised? What is considered as care for those who act and offer care, and for those who receive it?

In Greek, 'φροντίδα' (care) is defined as: (1) strong interest for someone or something; (2) concern, worry or trouble; (3) treatment; or (4) maintenance. In English, the term 'care' also has different shades of meaning. Within anthropological discussions and ethnographic examples, care remains a 'shifting and unstable concept' (Buch 2015: 297). For Martin (2013: 2), care is 'a complex, ambiguous and polysemous concept', understood as an obligation, a wish or a gift that may form or strengthen social relations. For Martin, Myers and Viseu (2015: 631), care is 'ambivalent, contextual and relational'; for Kleinman and van der Geest (2009), the term has various shades of meaning, with two basic constituents: that relating to emotion, in which care is an outcome and expression of concern, dedication and attachment, and that relating to technical or practical modes of supporting another person, through the physical care one person provides to another. In an effort to further explain these differences, Fisher and Joan Tronto suggest 'that caring be viewed as a species activity that includes everything that we do to maintain, continue, and repair our "world" so that we can live in it as well as possible. That world includes our bodies, ourselves, and our environment, all of which we seek to interweave in a complex, life-sustaining web' (cited in Tronto 1993: 101).

Street (2017) underlines the moral nature of care. She highlights the ways in which the object of care defines to a great extent the parameters of what we recognise as care, as well as the distinction between informal care practices, usually provided by and taking place with kin, and professional care practices. Along the same lines, Martin (2013: 3) states that 'there is often the implicit assumption that care is altruistic'; however, it 'carries a moralising connotation'. Who cares and who does not care, who should care and how care is expressed, are questions that point to the moral aspects of care and the difficulties that can arise when we seek to study such a morally loaded topic? How do we trace care and how do we recognise and study its absence?

According to Martin, Myers and Viseu (2015: 626), 'care looks and feels like it is both context-specific and perspective-dependent'. This means that if we want to study care in a particular cultural setting we must 'listen to those who are directly involved in it and by observing their

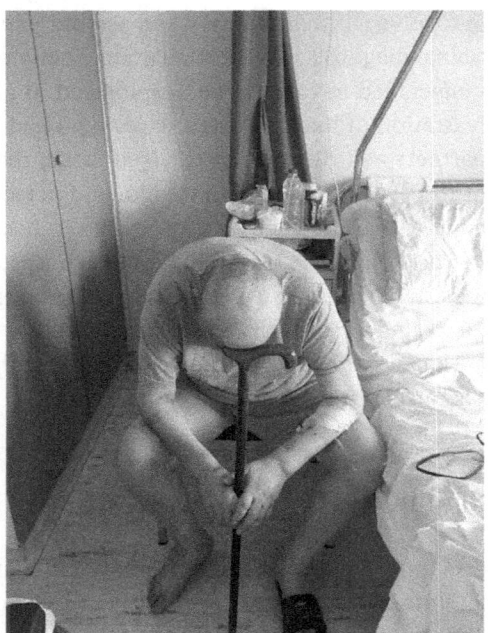

Figure 8.1   Moments in the cancer ward. Photo: Dr A.

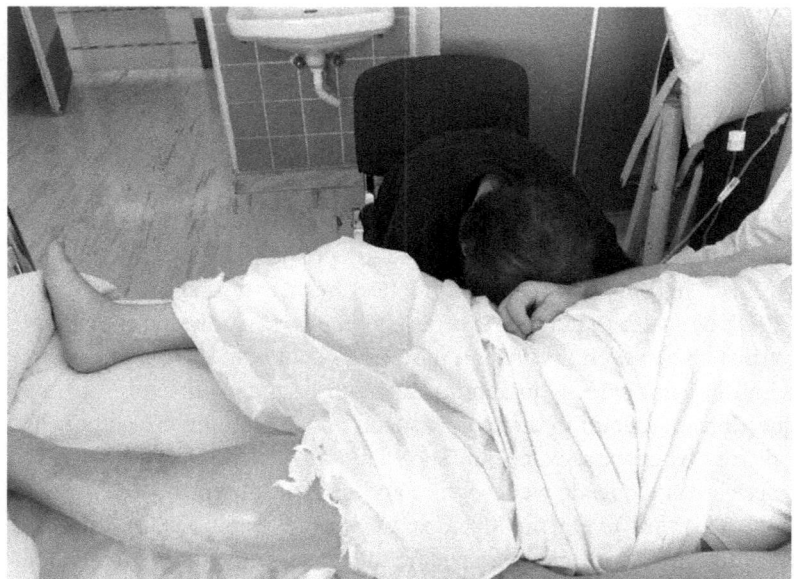

Figure 8.2 Not alone. Photo: Dr A.

actions' (Kleinman and van der Geest 2009: 160). Doing fieldwork in an oncology clinic involved my presence when people experienced the despair of a terminal diagnosis and the desolation when the illness or its treatment side-effects led to them to be hospitalised. It allowed me to witness the devastation of husbands and wives who had lost hope for their beloved partners and the tears of children facing the loss of their parents.[2] Out of respect for the highly intimate and personal nature of moments of pain or grief shared between loved ones, I chose not to make such experiences the focus of my research. Rather I chose to research the concept of 'care' from the perspectives of doctors and nurses. This means that I do not explore understandings of 'care' for patients or their families in this chapter. This methodological choice illuminates the concept of care within the medical setting of Ward A.

Improvisational practices

Though it is disappointing, Greece has no national cancer registry. Epidemiological data are estimates from pharmaceutical companies, which they collect for financial reasons. Another source is the Global Cancer Observatory, which also estimates data by using ratios derived from cancer registries in neighbouring countries. According to the Global Cancer Observatory, the estimated number of new cancer cases in Greece in 2018 was 67,401,[3] while in 2020 it was 64,530. This apparent trend in the decline in new cancers seem to be evident also in in cancer mortality. Lung cancer has the highest incidence for men and breast cancer for women; lung cancer has the highest mortality for both sexes. These numbers approximate the Greek reality where screening programmes and access to the healthcare system can be described as 'moderately satisfactory' at best.[4]

The healthcare system in Greece includes both public and private sectors. The national public health system operates within a social health insurance model, while the private sector includes profit-making hospitals, diagnostic centres and independent practices (Economou et al. 2017). In Greece, a country of almost 10.5 million people, there are four public cancer hospitals, three of them in Athens and one in Thessaloniki. My fieldwork took place in a public cancer hospital in Athens, located in the city centre. It was founded in 1935 and today is the largest cancer treatment centre in the country, with a bed capacity of 400 in a six-storey building. This hospital treats adults with all kinds of cancer, from across the country. The hospital's medical services are divided into three main departments: the medical oncology department, the surgical oncology department and the laboratory sector. The hospital administration gave me access to one of the two cancer wards of the medical oncology department and its associated outpatient clinic, which I refer to as Ward A. Here I spent almost one and a half years, undertaking participant observation and semi-structured interviews with patients, medical practitioners and nurses. Ward A is located on the third floor and has a bed capacity of 40 for adults diagnosed with all types of cancer. Admission to the cancer ward can signify many things: a three-day or more chemotherapy session,[5] disease progression, life-threatening chemotherapy side-effects and, for some, palliative care. The ward arrangement separates male and female patients, who are divided into seven rooms each with four beds, two rooms with two beds and three rooms with one bed. The ward is always full. Patients who have had surgery are admitted to the corresponding wards of the surgical oncology departments. Patients undergoing radiotherapy are not hospitalised and in public hospitals, radiotherapy, like other modes of treatment, is free of charge. According to the Medical Association of Athens, on 2 April 2019, in Greece there were 48 radiotherapy machines, 31 public and 17 private. However, understaffing of public hospitals results in insufficient use of their radiotherapy machines. This results in delays in radiotherapy initiation for up to three months and there are long waiting lists. Radiotherapy is easier to access in private hospitals, but the cost ranges from 1,500 to 2,500 euros.

One day, four ebullient and passionate young intern doctors invited me to drink coffee during their break and asked me to 'change roles' for a while and to let them interview me: 'Why are you really here?' Niki asked me laughingly. 'Be honest, why do you torture yourself? How can you follow us all day, watch all this cancers' ugliness, it must be very difficult for you', Minas said solemnly. 'Is it for you?' I asked him. He replied: 'Well . . . at the beginning it was very difficult for me. Patients under chemotherapy have terrible side-effects, especially those who are under long-term chemotherapy. Losing hair is nothing in front of [compared to] black nails or vomiting till your body is totally dehydrated.' 'Or when haematological toxicity threatens your life', said Zoe. 'Ascites can make your belly swollen', added Maria. 'Do you remember that woman? The one who admitted in the ward a week ago? Her face was so skinny, and the rest of her body was completely swollen. I have never seen something like that before', she added. 'I think the most difficult is the smell', said Niki. 'The smell of a body that has been eaten by cancer . . . The smell of decomposition . . .' And after a few seconds of silence, Minas said: 'Cancer eats you alive, eats your body and your soul. The most difficult for me is to watch patients becoming something . . . how can I describe it . . . it [cancer] makes you look like not human . . . It takes away your dignity, it takes away your ability to be human.'

During fieldwork, my daily research routine included attending the morning rounds in Ward A. Each day the whole team of doctors, specialists and interns,[6] along with the chief nurse and sometimes the clinic's secretary, conducted the morning rounds. I spent three to four hours, sometimes more, with them, as they visited and examined each patient of the ward. 'How do you feel today?' is the question that Dr Alexandris used to address each patient, while touching their hand or even hugging them.

'Unfortunately, we [the oncologists] are the only ones who can give some hope to the desperate eyes', he explained to me when I asked why he touches and hugs the patients; other doctors usually avoid doing so. Dr Alexandris continued:

> Because when you hug them [the patients] and kiss them, when you touch or brush them, you show them that you don't detest them. It means that you are not disgusted by the image or the smell of death. It is a way to show that you care and make them feel that they are not close to death.

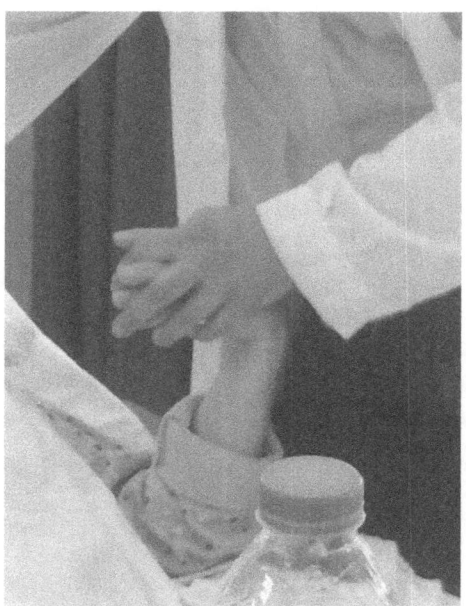

Figure 8.3 Touching hands – Dr A. during morning rounds.
Photo: Falia Varelaki.

As Puig de la Bellacasa (2017: 3) describes it, 'caring implicates different relationalities, issues, and practices in different settings'. For Dr Alexandris, caring for the 'altered body and subjectivities' comes through physically touching 'the wounded body and soul' during his daily morning rounds on Ward A. The practice of caring penetrates the corporeal boundaries while moving between different expectations regarding the provision and reception of care.

Another way to understand what 'care' means in the context of the cancer ward is to examine the services provided within Greece's public healthcare system. The 'patient's pathway' (Day et al. 2017: 150–151) in Greece is complex. The 'journey' usually begins either when the patient detects a change in her/his body or spots symptoms and gets tested,[7] or when she/he discovers the cancer by accident during routine screening or blood exams. The cancer diagnosis is followed by the first appointment with an oncologist in the outpatient clinic – either in a public hospital, which is free of charge during morning outpatient clinics but switches to a paid service during afternoon outpatient clinics, or in a private hospital which requires direct payment.[8] During the initial appointment, the cancer diagnosis will be 'validated' by the oncologist and the illusion of

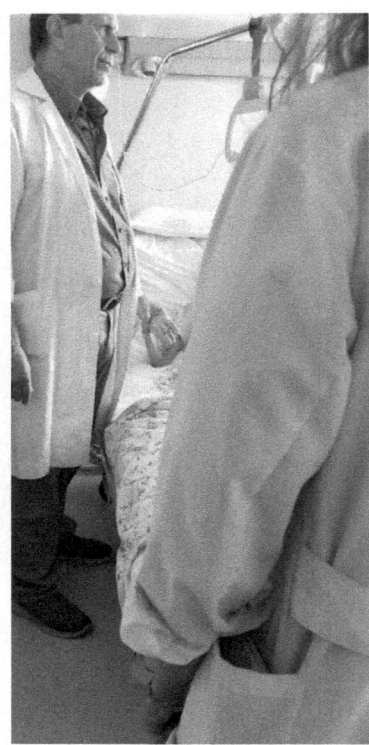

Figure 8.4 Fighting together. Photo: Falia Varelaki.

immortality shared by healthy people will be lost.[9] Then, the oncologist will refer the patient to a surgeon, in cases where the patient needs surgery, or the oncologist may order lab tests, imaging tests (scans) or other tests or procedures in order to more precisely diagnose and stage the cancer and plan the treatment. The patient will then begin treatment (surgery, chemotherapy and/or radiotherapy) and usually will be scheduled for another appointment in the outpatient clinic, with new screening and/or blood tests required during the treatment cycle in order for the oncologist to evaluate treatment progress. Another appointment will be scheduled at the end of the treatment session, again with new screening/blood tests ordered. In cases when the oncologist recommends that treatment ends, the patient will be monitored under a follow-up care plan every six months for the first five years and once a year after that. If, during a follow-up appointment, a reoccurrence is suspected, the oncologist will consider new treatment options.

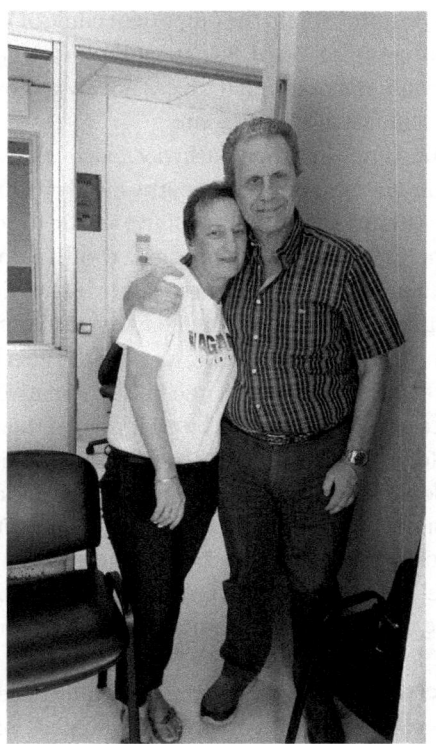

Figure 8.5 Dr A. and a patient, outpatient clinic. Photo: Patient, research participant.

The above description is a schematic and simplified form of the 'patient's pathway'. It is the 'formal' process to which a patient has access only through an appointment scheduled through the service 'Line for Health-1535', a management and service system that enables users to book an appointment either in a morning or in an afternoon outpatient clinic or with a doctor in any public hospital in Greece. The user can either call the number 1535 or use the website 1535.gr to book an appointment. As mentioned, the appointment in the morning outpatient clinic is free of charge, but the afternoon outpatient clinic offers the same range of services at a cost ranging between 36 to 64 euros depending on the seniority and specialisation of the doctor. Patients can choose the doctor they wish to meet, but the waiting period – mainly in the morning outpatient clinic – ranges from three to six months, sometimes even longer. These delays occur because, on the one hand, morning outpatient services are offered free of charge and therefore are preferable, while there are too few doctors – ten in the outpatient clinic of Ward A and eight in the outpatient clinic of Ward B – struggling to treat thousands of patients.[10] As a result, the outpatient offices are always overcrowded and the appointments almost always run late.

At the same time, another pathway exists that is parallel and unofficial. Patients participate in this pathway by visiting the morning outpatient clinic without an appointment and asking to see the doctor for 'just for a few minutes' because they are unable to afford an appointment in the afternoon outpatient clinic. In these short interactions or informal consultations, patients may receive their blood test results or their screening test results and so avoid the long waiting time for the next available formal appointment in the morning outpatient clinic. Alternatively, patients may seek informal access to their clinicians by asking to see their doctor because they need to inform him/her about the alarming side-effects of their chemotherapy. Some patients adopt the strategy of waiting until they see the doctor walking down the hall; they then run behind him or her and ask just them to quickly 'take a look' at their exam results and confirm that 'everything is fine'. Others chose to sit outside Dr Alexandris' office, waiting for hours until he manages to find some time to see them in between his daily responsibilities in Ward A.

One day, as I was walking to the canteen to buy coffee, I was stopped by an elderly woman. She was around 70, I assumed, with a face full of wrinkles, no eyelashes or eyebrows, with a scarf tied around her head. She wore an old and worn coat and, hanging from her cane, she carried a large bag with a logo on it from a well-known private diagnostic centre in Athens. She looked desperate. 'Are you lost?' I asked. 'Are you a doctor?' she said. 'I've seen you with Dr Alexandris. Can you please have a look at my exam results? I've finished chemotherapy, and I am still alive! Isn't that a miracle? My cousin unfortunately died during chemotherapy, that red drug was too strong for her. Here are my CT test results and my blood test results. No mammogram for me, you see . . .' and with her voice sinking to a whisper she said, 'the doctor removed both of them'. And then she continued:

> Now, I have these exam results, I've finished my chemotherapy sessions, what should I do? Will you give me those pills? I have a friend back in Aliveri who has a granddaughter.[11] She also had cancer and after chemotherapy her doctor gave her some pills . . .

I managed to interrupt her, and I said: 'I am so sorry, I am not a doctor. Are you here alone?' 'Yes', she said. 'I came here in the morning, by bus. I came to see the doctor. I first went to Ward A but they told me that I will find him in the outpatient clinic. I also went there but it is overcrowded.' 'Do you have an appointment?' I asked. 'No', she said, 'there was no available appointment for this week and the doctor told me to come right away after chemotherapy.' I didn't know what to say; I knew she was not the only one facing this situation. 'Well, would you please have a look?' she asked again. Feeling guilty, I reiterated that I was not a doctor. 'Oh . . . at least, can you read them? You are educated, you will understand if there is any cancer left . . .'

When I discussed this incident with Dr Alexandris, he described it as a 'liminal situation'. He explained that he often found himself in positions that were 'typically okay but still not legal enough' as he attempted to treat more than 50 people per day:

> Improvisational practices – This is what I call everything we do within the hospital in order to deal with this monster called bureaucracy. We improvise almost all of the time, and this is how we save both the healthcare system and the patient. Otherwise, people remain in a state of limbo. In fact, because of this inadequate system, the gaps that you can find within it, is what can save people. It is not only from the side of the doctors. Look at the nurses. Look at the staff. They treat patients humanely, while they struggle to overcome the system's inadequacies. But these inadequacies themselves help the weak and the uninsured patients and all those who would otherwise be unable to access the public hospital . . . Therefore, we improvise all the time.
>
> Let me give you some examples: we keep four different files for the same patient, one in the outpatient clinic, one in the archives, one in the cancer ward and one in the chemo-ward . . . This is how data circulates and how I am able to meet a patient who comes to me without an appointment . . . Because if I don't see the exam results early enough, maybe there is something there that the patient cannot recognise, (and so they do not know) how important it can be. It could be a reoccurrence. Or, in a different situation, someone can be upset after the exam results, but without reason to be. How many times do they come here in tears, and they leave with a smile on their face? How would they feel if I didn't accept them without an appointment and they try to book one, with the next available after six months?

When fieldwork began, I used to spend almost 12 hours a day on the cancer ward and its associated clinic, following the doctor's routine until

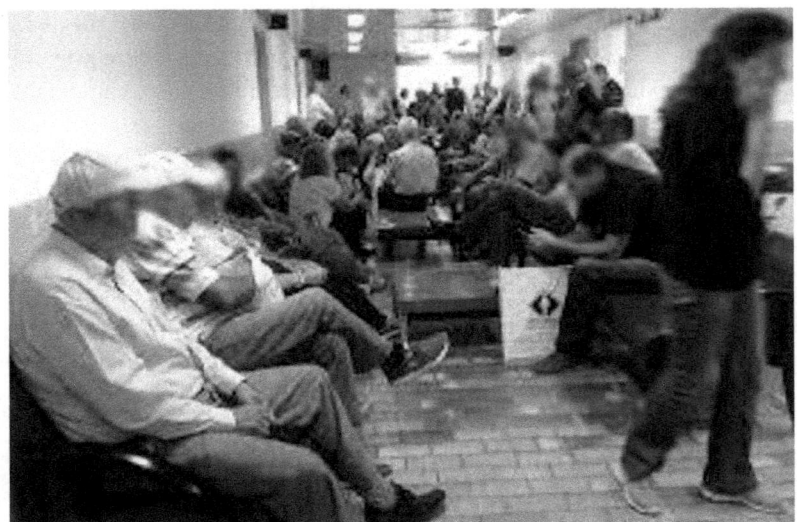

Figure 8.6 Monday morning, 9.50 a.m., outpatient clinic.
Photo: Falia Varelaki.

I was exhausted. Dr Alexandris was always the first to arrive at the hospital and the last to leave. I never heard anyone complain about the extra hours they were spending in the hospital; even the interns left late after a final visit to the patients of Ward A. Once, after a particularly long day, I asked Dr Alexandris how he was able to get through working so many hours every day. He replied:

> Did you count how many people we treated today? Did you count how many people left our office door relieved and smiling? Since the public health system doesn't care about poor people, who will? How can I go home and close my eyes tonight if I know that I refused to treat someone who was unable to book an appointment because of this rotten system?

The way Dr Alexandris responds to patient's efforts to reach medical care through the unofficial pathway can be interpreted as a levelling practice that improves access to the health system for the poor and socially marginalised. This levelling practice can be understood as a practice of care seeking to redress inequality, as it is aimed at securing the right to health for those who are otherwise structurally disadvantaged within the formal pathway for accessing care.

All of them need care

Cancer is a debilitating disease. Patients hospitalised on Ward A are usually in a critical condition. Some of them have been hospitalised in order to have chemotherapy three (or more) days in a row, with intolerable pain, nausea and vomiting. Others are hospitalised due to complications, such as a sharp drop in white blood cells or a recurrence of the disease. Anguish is reflected in everyone's eyes. Some are deeply depressed; others try hard to fight for their life; others consider any fight to be pointless. Some are surrounded by their family and friends; others are completely alone. Most of them die. But all of them need care.

In talking about care, Manolis, a 35-year-old intern, told me that 'if you want to understand what care means, you should talk to the nurses. In Ward A everybody cares about our patients. But nurses . . . they spend all day with patients and the patients in return surrender their body and sometimes their soul to them.'

Being a nurse in the cancer ward is a complicated endeavour, extremely important and extremely difficult. Only 13 nurses in Ward A were available to treat patients, making it difficult for me to talk with them during my fieldwork. They were always busy. One day I was standing at the nurse station observing a young nurse preparing the medical trolley. 'Can I help you?' Lisa, a 33-year-old nurse, asked me in a strict tone. 'I can feel you staring at me behind my back.' 'I am sorry, I didn't mean to bother you', I said, 'I was just looking at your hair, I like the colour.' She continued: 'Are you going to write a report about me? Are you here to evaluate us? I saw you yesterday, you were talking with my colleagues.' I told her about my research and we had a brief talk about care. She said to me:

> Well, my job is difficult because I am extremely busy. Too many patients for us . . . We do care for all of them, they need care. But you know, there is no such a thing 'good care' or 'bad care'. Either you care or you don't.

According to Livingston (2012: 96), nursing care in the ward 'is at once deeply personal and deeply social, and is a vital practical matter, crucial to patient well-being and survival'. On Ward A the nurse is the first one to say 'good morning' and to smile at the inpatients. They follow a strict daily schedule commencing from 6 am: blood and urine tests, administration of medications, procedures involving intravenous cannulation and preparations for chemotherapy, including the organisation and the

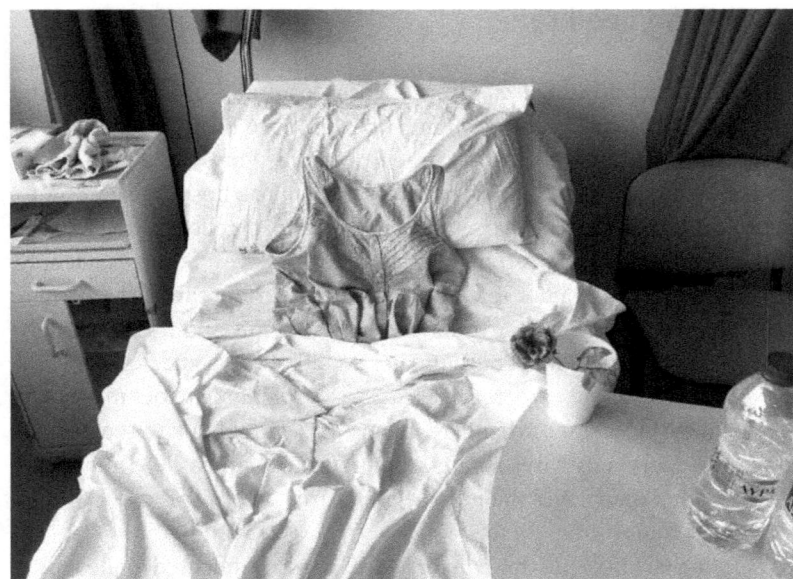

Figure 8.7   'I'll be back . . .'. Photo: Dr A.

necessary administration of medications. Nurses check each patient's blood sugar and vital signs, record data on each patient's chart, change their bedsheets and bathe them. The care work is continuous throughout the day and on Ward A it is largely performed by women. As everywhere, care work is gendered – 'mothers caring for the children, nurses for the sick, wives for the house, and the list goes on' (Martin, Myers and Viseu 2015: 628).

Maria, a 53-year-old nurse, explained:

> Taking care of patients is not always easy. The most important thing for us is to make sure that patients' dignity is always maintained. For example, we always make sure that we clean the patient behind drawn curtains. People always feel uncomfortable when they are unable to clean themselves and need help. They feel that their dignity is lost. Aside from the fact that they have cancer, they have to deal also with that [loss of dignity] . . . And it is the same feeling for both men and women. You have to . . . make them feel that you don't feel uncomfortable, that you are not disgusted by them, that you really care. Most of the times people understand, they accept it and appreciate the fact that you offer them care.

Drawing on Mary Douglas (1984), the sick body is viewed as polluted and its bodily fluids are considered as matter out of place. In Ward A all nurses are women. They are the caretakers of the passages between life, disease and death. They take care of the sick body, they treat the wounds, they try to make the body with cancer feel better and alive. The way nurses take care of the rotten flesh of cancer-affected bodies has similarities between the hygienic rituals of cleansing and symbolic purification rituals, as described by Douglas (1992). The process of cleaning the body and taking care of the body symbolically purifies it, pushing away everything that threatens the patient's humanity. Even the strict white uniform code of hospitals, according to Littlewood (2015), partly serves to emphasise the status of nurses as 'pure' and enables them to contain the pollution of disease and death. Thus, care as a social and an emotional practice can be perceived as a duty or a burden, but also as a pleasure or as a matter of course (Drotbohm and Alber 2015).

I had several conversations with Elena, a 42-year-old nurse. One day, as I followed her during her morning shift, she told me:

> I am a 'third floor nurse', do you know what that means? It means that we are not playing games here. It's not easy every day. You

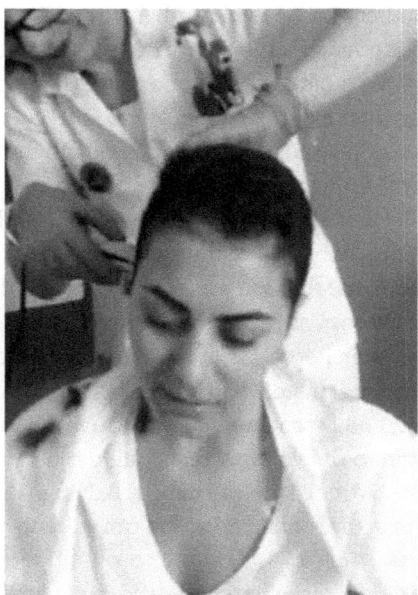

Figure 8.8 Preparing the patient for chemotherapy. Photo: Dr A.

know, people get angry with you, when you try to take care of them. But you should remain calm, you should be kind and smiling, and give them all the love you keep in your heart. The problem is that there are many people who we need to take care of, our ward is full all the time . . . But you know, most of the time people stay many days so you get to know them, you call them by their names, and they call you by yours . . . You will also hear the word 'thank you', even mumbled, but still, they appreciate everything you provide them. Of course, there are few who take it for granted, they even say 'it is your job', but rarely does a patient become ungrateful. But this is not a problem for us. The difficult part is that most of the time people die here. It's people who we take care of, and this is the most difficult part of our job. I try not to become friends with patients because it hurts when they are gone.

Intimacies: surrendering themselves to you

I'm sitting in the nursing station observing people in the ward. It is visiting time and the ward is crowded. The ward both looks and sounds different. There are people visiting patients, it's noisy, some of them are happy and laughing, some others try to say goodbye to their loved ones and cry because it's probably the last time they will see them alive. The nursing station is the perfect spot to be during visiting hours. It provides a kind of 'panoptic gaze'. Giannis, a young intern doctor, approached me, saying in a low voice: 'Let me guess, you sit here because you have nothing to do . . . again. Right? Let me help you, you can study what it means for the visitors to use the toilets during visiting time.' He walks away laughing. That could have been an interesting topic, but my attention was directed towards the chief nurse. It seems to me that she was walking around the ward worried. 'Something is wrong', she says to a young nurse, 'something smells wrong.' They enter Room N3 and approach an elderly man's bed. During the morning round, I had heard doctors saying that he is in the terminal stage, and I wondered if any relatives should be called. The chief nurse said to the younger one: 'Call the doctor and then come back to help me. We need to clean him, he is dying.' Then she addressed me: 'We will take care of him now. You can go', and drew the curtain.

This section of my fieldnotes among others, depicts how I would actively turn away when someone was dying or when nurses were taking care of a deceased body before the mortuary staff took over. Wondering about the cases of 'the alones' – the patients who pass away without family or friends, I asked Lisa what happened with them when it was time. She replied:

> This is not a problem. We are here for them and we take care of them. We will wash them; we will change their clothes; we will arrange everything for them. These people surrender themselves to us.

In an effort to better understand the relationship between the nurse and the dying patient, I asked the chief nurse what it meant to take care of a cancer patient?

> You mean 'what does it mean to take care of someone who surrenders themselves to you?' A cancer patient suffers from unbearable pain, fatigue and nausea. It is very difficult for them. Most of them have someone by their side to hold their hand, you know, just that can be the most precious thing for the patient... Our job is not difficult. There are just some difficult moments. Many patients 'externalise their pain', this is what I call it when someone gets angry and they lash out against you. At the end of the day, you must never forget that this is a cancer ward.

During this interview, the chief nurse identified the fact that patients 'surrender themselves to the nurse' with the concept of 'trust'. She explained:

> Most of them are practically unable to take care of themselves. Even those who have family members around them, a wife, a husband, or their children. They totally trust us to help them, surrendering to our care, we help them to perform the simplest and most basic human functions of the body. That means that they willingly left themselves to our discretion, though they have no other choice. But this is what we do when we take care of them. We respond to that trust.

According to Grimen (2009), trust within the context of healthcare systems is closely related to the concept of power. When the patient trusts nurses, it means that he/she transfers power to them. When patients are unable to walk to the bathroom by themselves, clean their own body or even feed themselves, they experience profound vulnerability and are necessarily dependent on nurses. The 'structurally inferior situation of patients' (Grimen 2009: 18) is the basis from which this power dynamic is established. While nurses seem aware of this power dynamic when patients surrender themselves to them, they chose to deploy this power through practices of care as a counterpoint to patients' vulnerability.

Interpreting care

In this chapter, I have provided insights into the day-to-day life of people on the cancer ward. Based on ethnographic experience, I argue that by analysing cancer as producing practices and discourses of care, we can interpret the relationships that are developed and performed between the medical staff and patients as a way to rehumanise the disease and those affected by it.

As described, practices of care in this specific cancer ward consist of daily routines. When cancer patients are threatened by dehumanisation, when cancer alters the body and removes human features and capabilities, care acts as an important social exchange The consequent rehumanisation is achieved through touch and the relationships that are developed, aiming at social 'healing' by mitigating social isolation and preventing the social death of the patient. Rehumanising bodies that 'are undergoing profoundly disfiguring processes of decomposition' becomes a practice of care, located at the place where 'the combination of technical skill, professional knowledge, and the sentimental work of cancer nursing concretises the humanistic promise of medicine' (Livingston 2012: 108). This ethnographic example illuminates the gaps that are created within the biomedical healthcare system and the practices of care that arise within it. The hospital, as a liminal space where human life meets human death, becomes the place where doctors and nurses perform these practices of care.

Ethnographic analysis provides us a pathway for achieving deeper insight into cancer care and the politics developed around it. Since care is both context and perspective dependent, it is important to understand the aspects of both those who perform care – and in this case their acts of humanising – and those who are care receivers – people who are threatened with or have already experienced dehumanisation. Ethnographic analysis offers multiple possibilities for deconstructing care and its politics, thus providing a context within which we can think more *care*fully about cancer. This ethnographic account responds to the wider call to 'humanise' our understanding of cancer and the politics of care. Paraphrasing Chatzidakis et al. (2020), rethinking care in this context is crucial for the politics of care today if we hope to foster a politics of tomorrow.

Acknowledgements

The research on which this chapter is based was funded by University of the Aegean through an Ypatia scholarship. I am grateful to Linda Bennett, Lenore Manderson and Belinda Spagnoletti for treating this chapter with such care. Their comments and insights helped sharpen my thinking.

Notes

1. Following the common anthropological practice, I use pseudonyms for my interlocutors, while I adopt a descriptive reference for my fieldwork site.
2. Ward A exclusively treated adult cancer patients and thus there was no opportunity to observe how loss was experienced or mediated in the context of parents losing children due to cancer.
3. See https://gco.iarc.fr/today/data/factsheets/populations/300-greece-fact-sheets.pdf. Accessed 2 July 2020.
4. For more detail regarding access to different levels of the Greek healthcare system, see Varelaki (2021).
5. Daily chemotherapy sessions are conducted in the hospital's One Day Clinic, a separate building that has operated since 2017. This day centre has three operating rooms and a 45-bed capacity.
6. Ward A of the medical oncology department is staffed by one scientific officer-director, nine medical specialists and eight interns.
7. This is not the only 'pathway', but it is the most common that I recorded during my fieldwork.
8. My fieldwork took place in a public cancer hospital; thus I am not familiar with the processes in private hospitals.
9. People usually come to the outpatient clinic for the first appointment with a medical oncologist. They already have a test with the cancer diagnosis, but they tend to seek the 'validation' of the diagnosis from the oncologist. By naming the entity, the doctor acquires the power of the creator and thus the entity has a name (cancer) and the power to exist. The verbalisation of the disease from the oncologist substantiates the diagnosis.
10. During a morning outpatient clinic, a doctor is allowed to see up to 25 patients, while during afternoon outpatient clinics doctors can see up to 12 only.
11. The distance by road between Aliveri and Athens is 120 km and it usually takes approximately two hours by bus.

References

Buch, Elana D. 2015. 'Anthropology of aging and care', *Annual Review of Anthropology* 44: 277–293. https://doi.org/10.1146/annurev-anthro-102214-014254.

Chatzidakis, Andreas, Jamie Hakim, Jo Littler, Catherine Rottenberg and Lynne Segal (The Care Collective). 2020. *The Care Manifesto: The politics of interdependence*. London and New York: Verso.

Day, Sophie, R. Charles Coombes, Louise McGrath-Lone, Claudia Schoenborn and Helen Ward. 2017. 'Stratified, precision or personalised medicine? Cancer services in the "real world" of a London hospital', *Sociology of Health & Illness* 39(1): 143–158. https://doi.org/10.1111/1467-9566.12457.

Douglas, Mary. 1984. *Purity and Danger: An analysis of the concept of pollution and taboo*. London and New York: Routledge.

Douglas, Mary. 1992. *Risk and Blame: Essays in cultural theory*. London: Routledge.

Drotbohm, Heike and Erdmunte Alber. 2015. 'Introduction'. In *Anthropological Perspectives on Care: Work, kinship and the life-course*, edited by Erdmunte Alber and Heike Drotbohm, 1–20. New York: Palgrave Macmillan.

Economou, Charalampos, Daphne Kaitelidou, Marina Karanikolos and Anna Maresso. 2017. 'Greece: Health system review', *Health Systems in Transition* 19(5): 1–192.

Grimen, Harald. 2009. 'Power, trust, and risk: Some reflections on an absent issue', *Medical Anthropology Quarterly* 23(1): 16–33. https://doi.org/10.1111/j.1548-1387.2009.01035.x.

Kleinman, Arthur and Sjaak van der Geest. 2009. '"Care" in health care: Remaking the moral world of medicine', *Medische Anthropologie* 21(1): 159–168. https://hdl.handle.net/11245/1.314817.

Littlewood, Jenny. 2015. 'Care and ambiguity: Towards a concept of nursing'. In *Anthropology and Nursing*, edited by Pat Holden and Jenny Littlewood, 170–189. London: Routledge.

Livingston, Julie. 2012. *Improvising Medicine: An African oncology ward in an emerging cancer epidemic*. Durham, NC: Duke University Press.

Makrinioti, D. 2008. 'Eisagogi: koinonikes kai politikes morfes diaxeirisis ths thnitotitas'. In *Peri thanatou. H politiki diaxeirisi ths thnitotitas*, edited by D. Makrinioti, 13–72. Athens, Greece: Nisos.

Martin, Aryn, Natasha Myers and Ana Viseu. 2015. 'The politics of care in technoscience', *Social Studies of Science* 45(5): 625–641. https://doi.org/10.1177/0306312715602073.

Martin, Jeannett. 2013. 'Rethinking care: Anthropological perspectives on life courses, kin work and their trans-local entanglements'. Paper originally presented at Work and the Life Cycle in Global History, Humboldt-Universität zu Berlin, 6–8 December 2012. H-Soz-Kult. Accessed 20 July 2020. https://www.hsozkult.de/conferencereport/id/tagungsberichte-4778.

Puig de la Bellacasa, María. 2017. *Matters of Care: Speculative ethics in more than human worlds*. Minneapolis: University of Minnesota Press.

Sevenhuijsen, Selma. 1998. *Citizenship and the Ethics of Care: Feminist considerations on justice, morality and politics*. London and New York: Routledge.

Street, Alice. 2017. 'What are we talking about when we talk about care? Reflections on the discussion'. Somatosphere. Accessed 27 July 2020. http://somatosphere.net/forumpost/what-are-we-talking-about-when-we-talk-about-care-reflections-on-the-discussion/.

Tronto, Joan. 1993. *Moral Boundaries: A political argument for an ethic of care*. London: Routledge.

Varelaki, Falia. 2021. '"Either you have money and plan your treatment, or you don't have money and plan your death": Tracing inequalities in breast cancer care'. In *Urban Inequalities: Ethnographically informed reflections*, edited by Italo Pardo and Giuliana B. Prato, 129–144. Cham, Switzerland: Palgrave Macmillan.

9
Practices of containment in the 'south-within-the-north': women with breast cancer in southern Italy

Cinzia Greco

In this chapter, I analyse the practices and patterns of containment among women with breast cancer in southern Italy. I show how, despite the neoliberal 'pink' discourse of breast cancer, which is present in Italy as elsewhere, the women I met had an approach to breast cancer which, while aimed at limiting its impact, was clearly distinct from the 'pink' approach. Instead, women's approach to their health was linked to and defined by their need to deal with other health and personal problems. I propose the concept of containment can account for this approach, which I argue can be understood by locating illness experiences in the broader context of southern Italy as a peripheral setting and as the 'south-within-the-north'.

Alonzo (1979: 399) proposed the concept of containment to describe the process of 'maintaining proper situational involvement while keeping bodily derelictions at the level of a side-involvement'. The concept contrasts with those of coping and adjustment, which emphasise the positive management of illness. While coping involves reducing the impact of the illness and adjustment describes reconfiguring one's life to manage the limitations introduced by illness, containment refers to the degree to which the illness is placed in the background by the need to deal with other aspects of life.

Alonzo initially used the idea of containment to explain delayed care-seeking, particularly for acute heart events (Alonzo 1979: 398), focusing on the microscale and the management of bodily sensations lasting less than a day. The concept was subsequently applied to understand delays in cancer diagnosis (Andersen et al. 2010). More recently, Hansen and colleagues (2018) extended the idea of containment post-diagnosis, focusing on the daily management of glucose levels and hypoglycaemic events to explore how people with diabetes manage their symptoms and monitor themselves during their work activities. Here, I extend the concept to analyse illness on a larger timescale. Following anthropological approaches of illness narratives, I consider what can be defined as 'biographic containment', that is, the process through which the illness is only afforded limited space in one's life, due either to the mobilisation of resources or to other issues which are more pressing. This analysis shares points of contact with previous studies of how, after an illness that has had a permanent impact, people try to build an identity that is not limited to their illness and its consequences (Manderson 2011). However, I use the concept of containment to focus on the limitation of space given to the illness as a result of external issues rather than as a means of (re)constructing one's own identity.

Applying the concept of biographic containment to cancer, and to breast cancer in particular, helps describe how women dealt with illness, as I encountered in my fieldwork. Breast cancer is at the centre of contradictory pressures. There is a general tendency in biomedicine to extend the medicalisation of illnesses and in some cases to medicalise risk factors such as being overweight or hypertension both through medical advice and lifelong treatments (see, for example, Dumit 2012; Manderson 2020). In the case of post-treatment breast cancer, the situation is one of a 'new normal', in which the return to 'normality' is hindered by long-term side-effects, the risk of relapse and bodily changes brought about by the surgery (see Manderson 2011: 173–206; Trusson, Pilnick and Roy 2016). At the same time, the public discourse about breast cancer is dominated by the strong positive-thinking rhetoric promoted by the 'pink' discourse. Such positivity discourses present attitude, strength and determination as personality traits essential for dealing with cancer. Several psychological studies conducted since the 1980s, but now shown to lack scientific validity (Pelosi 2019), popularised the idea that personality and attitude significantly influenced both cancer development and treatment efficacy (see in particular Grossarth-Maticek and Eysenck 1991). For breast cancer, the general imperative of optimism and positivity was developed in particularly strong terms around the 'pink' discourse. Originating in the United States, with the Susan G. Komen Foundation as its main promoter, the pink discourse has spread globally, in what has been termed 'pinkification' (Johansen et al. 2013), with several organisations following a common iconography and approach beyond the international activities of the Komen Foundation. A central point of the pink culture is a glamorised approach to breast cancer advocacy (King 2006; Sulik 2010). This involves asking for support from corporations, particularly in the fashion and cosmetics industries, and encouraging patients to resist the illness by engaging in practices that reinforce traditional femininity, such as wearing make-up and shopping. The survivor script for women with breast cancer includes maintaining an optimistic attitude and inspiring other women to assume the same attitude through activities such as festivals, fundraising runs and other sporting events, almost always with participants wearing iconic bright pink garments and pink lapel ribbons. Pinkification involves an image and ethos of survivorship reflecting neoliberal ideology. Two main critiques have been advanced against this approach. First, by individualising the illness and positioning survival as an outcome of a positive attitude, pink advocacy is particularly problematic for women who develop metastases and die from breast cancer, as their death is treated as a personal failure. Secondly, the approach has weakened breast cancer activism by emphasising individual involvement and corporate partnership to the detriment, among other things, of a critique of environmental pollutants and the corporations that produce them (King 2006; Klawiter 2008; Sulik 2010).

In Italy, along with the presence of a national Komen chapter, the pink approach has filtered into and is visible in many campaigns promoted by national and local health authorities and by some of the main Italian organisations working on cancer research and support. However, the women I met presented a vision of the illness that, while focused on containment, was clearly distinct from the pink rhetoric. Therefore, in this chapter, I aim to: (1) identify a theoretical approach that can account for these visions of the illness that do not fit in the pro- and anti-pink analyses present in literature; and (2) explain how these alternative visions developed in a country in which the pink rhetoric is present and visible.

By taking an analytical approach based on containment, I show how women develop ways to deal with the impact of breast cancer, without necessarily reducing their approaches to optimistic stories of victory. A few other studies (Salamonsen et al. 2016; Snell-Rood, Merkel and Schoenberg 2018) have shown how financial and familial issues can reduce the attention given to the illness, to the detriment of care and self-care. Containment is an ambiguous practice; it allows those who are affected to limit the impact of illness on everyday life, but it does not necessarily improve or promise to improve their situation. Containment can simply mean that the illness is minimised to allow for other problems to be juggled.

I focus on southern Italy, so to explore how responses to breast cancer are shaped by a specific context, which can be considered a 'south-within-the-north'. I argue that the marginality of southern Italy in relation to the north of the country, as well as to the rest of Europe, and the social position of the interviewees – predominantly women from working-class backgrounds living in semi-rural areas – can help explain their responses to breast cancer. The concept of 'south-within-the-north' has been used to describe areas within the global north which feature levels of poverty comparable to those prevalent in the global south (Gaventa 1998). This description does not completely fit southern Italy, where living standards are comparable to other areas of the global north and a national universal healthcare system offers Italians throughout the country good standards of care and treatment. However, the concept of 'south-within-the-north' usefully describes three dimensions of internal inequality. First, southern Italy is characterised by deprivation when compared to northern Italy:[1] incomes are lower and unemployment levels have been high for the whole of its contemporary history.[2] Consequently, migration to northern Italy and north-western Europe – and, in the past, to the Americas and Australia – has characterised much of the recent history of the south (see, for example, Pugliese 2006). Secondly, this relative deprivation can be linked to the broader economic disparity that structurally subordinates southern Italy's economy to northern Italy's – a situation that Gramsci (1966) described as the result of an 'alliance' between the factory owners of the north and the landowners of the south. Finally, since the country's unification in 1861, the south has been subject to stigma, whereby southern Italians are described as backward and lacking civility and civic sense, and which attributes regional inequalities to culture, corruption and criminality (Schneider 1998). Structural economic asymmetries between north and south Italy are downplayed.

The disparity between north and south carries health implications. For example, environmental cancers in highly impacted areas in southern Italy have been framed as lifestyle cancers.[3] The stigmatisation against people in the south, and the assumption that this correlated with poor quality of care and services, meant that many women I interviewed felt the need to either move to northern Italy for treatment for breast cancer or to justify being treated locally (Greco 2019). Both social conditions and stigma can make cancer in southern Italy especially problematic, producing recursive cascades in which social and health problems reinforce each other (Manderson and Warren 2016).

However, in this chapter, I focus on a different dimension: the ways in which the social and cultural context of this 'south-within-the-north' redefines the experience of breast cancer and, in particular, the kinds of containment mobilised by women with breast cancer in this context. The idea of the 'south-within-the-north' positions southern Italy as peripheral both symbolically and structurally and for most of the interviewees on whose experiences I draw here, this condition adds to the fact that they lived in semi-rural centres and came from working-class backgrounds. Despite the visibility of the pink rhetoric in Italy, the local specificities of southern Italy (and the social background of most interviewees) redefined this vision. Underlining the structural basis to the peripheral profile of southern Italy helps us avoid interpreting local differences in perceptions and experiences of breast cancer as mere cultural alterity or, worse, as backwardness and helps link these differences to specific social conditions.

In this chapter, I consider the different containment practices that women described in their illness narratives. While containment approaches are strongly interwoven, I distinguish between moral strength and religion, family and community and the positioning of breast cancer as one among other diseases.

Methods and context

The field research on which this chapter is based was conducted in the provinces of Lecce and Brindisi, in Salento, the southern part of the Apulia region of southern Italy.[4] Geographically, Salento is often described as the 'heel' of the Italian 'boot'. Here I draw on 15 interviews with women aged between their 30s and late 60s, the majority post-menopausal. This roughly matches the epidemiology of breast cancer, as the disease usually develops after menopause. All interviewees were locally born and resident and the majority were from working-class backgrounds. While I draw primarily on formal interviews conducted between 2012 and 2014, I have continued to talk about breast cancer with women in Salento since then on an informal basis. While some interviews were conducted in Salento's larger urban centres, most were in small semi-rural centres varying in size from 2,000 to 10,000 inhabitants, where agriculture was the main economic activity until the 1980s. A significant part of the population remains involved in agriculture. Given the high level of homeownership in Italy and the relatively low cost of real estate in these centres, most interviewees lived in nuclear family houses, with their adult children often residing in the neighbourhood. Although many had relatives who had migrated, especially to northern Italy, all women had relatives living locally. The interviewees usually drove (or were driven by relatives), for all treatments and follow-up care, to the hospitals in Lecce and Brindisi, but also to other hospitals in mid-sized centres. A single therapeutic pathway, even if local, could be distributed over up to three different centres, with driving distances between half an hour and an hour. Beyond local mobility to access healthcare, long-distance travel to the regional capital Bari or to northern Italy was also common (Greco 2019).

The interviewees were contacted through my own personal networks and snowballing and the interviews were conducted in a mix of standard Italian and the local dialect, which I understand and speak. All translations are mine and I have tried to convey in English some of the particularities of the mixed-language speech in the interviews. All names used are pseudonyms and minor biographical details have been altered to safeguard privacy. While I focused on the experiences of breast surgery, I collected extensive illness narratives which included previous health issues, the experience of breast cancer from diagnosis to completion of treatment and the interviewee's relationships with medical professionals and personal support networks. Women often also talked about other related themes.

My analysis was based on a biographic and comparative approach. I explored narratives in depth and across interviews. I also linked women's narratives to the broader structural context of southern Italy using the extended case method approach (Burawoy 1991), in which ethnographic data are connected to phenomena at a larger scale than the one observed.

'Io so' tosta': moral and religious values as strategies of containment

One strategy through which women tried to contain the impact of the illness was by embodying an attitude of moral strength. A breast cancer diagnosis is a difficult moment and many women experienced anxiety and uncertainty. Lucrezia, a woman in her 40s, told me that she had been very anxious before deciding to undergo a mammography. However, upon discovering she had a tumour, she tried to be courageous – she told me she thought *Già che sono in ballo, balliamo*.[5] The saying, used mostly in southern Italy, indicates the need to give one's best even in the most difficult life circumstances. Although Lucrezia underwent multiple interventions for her cancer, she told me she had 'an incredible desire to get back immediately on [her] feet' and that her approach was to minimise the role of the illness and treatments in her life (compare Manderson 2011 for similar accounts). A number of other women emphasised their 'strong character', suggesting that this helped them to deal with the diagnosis. Carola, a woman in her 60s who maintained a cheerful tone throughout the interview, told me *io so' tosta* (I am tough) and described her relationship with her doctors as follows:

> They have to give you some confidence, although I am not the kind of person to lose heart, to get scared, not at all. I didn't even take it that badly, this thing. As I say 'whether you take it bad or good, you have it and you have to take it out and you have to continue keeping on'.

While she mentioned patients' need for reassurance from their doctors, Carola underscored her strength in explaining how well she reacted to her diagnosis. This strength was mixed with fatalism: Carola thought that a negative attitude would have no impact on the outcome of the illness and that it was important to go on.

Luciana, a woman in her 50s, underlined how relaxed she was towards the illness by insisting that it had no impact on her work. Luciana had several physically demanding jobs, including providing home care for seniors. She described how, immediately before her surgery, the son of one of these seniors asked about her health, telling her, 'I forget [about your health problem] because I see you are so calm that it doesn't seem like you're dealing with this kind of thing.' Luciana considered her strength and her calmness to be assets in confronting the experience. The fact that women established their social role by emphasising their physical strength and their capacity to do physically demanding work has been identified in other southern European contexts (Roseman 2002). The capacity to directly contribute to their family's needs was also important for the identity of the women I met in Salento. Luciana, Carola and most other women I met were working class, doing manual jobs that were often intermittent but critical in financially supporting themselves and their families. In some cases, women had to deal with both the illness and the economic problems brought about by it through direct and indirect costs such as loss of income.

Women may be required to support members of their family and others close to them. Celeste, a woman in her 60s, for example, underwent breast surgery without knowing beforehand whether her breast would be totally or partially removed. Only several hours after surgery, when she woke up to go to the bathroom, did she discover that her breast had been removed. Celeste was not alone at the time; her sister was spending the night with her:

> The night I got down – my sister, the little one, spent the night with me – 'You stay put', I said, 'I have to go to the bathroom.' I went in front with her behind me, I got there, there was a mirror in the bathroom, I look at myself; I say 'but don't you see that they took it off [the breast], no?' My sister was a bit like this [surprised], and then said 'they took it off'. [I answered:] 'So what? Are you crying? We will manage, what are you worrying for?'

Celeste's first reaction upon seeing that her sister was upset by the mastectomy was to minimise the impact of the surgery. Women's reference to the need for strength was linked to their perceived need to protect their family from the impact of the illness. Ida, a woman in her early 60s, found herself in a similar situation when, after her mammogram, the doctor told her the identified lesions were probably cancerous. Her thoughts moved directly to her family, and she told herself: 'I have to be strong for the family, I have to be strong for myself.' When she returned home from the mammogram and preliminary diagnosis, she tried to put aside the news while preparing dinner for her family as usual. However, her sons realised something was wrong and when Ida finally told them the truth they pressed her to immediately call an oncologist to make an appointment. Celeste's and Ida's cases both indicate gendered feelings of duty to continue to care for the rest of the family, even during illness (Sulik 2007b).

As mentioned, the idea that a positive and determined attitude might aid recovery is very common. This is also expressed by metaphors in campaigns and media representations of cancer as a war and of those who die of cancer as losing their battle (see, for example, Garrison 2007). This military terminology has been criticised as dangerous for patients dealing with the disease and the side-effects of treatments (Haines 2014). The attitudes of my interviewees and the vocabulary they used might superficially resemble this rhetoric. However, the idea of fighting a battle against an enemy suggests an individualistic form of heroism absent from the Italian women's accounts. The strength women mentioned was linked to the need to be strong for oneself but also for the people around them – their families – who might depend on them practically and emotionally. Instead of fighting the disease, women's stories emphasised strength to face the disease, reflecting not an individualistic vision of the disease as demanding a heroic attitude but as just one more problem in a life scattered with hardships and difficulties. Mentions of strength alluded to the resilient behaviour of people used to integrating problems and difficulties into their life. The ambiguous role of containment is visible here: although the practice was a resource for my interviewees to manage their illness, their strength was also necessary to avoid others' anguish. It is not clear to what degree this might have hindered their self-care.

Many interviewees found comfort in religion. Italy is a predominantly Catholic country and religiosity is strong in the smaller, semi-rural centres of southern Italy, such as those in which I conducted much of this research. In these locales, many social activities revolve around Catholic rituals, celebrations and institutions. For many women, faith and participation in their community's religious life gave meaning to their illness experience and was a source of support. Annamaria, a woman in her 60s, for example, told me she considered the Virgin Mary to have brought her to undergo a mammography: 'I really believe in the Madonna, I am very devoted and . . . now even more, because I really saw her hands, that she got into [my health].'

In some cases, religion was mixed with fatalism. Carola told me that her calmness in the face of illness reflected her belief that a negative attitude would not have changed the situation: 'The Lord sends it to you as he wants.' Fatalism has often been presented as a dominant trait of southern Italy, one of the factors hindering its development and a feature of the Orientalism directed at the region (see Banfield 1958; Cancian 1961; for a recent critique, Huysseune 2020). Drew and Schoenberg (2011) have argued the need to deconstruct the concept of fatalism in health, particularly when it is assumed to be the reason for non-adherence to cancer screening. They argue that fatalist rhetoric can coexist with very different health-related behaviour patterns. Among my interviewees, fatalism was not linked with any avoidance of screening or treatment, nor was it associated with a passive attitude towards the diagnosis. Instead, it was used to emphasise their perception of a negative attitude as useless. Faith was used as a cultural tool to fully include breast cancer in their life as one incident among others.

Ambivalent forms of containment: family and community

Women often discussed the moral and material support they received from community members. Lucrezia told me that she did not want to upset her elderly mother with her diagnosis, but she was supported by her brothers and her sister-in-law, who 'assisted her as a sister would do'. Lucrezia also discussed her situation with her closer male and female friends, who were very helpful:

> My [female and male] friends have been extremely close to me, also because when I left the hospital and went home I wasn't good for anything [she laughs]. [They helped me] with everything, they took me to the hospital for the follow-up appointments in the early morning. I have received very good assistance [from them].

Lucrezia said that one positive aspect of cancer was discovering how many people cared about her and were there to help her. She was one of the youngest women I met, a professional with an extensive friendship network as well as her family and the support of both family and friends was intertwined. Other women frequently mentioned the help of nieces and nephews, sisters- and brothers-in-law, while others discussed the particular role of close family members, including spouses and adult children. Ida, a woman in her 60s, told me that when she received the invitation to take part in a breast cancer screening programme, her husband insisted that she go. During treatment, her husband and two adult sons were a major source of support:

> The relationship with my family in this situation has been wonderful. I wish for all mothers' daughters [*le figghie de le mamme*], if they have problems, [to have] a husband and children who help. I had a wonderful family, a sister who helped me, all the people within the community, whoever could help me did so. But my husband and my sons were my support [*l'arcu familiare* – literally, 'the family arch']. My husband cleaned the house, better than this the Lord could not send them to me, and they did not know how to do anything [any domestic chore] before this, none of these three.

Ida told me that her community – neighbours, friends and other family members – all helped, but her husband and sons supported her through the most difficult side-effects of the chemotherapy when she was barely able to leave the bed. As she emphasised, before her illness they had never undertaken any domestic work and had never taken care of a sick person. Domestic and care work are considered to be female duties, in particular in rural southern Italy; thus, the men's lack of experience was a way for

Ida to emphasise that before the diagnosis she fulfilled normative gender role expectations.

The women I met not only received care but also provided care to their family members. This two-way dynamic illustrates the relational and reciprocal nature of care, that is, how the vulnerability inherent in human nature means that each of us needs care. However, the women did not benefit unequivocally from the dynamic of care. Breast cancer can be said to question gender expectations that women should do most of the care work – expectations that are common in most families, especially among older couples. Sulik (2007a, 2007b) identified the ways breast cancer disrupts gendered norms of care and redefines care relations to enable support for women with breast cancer. She has also demonstrated how this rebalancing could be limited, characterised by tensions or carry a sense of guilt for the women. Following Sulik, we can further say that a politics of care which addresses everyone's vulnerability, rather than being a gendered burden, is possible only if care is 'defeminised'. That is, if gender asymmetries are redressed and if we stop linking the value of women to their inclination towards care.

In this context, the support that my interviewees received from the men in their family was highly appreciated and often unexpected. The hegemonic masculinity (compare Connell and Messerschmidt 2005) that characterises men in rural and working-class contexts in southern Italy, according to which men should not be involved in care and domestic work, can be redefined by illness. In Ida's case, the versatility of the men in her life, described as being capable of taking a care role, was highly valued. Furthermore, this redefinition of roles seemed to be lasting in many cases. In Ida's case, for instance, the surgery to remove the breast and lymph nodes significantly reduced her arm strength and for a long time after the surgery her husband continued to help to clean their house.

However, families can be deeply ambivalent, as Giulia, who was in her late 60s, described it. She told me that she had felt a lump for quite some time but was reluctant to go to the doctor because she did not want to 'turn [her] house upside down' (*mettere la casa sottosopra*); that is, she did not want to trouble her family. It was only when she noticed the lump was getting bigger that she eventually decided to have it checked. In this case, the need to protect her family pushed containment to dangerous limits. The ambiguity surrounding the family and the larger community can manifest itself in other forms. For example, the attention of a small community can invade privacy and overturn autonomy, as Annamaria experienced. Annamaria, in her 60s, started wearing a wig during chemotherapy because her short hair and scarf were attracting too much attention and people were asking questions she did not want to answer. A strategy that she used during undesired conversations was to control the narrative by, for example, switching the focus from her personal situation to the importance of getting screened. Annamaria added that the disease – in particular the mastectomy and the subsequent changes to her body – had negatively impacted her intimate relationship with her husband. Like Ida, Annamaria was comforted by her relationships with her adult children. She told me that her eldest daughter had taken leave from work to help her during treatment. Annamaria was moved when describing how her daughter helped her to overcome the hair loss caused by chemotherapy:

> I had long hair and when my hair fell out . . . an oncologist had already said to me, 'Madam, I advise you to cut it, because otherwise you will end up with locks in your hand', and OK, I cut it short [but my hair was still falling out], then my daughter took me once and said 'come here, come here, [I will cut your hair]' because I was going to wash my hair. I am rather strong, I try to take things in good humour, let's say, but it's a trauma to see this hair that fell out.

Although Annamaria, like other interviewees, described herself as strong, she was also moved and grateful for her daughter's support. Celeste, who was not married and did not have children, mentioned being helped by her nieces. For most interviewees, family was the main source of support, especially practical help. Women's larger friendship networks were more likely to offer moral support; that is, people to confide in and perhaps to vent to. The interviews I conducted reveal the ambivalent role of the family as both a source of support and an institution that can limit agency. Many women found solace and support within their family, while simultaneously enacting strategies of containment to limit the disease's impact on them.

Drawing on Marxist theory, the nuclear family is often seen as the fundamental institution upon which capitalism has built its exploitative power while also providing a space for patriarchy and gender oppression to thrive, where women have to bear the burden of domestic and reproductive labour (Federici 2012; O'Brien 2020). Family can also be a source of care, love and support, especially in weak welfare states with limited collective support mechanisms. Recently, scholars, while continuing to underscore the demerits of the family, particularly the nuclear family, have also called for the creation of new collective forms of support and care; such forms would redefine family roles to offer the same protections without reproducing capitalistic and gendered forms of exploitation (compare Lewis 2019; O'Brien 2020). Family in southern Italy has been associated with the concept of amoral familism, as proposed by the US sociologist Edward Banfield (1958). In Banfield's view, subject to long debate and criticism (for a recent synthesis, see Huysseune 2020), family relations in southern Italy are pivotal in shaping local society and maintaining the perceived characteristics of a 'backwards society'. According to Banfield, the strong focus on family led people to maximise advantages for their immediate family while ignoring the welfare of the larger community and the values of justice and meritocracy that Banfield considered the basis of modern societies. While largely discredited, these ideas continue to influence images of southern Italy. In my research, the family and the wider community constituted a terrain of gendered conflict; women were aware of this, but they were also aware that, in a society with limited services and support mechanisms, the family was their only safety net.

One disease among others

For many interviewees, the strength and acceptance they showed when dealing with breast cancer were linked to previous experiences of illness. Some interviewees, especially older women, showed me the boxes of drugs they regularly used, emphasising that only some of the drugs were for breast cancer. They located their cancer experience within a broader conception of illness that included their other health problems and the experiences of cancer of other people in their community. This context changed the meaning of their illness. Many women had negative experiences of the medical system prior to their cancer diagnoses and were used to long waiting times and the paternalism and brusqueness that can characterise interactions with medical professionals. These experiences lowered their expectations, such that they were positively surprised when the medical system worked efficiently. Alongside the social experience of cancer and illness, many interviewees had embodied experiences, including the struggle with long-term treatments and their side-effects that limited their quality of life. In this context, they tried to wield knowledge of the uncertainty deriving from the illness to contain the effects of diagnosis.

In the middle of telling me about her breast cancer experience, Sara, a woman in her 50s, deviated to explain how, several years earlier, she had undergone another operation to remove a nodule, ultimately benign, from her tongue. Sara noted the difficulty of the operation: 'Eh, but I had more problems with the tongue, for that I did go through a lot, I was twenty days in Bari, with a fever, I was not drinking, I was not eating.' What appeared to be a sudden change in the narration, apparently irrelevant, functioned to localise the diagnosis and the experience of breast cancer along a continuum of medical problems that Sara considered equal to or more serious than breast cancer. This kind of discursive presentation did not deny the impact of the disease, but highlighted its similarities with past experiences.

In many cases, women's experiences of long-term illness extended to others. Many women had cared for relatives with illnesses, taken them to hospitals and to see doctors and spent nights with them in the hospital. These factors influenced women's own experiences and they often intertwined narrations of their own illness and those of others. When I asked Apollonia, a woman about to turn 70, about her experience with doctors, she mentioned her frequent visits to the hospital for her son and her siblings. All four brothers had had tumours, although in different organs. Apollonia compared her breast cancer experience, which included a mastectomy and chemotherapy, with that of her sister, who had died from stomach cancer. Similarly, Carola often compared her experience with that of her mother, who had died from uterine cancer. When she knew she had to undergo radiotherapy, Carola remembered how hard this had been for her mother. Fortunately, Carola experienced few side-effects. This might reflect improvements in radiotherapy in the years between her mother's treatment and her own. Still, her intimate knowledge of radiotherapy helped Carola to accept the impact of the treatment, which she described as tolerable. Carola's mother was not the only family member to have experienced a serious illness:

> I have a storied family (*una famiglia de storia*) . . . my father died of a tumour, my mother died of a tumour, my husband was operated on twice for a tumour, three times, as then he had polyps in the intestine. My son was operated on because he had a bicuspid valve, and they took out his valve and he has a bypass. I have a tragedy family [she laughs]. Now my husband has had an intervention to the spine because all the vertebrae have gone down, it was a bit of a difficult intervention. In addition, after the intervention he had a paresis to the leg.

Every member of Carola's family had an illness story; some closest to her had had cancer, some had died from it. Apollonia and other interviewees also told me about cancers in their families. Although some women hypothesised vaguely that their cancer could be a 'family problem', neither genetic predisposition nor environmental factors were explored in their medical pathway. The description of cancer as a 'family problem' expressed more the feeling that cancer was a problem with which their families had lived (and supported each other through) for a long time.

Some recent research has emphasised the ways multi-morbidity can introduce cascades; that is, different illnesses and social problems reinforce and provoke each other (Manderson and Warren 2016). Looking beyond the individual to consider the illnesses of others within their family network, it is apparent that although the family can provide a resource for managing one's illness, it can also generate requests for care that can limit an individual's capacity for self-care (Snell-Rood, Merkel and Schoenberg 2018). Salamonsen and colleagues (2016) have shown that, as in the cases I present here, cancer might consequently not be a patient's main concern, either because other illnesses are a greater problem or because the main concerns are derived from illnesses of other individuals in the family network, including responsibilities to care for those individuals. Again, containment is not always a way to solve the problems linked to the illness; it can simply mean that the attention given to one illness is limited because of the presence of other illnesses, whether the patient's or another family member's. Multi-morbidity, whether individual or across a family network, is a challenge for healthcare systems because, even when such systems function efficiently, they are structured to treat each disease separately (Manderson and Warren 2016; Salamonsen et al. 2016).

For my interviewees, the experience of illness intersected with their class position and with their relationship with a healthcare system that is advanced and universal but still features significant problems in terms of waiting times and doctor–patient relationships. The interviews show how these women had tried to transform their experiences – both personal and within their network – as a resource to help them practically and emotionally manage the illness.

I have mentioned how, in Carola's case, most of her family had experienced severe health problems. In her interview, she maintained a calm, undramatic tone and punctuated her account by laughter as she described her own suffering intertwined with that of her family. This does not mean that Carola was unaware of difficulties – she told me that she could write a book on her experiences of illness, both as a caregiver and as a patient. But such experiences rendered illness a known event for Carola and other women, enabling them see it as an unavoidable event that nonetheless must be managed. Further, in the majority of the cases, such suffering was not limited to a single occurrence. The containment of the disease thus was a necessary practice; otherwise, they might be overwhelmed and 'crumble' (*accasciarsi*) in the face of adversity.

Conclusions

In this chapter, in exploring forms of containment of breast cancer, I have focused on three aspects: the positive evaluation of moral strength, also linked to religion and fatalism; the role of the family and the community; and the role of other illnesses – experienced by both the woman and members of her family network – in pushing breast cancer diagnosis and treatment at least in part into the background of their lives.

For the southern Italian women with whom I worked, containing an illness means limiting its weight on the woman's life and the lives of those in her network. Conceptualising this procedure as containment, rather than as coping or adjustment, allows us to emphasise that this process is not only about a positive – let alone heroic – overcoming of the illness. Many women use containment strategies because other problems demand their attention; whether these problems are personal, economic or family-related, the women would not have been able to attend to them if they had not reduced the space breast cancer occupied in their life. Containment does not mean that breast cancer has been overcome, but rather that it is minimised to deal with other aspects of life.

Defining illness and its treatment as tolerable or manageable is a necessary strategy to allow women to continue working through the treatment and manage its aftermath, as was the case for Luciana. The approach was made necessary because the women I interviewed played an important role in the material and moral support of their family. In some cases, illness partially redefined gender roles within the family, pushing men into domestic work from which they were previously exempt. However, the containment process also closed off possible alterations to dominant gender roles. Almost all interviewees had previous illness experiences both as a patient and a caregiver. This two-way dynamic of care was a resource for these women and their families, but it also involved ambiguity. Women in southern Italy care for other family members and, in a context in which care services outside the hospital are rather limited, this can become a full-time activity. With most care work weighing on women, containment becomes necessary to avoid having one's life absorbed by illness, whether their own or that of a family member.

As noted at the beginning of this chapter, cancer, and breast cancer in particular, are dominated by a pink cancer culture that demands that patients take on a heroic role based on consumerism. This culture is strongly individualistic and rooted in neoliberal consumerist ideology. The containment strategies pursued by the women I met in southern Italy, while sharing some aspects with the heroic image of the survivor, such as strength of character, presented a different profile. As described, this different profile can be linked to southern Italy's peripheral status and to the social background of the interviewees. Among the women I met, practices of containment were anchored in collectivistic understandings of illness, in which the experience and the impact of the illness extended beyond the individual patient. Family, religion and the shared experience of illness shaped the ways women contain breast cancer, while at the same time offering them some help to limit the problems that breast cancer introduces to their life.

Acknowledgements

The research on which this chapter is based was made possible by a PhD scholarship in Social and Human Sciences from the Cancéropôle Île-de-France. The chapter was written while I was a Wellcome Trust Research Fellow in Humanities and Social Science (grant number: 212736/Z/18/Z).

Notes

1. There are different definitions of which Italian regions can be defined as part of southern Italy. One approach is to include the regions that were part of the historical Kingdom of Two Sicilies – that is, Abruzzo and all the regions south of Abruzzo, but not Lazio, the region in which Rome is situated. Sardinia, which was historically not part of the Kingdom of Two Sicilies, is usually grouped within southern Italy.
2. The I.Stat estimate of average available income (from economic activities and house ownership) per inhabitant for 2018 was of 22.147 euros in northern Italy and 13.968 euros in southern Italy – see http://dati.istat.it.
3. This is the case for a cluster of lung cancers in Taranto, which have been linked to the presence of large steelworks, and a cluster of stomach, liver, bladder and kidney cancers north of Naples, which have been linked to the presence of illegal toxic dumps – see Greco (2016) for a larger discussion.
4. The interviews were conducted as part of a larger research project on breast surgery that also included fieldwork in northern Italy and the Île-de-France region, as well as interviews with cosmetic surgery patients and medical professionals working in oncology and reconstructive and cosmetic surgery.
5. A literal but imperfect English translation would be 'Given I am at the ball, let's dance', but in Italian there is also the meaning of 'being in the ball' as 'being at stake'.

References

Alonzo, Angelo A. 1979. 'Everyday illness behaviour: A situational approach to health status deviation', *Social Science & Medicine. Part A: Medical Psychology & Medical Sociology* 13: 397–404.

Andersen, Rikke Sand, Bjarke Paarup, Peter Vedsted, Flemming Bro and Jens Soendergaard. 2010. '"Containment" as an analytical framework for understanding patient delay: A qualitative study of cancer patients' symptom interpretation process', *Social Science & Medicine* 71(2): 378–385.

Banfield, Edward C. 1958. *The Moral Basis of a Backward Society*. New York: Free Press.

Burawoy, Michael. 1991. 'The extended case method'. In *Ethnography Unbound: Power and resistance in the modern metropolis*, edited by Michael Burawoy, Alice Burton, Ann Arnett Ferguson, Kathryn J. Fox, Joshua Gamson, Nadine Gartrell, Leslie Hurst et al., 271–290. Berkeley: University of California Press.

Cancian, Frank. 1961. 'The southern Italian peasant: World view and political behavior', *Anthropological Quarterly* 34(1): 1–18.

Connell, R. W. and James W. Messerschmidt. 2005. 'Hegemonic masculinity: Rethinking the concept', *Gender & Society* 19(6): 829–859.

Drew, Elaine M. and Nancy E. Schoenberg. 2011. 'Deconstructing fatalism: Ethnographic perspectives on women's decision making about cancer prevention and treatment', *Medical Anthropology Quarterly* 25(2): 164–182.

Dumit, Joseph. 2012. *Drugs for Life: How pharmaceutical companies define our health*. Durham, NC: Duke University Press.

Federici, Silvia. 2012. *Revolution at Point Zero: Housework, reproduction and feminist struggle*. Oakland, CA: PM Press.

Garrison, Kristen. 2007. 'The personal is rhetorical: War, protest, and peace in breast cancer narratives', *Disability Studies Quarterly* 27(4). http://dx.doi.org/10.18061/dsq.v27i4.52.

Gaventa, John. 1998. 'Poverty, participation and social exclusion in north and south', *IDS Bulletin* 29(1): 50–57.

Gramsci, Antonio. 1966. *La questione meridionale*. Rome: Editori Riuniti.

Greco, Cinzia. 2016. 'Blaming the southern victim: Cancer and the Italian "southern question" in *Terra dei fuochi* and Taranto', *Anthropology Today* 32(3): 16–19.

Greco, Cinzia. 2019. 'Moving for cures: Breast cancer and mobility in Italy', *Medical Anthropology* 38(4): 384–398.

Grossarth-Maticek, Ronald and Hans Eysenck. 1991. 'Creative novation behaviour therapy as a prophylactic treatment for cancer and coronary heart disease: Part I – description of treatment', *Behaviour Research and Therapy* 29(1): 1–16.

Haines, Ian. 2014. 'The war on cancer: Time for a new terminology', *The Lancet* 383(9932): 1183.

Hansen, Ulla Møller, Bryan Cleal, Ingrid Willaing and Tine Tjørnhøj-Thomsen. 2018. 'Managing type 1 diabetes in the context of work life: A matter of containment', *Social Science & Medicine* 219: 70–77.

Huysseune, Michel. 2020. 'Theory travelling through time and space: The reception of the concept of amoral familism', *International Journal of Politics, Culture, and Society* 33(3): 365–388.

Johansen, Venke Frederike, Therese Marie Andrews, Haldis Haukanes and Ulla-Britt Lilleaas. 2013. 'Symbols and meanings in breast cancer awareness campaigns', *NORA* 21(2): 140–155.

King, Samantha. 2006. *Pink Ribbons, Inc.: Breast cancer and the politics of philanthropy*. Minneapolis: University of Minnesota Press.

Klawiter, Maren. 2008. *The Biopolitics of Breast Cancer: Changing cultures of disease and activism*. Minneapolis: University of Minnesota Press.

Lewis, Sophie. 2019. *Full Surrogacy Now: Feminism against family*. London: Verso.

Manderson, Lenore. 2011. *Surface Tensions: Surgery, bodily boundaries, and the social self*. Walnut Creek, CA: Left Coast Press.

Manderson, Lenore. 2020. 'After illness, under diagnosis: Negotiating uncertainty and enacting care', *Medicine Anthropology Theory* 7(2). https://doi.org/10.17157/mat.7.2.685.

Manderson, Lenore and Narelle Warren. 2016. '"Just one thing after another": Recursive cascades and chronic conditions', *Medical Anthropology Quarterly* 30(4): 479–497.

O'Brien, M. E. 2020. 'To abolish the family', *Endnotes* 5: 360–416.

Pelosi, Anthony J. 2019. 'Personality and fatal diseases: Revisiting a scientific scandal', *Journal of Health Psychology* 24(4): 421–439.

Pugliese, Enrico. 2006. *L'Italia tra migrazioni internazionali e migrazioni interne*. Bologna, Italy: Il Mulino.

Roseman, Sharon R. 2002. '"Strong women" and "pretty girls": Self-provisioning, gender, and class identity in rural Galicia (Spain)', *American Anthropologist* 104(1): 22–37.

Salamonsen, Anita, Mona A. Kiil, Agnete Egilsdatter Kristoffersen, Trine Stub and Gro R. Berntsen. 2016. '"My cancer is not my deepest concern": Life course disruption influencing patient pathways and health care needs among persons living with colorectal cancer', *Patient Preference and Adherence* 10: 1591–1600.

Schneider, Jane, ed. 1998. *Italy's 'Southern Question': Orientalism in one country*. Oxford: Berg.

Snell-Rood, Claire, Richard Merkel and Nancy Schoenberg. 2018. 'Negotiating the interpretation of depression shared among kin', *Medical Anthropology* 37(7): 538–552.

Sulik, Gayle. 2007a. 'The balancing act: Care work for the self and coping with breast cancer', *Gender & Society* 21(6): 857–877.

Sulik, Gayle. 2007b. 'On the receiving end: Women, caring, and breast cancer', *Qualitative Sociology* 30(3): 297–314.

Sulik, Gayle. 2010. *Pink Ribbon Blues: How breast cancer culture undermines women's health*. Oxford: Oxford University Press.

Trusson, Diane, Alison Pilnick and Srila Roy. 2016. 'A new normal? Women's experiences of biographical disruption and liminality following treatment for early stage breast cancer', *Social Science & Medicine* 151: 121–129.

10
Noisy bodies and cancer diagnostics in Denmark: exploring the social life of medical semiotics

Rikke Sand Andersen,
Sara Marie Hebsgaard Offersen
and Camilla Hoffman Merrild

Sofie lives with her husband, Christopher, in a small terraced house on the outskirts of a provincial town. Merrild was conducting ethnographic research on social differences in health and visited the couple shortly after Sofie was diagnosed with cancer for the second time. Eighteen years had passed since Sofie's first diagnosis and now the cancer has spread to her bones. When asked how her new diagnosis came about, Sofie embarked on an extended explanation:

>Sofie: Well, for a long time I had really been in pain. But they [the doctors] did not really believe that it might be cancer in my bones. So, I was sent to phys [physiotherapy] and training, rehabilitation and what not. And then I was sent to another hospital, and I asked the doctor up there, if they could not damn well investigate whether it was cancer that had spread.
>Merrild: You simply said that to them?
>Sofie: Yes, well, they said that then it would be a completely different situation we were in. And I said to them, I know that. That was also the time when I was told that the pain

was a fictitious thing, you know. It cannot be measured, they said. But my daughter was there with me, and she says to him: 'When my mother says she is in pain, then she is in pain.' I asked them again if they would investigate, and he agreed, and sent me to yet another hospital that could do it fast, and I was scanned. The next day I was called up by our own doctor, and she told me that it was a cancer that had crumbled away the bones in my neck.

Social inequalities in health are intricate and rooted in complex configurations of social, cultural and biological differences that we are only beginning to understand and conceptualise (Nguyen and Peschard 2003; Seeberg and Meinert 2015). In the global south, structural violence in the forms of poverty, gendered inequalities and race- and caste-based discrimination limit access to healthcare (Farmer 1999). In such settings, inequalities in health increase and capitalise on structural vulnerabilities such as cramped living conditions, malnutrition and co-morbidities (Biehl, Good and Kleinman 2007; Farmer 1999). In comparison with countries in the global south, Danish society is characterised by a high degree of social equity and operates under the ideal of free and equal access to healthcare ideally available to all people living in Denmark. Yet health inequalities have always been evident and are increasing (Udesen et al. 2020). Among people diagnosed with cancer between 2005 and 2013 (most recent data, 2022), only 53 per cent of those from the lowest income bracket had survived after five years (2010 and 2018), compared with 69 per cent of those from the highest income bracket (Olsen, Kjær and Dalton 2019). For males, life expectancy may fluctuate by as much as 10–13 years between those at the top and the bottom of the income ladder (Brønnum-Hansen and Baadsgaard 2008). These trends emphasise that welfare societies are not immune to the deepening social inequalities occurring globally. In Denmark, despite growing investment in cancer control programmes, the gap in life expectancy rates has been widening since the 1980s, while differences in relative survival for most cancers are becoming increasingly apparent (Dalton et al. 2019).

Looking closely at Sofie's life helps us to better understand what lies behind these numbers. She grew up in a poor family. She started working at the age of 13, first as a seamstress and then as a shop assistant. Her husband Christopher suffers from diabetes, irregular heart rhythms and liver disease after many years of heavy drinking. Sofie has three children from a previous marriage and her youngest

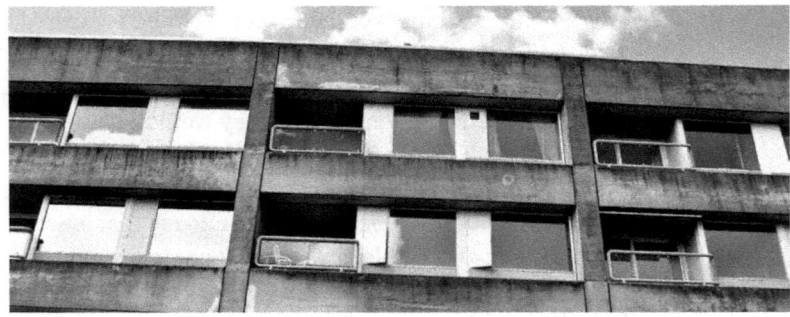

Figure 10.1 Picture of a social housing association in Denmark. Photo: The Danish Cancer Society.

son is mentally ill and lives in sheltered housing. Now, at 66, Sofie's bodily condition is a testimony to the adversity of her life (Kleinman and Kleinman 1994). Often racked with pain and enduring stiffness in her joints, she moves slowly around her small apartment, relying on a seat walker and sporadic assistance from Christopher. For several months before she was diagnosed with cancer, Sofie had endured diffuse and indistinct pain, but she was unable to convince her doctors that she did not need more physiotherapy, as they failed to see the distinction between Sofie's previous discomfort and her more recent pain. Now, after several major operations, Sofie's bones have crumbled and her backbone is held together by metal screws that enable her to hold her upper body somewhat upright.

Danish researchers have often pointed to gendered or social bias on the part of practitioners, as well as lifestyle differences and social and cultural differences in health-seeking behaviour and decision-making, including in relation to cancer (Ibfelt et al. 2013; Vilhelmsson and Östergren 2018). People with lower incomes and low levels of education are less likely than wealthier, better-educated people to seek medical care or recognise cancer symptoms and are more likely to have negative beliefs about cancer treatment (Hvidberg et al. 2015). While these studies are sensitive to how local actors embody meaning-making and engage with the healthcare system, more recently, clinical ethnographers have advanced the hypothesis that biomedical knowledge is 'biased', not in the sense that it is 'wrong', but in the sense that it is partial knowledge constructed from prevailing understandings of the body and society (Manderson and Ross 2020; Nguyen and Peschard 2003). For instance, if biological norms and diagnostic tests are standardised on middle-class, white populations, they may not perform accurately in groups that differ biologically or in the way they articulate and embody changes. Dominant forms of knowledge of the body, and the care politics (Tronto 2012) and therapeutic practices through which the body is made visible or attended to, are central to our understandings of social inequalities in health (Manderson and Ross 2020). In some ways, by virtue of its efficacy, medicine has 'become an unwitting accomplice to biological inscription of social hierarchies', as noted by Nguyen and Peschard (2003: 457).

In this chapter we suggest that medical representations of cancer symptoms, or what we refer to as medical semiotics, and the promise of bodily distinctions that these representations bring into diagnostic infrastructures, are imaginaries that augment the deepening of social inequalities in health in Denmark. Through detailed examination of ethnographic cases, we explore what we call 'the noisy bodies' (Merrild, Vedsted and Andersen 2017: 14) of people who live on the margins of the Danish welfare society. We ask how they experience, attend to and represent their bodies and we describe the limitations they face in making the kinds of bodily distinctions that are encouraged by contemporary cancer care politics advocating 'early diagnosis' and 'do not delay' messages (Andersen 2017).

Material and methods

In this chapter we draw on data from interlinked ethnographic field studies conducted by Merrild, Offersen and Andersen on cancer diagnostics between 2012 and 2019. The studies were part of a research portfolio carried out in a multidisciplinary research centre at Aarhus University, in Denmark, observing ongoing changes in cancer control. All studies explored everyday forms of embodiment, people's perceptions of cancer, cancer symptoms and healthcare-seeking practices. Intermittently from 2012 to 2019, Merrild and Offersen worked in different sites in suburban and rural areas in Jutland, Denmark, among different social classes. Merrild carried out fieldwork among people who lived in socially deprived areas, who had little or no education and low levels of income and who may be described as coming from disadvantaged backgrounds. Some of Merrild's interlocutors were suffering from cancer, and some were not (for example, Merrild and Andersen 2019). Offersen conducted fieldwork in two local communities: one could be characterised as middle class with ready access to regional services and one could be characterised as rural and 'remote' in terms of geography and access to healthcare services. Her interlocutors were not suffering from cancer but did participate in national cancer screening programmes and would occasionally seek care on suspicion of cancer, along with other worries (Offersen et al. 2018). Andersen conducted fieldwork in suburban areas of Jutland, exploring clinical encounters and care-seeking practices in four general practice clinics between 2012 and 2018 and visiting people in their homes; all her interlocutors had sought care on the basis of suspected cancer (Andersen 2017). In total, we conducted 89 interviews with potential patients on healthcare-seeking experiences and everyday embodied experiences of cancer risks and symptoms and more than 50 interviews with healthcare professionals in GP clinics – nurses, receptionists and GPs – on their experiences of diagnostic encounters. Although we worked with some people who were suffering from cancer, the majority of our interlocutors were not. This meant that we relied on prospective empirical material on embodied experience and diagnostics when exploring peoples' notions of cancer symptoms and healthcare seeking. People with migrant backgrounds (such as Kurds, Somalis or Arabs) were present in our fields, as patients or health professionals in GP clinics or as neighbours and community members in the local settings where Merrild and Offersen worked. None of our key interlocutors or interviewees represented these migrant groups, however. We realise that this is not an innocuous decision; it somewhat speaks to a conceptualisation of the existence of bounded cultures or an imagined sameness among 'indigenous Danes' (Rytter 2019). However, as suggested in the literature on inequalities in health, people with migrant backgrounds, particularly people from Arab and African countries, may face particular language- or stigma-related problems when engaging with the Danish healthcare system (Rosenkrands et al. 2020). Also, due to their experiences of replacements, racism and economic hardships, their health status and the social sufferings that mark their lives may differ from that of people with non-migrant backgrounds (Ølholm et al. 2016). Due to these potential differences in life experiences and health status, we decided not to include them as interviewees and key interlocutors in our studies.

In writing this chapter, we draw on cases from our respective fieldwork, focusing on people who may be characterised as living less privileged lives in relation to income, education and social status, illuminating the embodiment of social inequalities observed across our data. In this chapter we present the lives of Jenny and Sofie, both of whom Merrild followed for more than a year.

Cancer care politics and an expanding medical semiotics

Medical semiotics, or what by medical convention is considered the symptoms and signs of underlying disease, have, as eloquently shown by Angel Martinez-Hernandez (2000), historically played an important role in how physicians order and interpret patient bodies. Symptoms such as pains or dizziness have traditionally in biomedicine been considered 'a patient's subjective illness complaint', which, through the inference of a physician, are either assigned to pathological categories or deemed subjective and clinically irrelevant (Martinez-Hernandez 2000: 5–7). Signs such as blood or lumps, on the other hand, were considered to constitute more direct semiotic references to biology and the diseased body (Martinez-Hernandez 2000). Since the publication of Foucault's (1994) *The Birth of the Clinic* (first published in the late 1960s) social scientists have debated the continuing importance of signs and symptoms in medicine, some suggesting that the role of medical semiotics, and particularly symptoms, has been pushed to the background because of the increasing reliance on technology. It has been suggested that the patient is now scanned rather than listened to (Martinez-Hernandez 2000).

As Andersen (2017) has proposed elsewhere, however, the role of medical semiotics is increasingly important in building diagnostic infrastructures. Diagnostic infrastructures rely on people moving around (seeking care or being referred) and medical semiotics are important indictors of action in this process. This is also the case in contemporary cancer diagnostic infrastructures. In order to reap the benefits of biotechnologies such as PET and MRI scanners that can make early disease stages visible, it is essential that potential patients respond to 'early' signs and symptoms of disease. While Foucault (1994) predicted that medical practice of diagnosis by symptoms would vanish with the birth of anatomical pathology, we suggest that the biotechnologies that make the interior of bodies visible have not lessened the importance of symptoms to medicine, but they have somewhat changed their status from a signifier of disease (or risk) to a signifier of action. Contemporary care politics are directed towards the governing of the tactile, sensorial body.

This change in status, and the importance of medical semiotics to building diagnostic infrastructures, are evident in the cancer politics that have dominated the Danish healthcare system since the early 2000s. In the late 1990s, in contrast to other high-income nations, Denmark was struggling with high cancer morbidity and mortality and cancer epidemiologists and health promoters pointed to delay in diagnosis and treatment as the main culprit (Jensen, Mainz and Overgaard 2002).

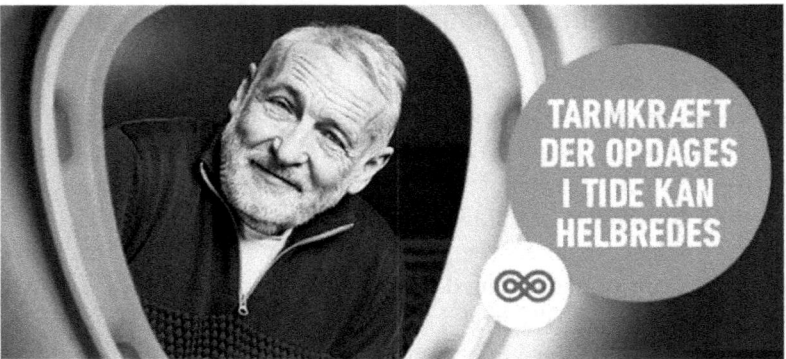

Figure 10.2 'Colon cancer detected in due time can be cured'. Poster from a cancer-awareness campaign run by the Danish Cancer Society in 2014.

This brought about unparalleled regulation of the healthcare system, with an explicit focus on timely cancer diagnosis and treatment. The public and healthcare professionals were subject to several campaigns promoting 'do not delay' messages, which urged people to act on any perceived anomaly, such as a persistent cough, blood in stools or unexplained pain. Reference to cancer symptoms was also central in the clinical guidelines that serve as a reference point between general practice clinics and hospitals. In order to produce knowledge of relevance for early diagnosis initiatives, cancer epidemiologists and health promoters turned towards cancer symptoms (for example, Hamilton 2010), seeking to identify those 'early symptoms' through which 'early stage cancer tumours' make themselves perceptible to the sensing tactile body.

Epidemiological knowledge on the classification of symptoms of cancer is based on probability theory and provides quantified probabilities regarding the risk of having a cancer when experiencing a specific bodily sensation. From epidemiological as well as clinical perspectives, knowledge on what may be classified as a cancer symptom rests on the assumption that the ill body speaks to us through symptoms. Following this logic, symptoms may be identified in empirical research and grouped into taxonomies according to the underlying cancer thought to cause them. Although cancer risk as indicated by particular bodily sensations increases with age and when symptom categories cluster, it is assumed that a colon cancer (for example) will reveal itself in the same ways across humans of different ages or cultures, depending on the stage of the tumour growth.

Some early papers and discussions within the cancer epidemiological community suggested pursuing a 5 per cent risk strategy, meaning that people presenting in the clinic with symptoms indicating a 5 per cent risk of an underlying cancer should be further investigated. Leading epidemiologists and clinicians, however, quickly realised that this would result in a rather short list of cancer symptoms, which would not solve the problem of delay in presentation for diagnosis and treatment (see Andersen 2017). As an example, haemoptysis or coughing, which may indicate lung cancer, has predictive values of approximately 0.4 and 2.4 per cent when occurring as a single symptom among people seeking care. The same low risks are reproduced when exploring relations between rectal bleeding and colon cancer, or post-coital bleeding and ovarian cancer (Hamilton 2009). During the past decade, as early diagnosis and 'do not delay' messages have gained increasing political and public momentum, we have seen a vast expansion of what clinicians and epidemiologists now classify as cancer symptoms (Andersen 2017). Today, the lists of cancer symptoms in guidelines and awareness-raising campaigns are extensive. People are encouraged, for example, to seek care (and doctors are encouraged to raise cancer suspicion) if they experience tiredness, feel bloated, lose weight, if their digestive habits change, if they experience unexplained pain, if stiffness lingers for too long, if they cough or have an itch and so forth.

As noted by Offersen and colleagues (2016), this list of symptom categories feeds into the production of a cancer discourse that teaches us that a cancer may be hiding in silence within our bodies and it reminds us that bodies, in our contemporary world, are heavily invested with meaning. Medical semiotics carry social meanings, and contemporary biomedicine encourages self-conscious and hyper-vigilant forms of embodied attention and meaning-making (Jain 2013; Nichter 2008). Moreover, as we now describe, the medical semiotics of cancer does not consider the biological human body as a site of both considerable commonality and difference (Lock 1993; Lock and Nguyen 2010). Nor does it take into account that that people's perceptions of potential illness are continually altered from the standpoints of different bodies embedded in a world of practice and future.

Attending to noisy bodies

The interpretation of embodied sensations as symptoms of potential disease is always a social process, as are the movements (such as care seeking) that follow the recognition of symptoms (Merrild, Vedsted and Andersen 2017; Offersen et al. 2016). Hinton, Howes and Kirmayer (2008) describe sensations as social and cultural schemas, while Hay (2010) emphasises the need to understand how bodily representations are formed and when sensations are perceived as 'symptoms of underlying disease'. Such perspectives emphasise that the processes by which bodily representations occur must be studied across cultural and historical contexts (Hinton, Howes and Kirmayer 2008). With the concept of the noisy body, we would like to take the discussion further, to emphasise what Kleinman and Kleinman (1994: 710) called 'the unfolding of culture into the body' and what Lock (1993: xxii–xxiv) has described as 'local biology'. Lock posited the idea of local biologies to account for ethnographic findings that symptom experiences at the end of menstruation differed significantly between women in Japan and women in North America. Lock insisted that this difference was not merely due to cultural differences in bodily representations, but was also material, in the sense that female bodies in Japan and in North America should not be considered as similar specimens of a universal body (Lock 1993). She asserted that the concept of local biologies accounts for the way in which 'the embodied experience of physical sensations, including those of well-being, health, and illness, is in part informed by the material body, itself contingent on evolutionary, environmental, social and individual variables' (Lock 1993: 39).

While the Kleinmans did not conceptualise the biological basis of embodied experiences in the same way as Lock, they share the idea of the biological body as both culturally inscribed, and – as critical for understanding our argument – consequential to social practices, such as the making of bodily distinctions. Reflecting on empirical work on the effects of decades of trauma in China, since pre-World War II revolutions through to Tiananmen Square, they describe symptoms as 'lived memories' (Kleinman and Kleinman 1994: 713–715), bridging troublesome social contexts of their interlocutors and their bodily selves. They state that the body responds to trauma with bodily symptoms, hence bodies and cultures are interwoven, with this 'interweaving' situated in the body-self, which they define as the 'transpersonal moral-somatic medium of local worlds' (Kleinman and Kleinman 1994: 716). These concepts suggest that embodied experiences, and the ways in which they are attended to and interpreted, are informed not only by cultural understandings of physiology, health and illness, but also by the ways that medicines, foods and social hardship may act in and on the biological body. The cultural representations of bodies and the transformation of sensations into symptoms differ across cultural and historical settings, but in addition, the flesh (Frank 1995) or the material biological bodies (Lock 1993) differ. We emphasise this interweaving of social inequality and embodied experience through the concept of noisy bodies. The notion of noisy body reminds us that bodies are flesh, and flesh cannot, as Frank (1995) insisted, be denied. But as body-selves, people experience and make sense of their material bodies in particular ways and this has implications for healthcare seeking and how, when or if people engage in diagnostics (Andersen, Nichter and Risør 2017).

Sofie

In Denmark people rarely speak about social class. Danes, like other Scandinavians, like to think of themselves as living in a 'classless society' (*klasseløst samfund*). This does not mean that differences or social hierarchies do not exist. As suggested by the Danish anthropologist Steffen Jöhncke, it more likely reflects dominant cultural ideals that equate being middle class to being Danish. These ideals 'veil rather than remove class as a structural principle' (Jöhncke 2011: 46). As described, inequalities in health are deepening, as are differences in income and social hierarchies. The Danish welfare state is built on the ideal of universal coverage, with healthcare services, subsidised childcare, education and student grants and social security schemes all financed through income tax; access to most services is not means tested. Since the 1980s, however, neoliberal ideologies of governance have emerged with accompanying welfare state retractions and the consequences of this are unevenly distributed (Merrild and Andersen 2019; Vallgårda 2019). Housing reforms, workforce reforms, restricted access to social benefits and the introduction of less generous unemployment benefits have made lives increasingly difficult for those most disadvantaged. The translation of inequality into precise figures is difficult, but conservative estimates suggest that 250,000 Danes (of a total population of 5.8 million) live in poverty. Despite Denmark's publicly funded healthcare system, co-payments for medication and other out-of-pocket costs such as transport pose significant burdens on those from low-income households (Bakah and Raphael 2017). Moreover, circumstances such as being unemployed, being overweight or suffering from so-called lifestyle-related diseases increasingly function as social markers of failure and intensify stigma (Dencker-Larsen and Lundberg 2016).

Sofie and Christopher affirm these inequalities. They have both worked in unskilled jobs and unlike most of the Danish population, they live in a rented house instead of owning their own property. Before her first experience of cancer 18 years ago, Sofie undertook physically demanding, low-paid work. However, she has spent the past 13 years reliant on social benefits. Christopher, who used to work in a warehouse, also lives off early retirement benefits. He has been drinking heavily for many years, which has severely damaged his liver. He also suffers from diabetes, which is worsening as he does not follow the dietary recommendations. Early retirement and social welfare benefits are intended to support people who, due to health-related problems, are unable to work. Recently, however, the criteria to qualify for these benefits has changed, causing great concern to many who are dependent on them. Sofie and Christopher often complain about the ongoing assessment of their health by the state 'to make sure that they are still too sick to work', as Sofie says.

Despite changes in the distribution of social benefits, Sofie and Christopher enjoy free access to medical services, with their GP serving as the primary entry point. They are both experienced users of the healthcare system. Christopher has a home nurse who visits fortnightly to check his medications, discuss lifestyle issues and engage in acute consultations due to falls, pains or other concerns. Sofie rarely contacts healthcare providers outside her scheduled appointments. She only consults with her GP when she needs to adjust her medications for cancer control and chronic pain and she is in regular contact with the hospital department which is monitoring the progression of her cancer.

Sofie likes to spend most of her time at home, trying to keep the house in order. She worries about how she is going to manage it as she easily tires and her joints are painful. Simple things like cleaning the top shelves in the kitchen cabinets are difficult and to do so, she has to ask her neighbour or her daughter for help. Christopher does not really help much. He sometimes vacuums the floor and Sofie does not think that she can expect more from him. 'He has not been used to doing that sort of stuff', she says. Sofie struggles to manage her and Christopher's day-to-day care and their failing, unstable bodies without relying too much on others. She does not complain, having grown up in a poor family where she had to contribute from an early age. Before meeting Christopher, she lived for many years as a single mother with three small children, so she is used to 'getting along' (*klare sig selv*), moving uncomfortably around using the walking chair, trying to position her body in a way that causes her least pain.

On several occasions before cancer in her neck was diagnosed, Sofie made attempts to voice her embodied experiences of pain and tiredness and to articulate them in a way that would make sense to her GP, on whom she knew she had to rely in order to get the scan that she believed she needed. When asked how long she had experienced her pains, she answered: 'I tried to tell them about my pains, for almost a year I tried to explain. But they, well nobody really, wanted to accept that it hurt as much as it did.' Sofie finally decided to raise her voice, which, for her, was unusual: 'I was sure that it was cancer. But they didn't think so. To them it did not fit the pattern.'

If we think of the noisy body as a kind of body-self (Kleinman and Kleinman 1994) that expresses underlying diseases, traumas or memories of loss through sensorial changes, it becomes clear how people such as Sofie, who live difficult lives, do not benefit from an expanded medical sign system that feeds on clear associations between the specifics of bodily sensations and the classification of underlying disease and which considers cancer a standard disease, similar across biological bodies. Such a sign system does not enable Sofie to share her sentience or to 'recognise the early cancer symptoms'. Her pains could have 'just' been her old pains, not pains signifying new kinds of diseases; her tiredness could have 'just' been caused by her daily struggles to make ends meet. Sofie's situation thus exemplifies how lives marked by distress and illness shape noisy bodies that bear poor witness to the subtle sensorial changes that an early stage cancer might have produced. But it also shows how bodies are always, already, embedded in a series of culturally shared forms of knowledge that help organise them (Nichter 2008). Sofie had to raise her voice in order to be heard. Many of our interlocutors, living in difficult life circumstances, share this experience; often they must present their complaints several times to doctors and their symptom experiences are explained with reference to already identified diseases.

Noisy bodies are thus easily rejected in the clinical setting, because suitable explanatory models are already in place. Simply thinking of symptom awareness as a cognitive or informational act does not take into consideration that embodied experience is an assemblage of social processes, which flows back and forth through the social spaces of institutions and the body-self (Kleinman and Kleinman 1994).

Jenny

Jenny is 65 years old. She lives together with her husband and their adult daughter, Christina, in a small apartment in a poor suburban area in Jutland. The apartment seems cramped, perhaps because it is packed with stacks of newspapers and large furniture and the TV is always on. During one of Merrild's visits, Jenny has a cast on her arm. She suffers from tenosynovitis, caused by the strain of carrying Christina up and down the stairs after she suffered a complicated fracture in her leg. Christina suffered brain damage during birth and she has ADHD and non-verbal learning difficulties; she still lives at home due to her disabilities. Jenny spends most of her time at home caring for Christina, the youngest of her seven children. Like Christina, Jenny's other children all suffer from physical and cognitive disabilities and all of them live on social benefits. Her husband is away at work all day and she has few friends. 'I have become lazy, and watch too much television', she sighs when Merrild asked her about her everyday life. There is a sense of stillness in her life, a sense of detachment and little motivation; she just manages to get through each day. Jenny has spent most of her life at home taking care of her children. She worries about Christina, who has attempted to take her life several times, and she is concerned about her if one day Jenny is not able to care for her.

Jenny worked as a social and healthcare worker for about 12 years, but due to her asthma and COPD (chronic obstructive pulmonary disease), her retirement pension kicked in when she was in her late 30s. This was long before it became so difficult to qualify for it. Much like Sofie, Jenny does not seem to complain. Almost to the contrary. When asked if she has other things that she struggles with, apart from her asthma and COPD, she replies, 'well, not more than other people are dealing with . . . high blood pressure, cholesterol. And then my ADHD of course.' As she talks, however, it seems that she has more to deal with than most people. She suffers from chronic pain stemming from her osteoarthritis. Some years back she suffered from a blood clot. 'Oh yeah, and I also have depression and get anti-depressants for that', she casually remarks. As a result of her many conditions, she takes a lot of medication, which comes prepacked from the pharmacy. She can name the different drugs she is taking and she is aware of their possible side-effects. The anti-depressants make her tired and the drug that keeps her blood pressure 'in the range of the normal', as she describes it, sometimes makes her dizzy and gives her a headache.

There is no doubt that life is hard for Jenny. She manages most things on her own and she is used to getting things done without help. When we talk about friends and family, she goes quiet, as if pondering. She has few friends. And she is often tired, so it is easier just staying at home. It is clear that she is trying to keep her life, and that of her daughter, her health and her body, afloat and much of the time she does this while lying on her bed, alone in her apartment watching the TV.

Jenny tries her best to manage the many side-effects of her medications and she elaborately explains how much she can take and when it is best for her to take what drugs. When asked how she knows all this, she tells Merrild about a variety of Facebook groups and websites where there is considerable information about her conditions. Jenny is a member of several online groups where members share their predicaments, their knowledge of bodily experiences and new forms of treatment.

Jenny knows the healthcare system well. She regularly visits her GP and she sees a lung specialist three times a year. When she talks about the healthcare system, she seems frustrated, like Sofie. 'In the old days, when you went to see the doctor, they would take care of your problems, but now you can only bring one thing to each consultation', which is often the case in GP clinics who operate on tight time schedules. But for Jenny, 'there is never just one thing' and last time she saw her GP she also raised the concern that she might have cancer. Almost a year earlier she noticed a birthmark on her back, which was itching and annoying her. So the week before she met with Merrild, she consulted her GP: the pain in her arm was becoming unbearable and the combination of painkillers and anti-depressants were making her tired. Just as she was leaving, she asked the doctor if he would mind taking a quick look at her back. She knew quite well that this was not the proper process, 'they want you to make separate appointments for stuff like that, but usually they agree to take a quick look', she says with a sneaky smile. She continues to talk about her arm and how it is difficult to help Christina while it is in a cast. Merrild asks what happened with the thing on her back. 'He [the doctor] said it was fine. He could remove it another time, if I wanted him to. But you know there is all this talk about skin cancer and stuff like that so I figured I might as well ask. And it had been so annoying on my back, and also, you know, I was feeling tired due to the drugs and all.'

Jenny may be what is often referred to as a 'frequent attender' in public health terms, meaning that she has contact with her GP more than eight times a year (Sundhedsdatastyrelsen 2020). The frequent attender label is perceived negatively by the Danish public. Using the healthcare system in a sensible manner is culturally condoned. People are often eager to emphasise that they do not misuse the healthcare system and our interlocutors often maintained 'I rarely or ever go to see my doctor' or 'I only go when it is necessary.' However, an expanding medical semiotics, and the noisy body of Jenny, which bears the memories of pharmaceuticals and her depression, her respiratory illness and her hardships carrying

Christina around (figuratively and literally), makes it difficult for her to be sensible and to make the kinds of bodily distinctions that would ensure an 'early diagnosis' if cancer were growing inside her body. Jenny's noisy body is an assemblage of the ingestion of drugs and social and mental hardships, which stimulate her sensations 'concordant with cultural norms' (Nichter 2008: 163). Jenny is expected to be tired.

Jenny's hardships make clear how different life experiences enable and constrain different kinds of embodied experiences, actions and care-seeking decisions. If we follow the idea that symptoms may be the 'lived memories of past trauma' (Kleinman and Kleinman 1994: 716) and that the material body is contingent on environmental variables such as alcohol or drugs, then Sofie's pains and Jenny's tiredness are not just 'the symptoms that make up' their noisy bodies, but also the phenomenal point of departure from which they experience their worlds (Merleau-Ponty 2012: 100). How people engage in cancer diagnostics depends not only on how they interpret their bodies but also on the culturally embodied possibilities they have for distinguishing feeling fine from being sick (Hay 2010). The limitations of Jenny's and Sofie's (and their doctor's) possibilities to 'hear their body speak' (Frank 1995: 29) thus reveal the failed promise inherent in contemporary cancer semiotics and exemplify how medical disease representations may add to the production of inequalities in health. The vague and expanding medical semiotics that constitute contemporary cancer diagnostic infrastructures do not easily translate into useful sensorial distinctions for people living with noisy bodies. The noisy body is thus a poor phenomenal point of departure to detect an early cancer. This compounds the effects of a clinical culture that values efficiency (only one problem at a time operated in tight time schedules) in the cultural figure of 'the sensible patient' and, in the Danish context, a sensible middle-class patient (Offersen et al. 2016).

Conclusion: the failed promise of contemporary medical semiotics

In the late 1990s and early 2000s when cancer diagnostic infrastructures in Denmark were readjusted in order to avoid the long waiting lists that had long characterised the health system, symptom awareness was coined as a key strategy to accelerate diagnostic procedures. Since then, changes in diagnostic infrastructures have solved some problems: people do not wait for months before undergoing diagnostic investigations and patients are increasingly diagnosed with cancers that are curable (Jensen, Tørring and Vedsted 2017). The social inequalities in cancer, however, have not been addressed; rather they seem to have widened (Dalton et al. 2019).

Within health promotion circles, in Denmark and beyond, inequalities in cancer survival are often explained with reference to lack of recognition of cancer symptoms and delays in care seeking (Davies et al. 2018; Ibfelt et al. 2013). In a recent report on early cancer diagnosis, the World Health Organization highlighted the importance of awareness of cancer symptoms as key to improving diagnosis: 'Patients must be aware of specific cancer symptoms, understand the urgency of these symptoms, overcome fear or stigma associated with cancer and be able to access primary care' (WHO 2017: 13). While such statements may work to encourage countries to improve access to care, they do not reflect the complex assemblage of biological, social and cultural dimensions that converge in the embodied practices of awareness and care seeking. This situation becomes infinitely more complex in local settings where the western scientific tradition of 'symptoms and cancer' has been imported and grafted onto local knowledge and forms of life (Livingston 2012). Simply thinking of symptom awareness as a cognitive or informational act does not take into consideration the way in which embodied experience is 'an assemblage of social processes that come together as a medium of interaction that flows back and forth through the social spaces of institutions and the body-self' (Kleinman and Kleinman 1994: 712).

In this chapter, we have explored the social life of medical semiotics and, specifically, how cancer symptom representations are produced and how people give meaning to bodily sensations within specific individual, social and biological contexts. This approach allows us to understand how disease representations bring new possibilities of perception and embodiment to social life. We have also shown how these fail to deliver useful distinctions for people living difficult lives at the margins of the Danish welfare state, illustrating the interconnections between health, institutions and bodily experiences. By viewing symptom experiences as embodiments of biological, social and cultural contexts, we have emphasised how (potential) failures to make distinctions between bodily sensations (as symptoms of underlying disease or as part of the everyday 'normal') are not merely attributed to errors of judgement but to aspects of local biology; or how culture and the biological body are interwoven (Kleinman and Kleinman 1994). Following Nguyen and Peschard (2003: 254), we suggest that 'the inequality – disease relationship is enhanced through the classificatory rationalities that dominates contemporary medicine'. Medical representations of cancer symptoms, and the promise of embodied distinctions they bring into the building of diagnostic infrastructures, are thus imaginaries that augment the deepening of social inequalities in health in Denmark. By paying attention to the social life of medical semiotics, we are reminded that there exists what Rose (2007: 254) might have called 'a biopolitical vocation' to sensorial experience and bodily attention that adds to the production of differentiating social statuses and privilege.

The notion that culture 'unfolds into the body' (Kleinman and Kleinman 1994: 710), or the idea that the material body should not be left unattended when researching embodied experiences such as symptoms or sensations, is not new to anthropology. Scheper-Hughes and Lock (1987) used the concept of the 'mindful body' in their initial attempts 'to problematise the body' in anthropology and other social sciences. Recently, focus on violence and trauma, coupled with the subjectivity, has generated interdisciplinary conversations threading together the processes of individual experiences within specific cultural, social and biological contexts (Biehl, Good and Kleinman 2007; Hinton and Good 2009; Meinert and Whyte 2017; White et al. 2017). Hinton and Good (2009), for example, found that strong emotional states, including states of anxiety, are often re-experienced as a cascade of embodied sensations associated with evocative memories, triggered by particular spaces, times and breaches in social relations, as well as by states of uncertainty and threats to the future. Lock (2018: 458) has further conceptualised environmental and human entanglements through critical discussions with epigenetics, reminding us of the complexity of the questions raised once we take the material body seriously in anthropological analysis. As these insights gain momentum, a research agenda on the social life of medical semiotics will continue to improve our understandings of the relationship between social inequality and embodied experience. Overall, we know little about how social response and the experience of sensations are changing in socio-political cultural contexts exposed to new types of medical semiotics, produced and developed in response to new medical ideologies and technologies (Nichter 2008). If we glimpse into the future, the convergence of big data and vast resources to build artificial intelligence based diagnostic technologies will most likely result in diagnostic imaginaries where biographical and biological details, behaviours and sensorial experiences are transformed into new kinds of medical semiotics. How will such kinds of medical representations or visions of diagnostics transform into bodily experiences and how or when people ask themselves: Am I sick? Should I seek care? And, critically, how will they alter or exacerbate global inequalities in health?

Acknowledgements

We would like to thank our interlocutors who have patiently worked with us, sometimes for months on end. Also, our research would not have been possible without funding for research projects on healthcare seeking, social inequality and cancer diagnostics from the Danish Cancer Society (R82-A5456-B1478, R48-A2686-B1478, R85-A5678-B1478) and Helsefonden (Health Foundation). The foundations have not been involved in the preparation of this chapter nor in the underlying research. Data collection and management followed Danish data protection laws and guidelines and was approved by the internal review board at the authors' place of employment, which holds a permanent authorisation to gather research data in Denmark. The idea and initial writings for the chapter was developed in collaboration among the authors with inspiration from work published by Merrild, Andersen and Vedsted (2017) and from a paper by Offersen and Andersen in the panel about 'Anthropological Contributions for Understanding the Global Cancer Divide' at the conference of the Association of Social Anthropology (UK), University of East Anglia, Norwich, September 2019. Andersen wrote the first draft, and when it was decided to represent empirical material from Merrild's fieldwork in the chapter she wrote the first storylines with detailed insights into the lives of Sofie and Jenny. All authors contributed to the analysis, theoretical conversations and the final writing of the chapter.

References

Andersen, Rikke Sand. 2017. 'Directing the senses in the contemporary orientations to cancer disease control: Debating symptom research', *Tidsskrift for Forskning i Sygdom Og Samfund* 26: 145–167. https://doi.org/10.7146/tfss.v14i26.26282.

Andersen, Rikke Sand, Mark Nichter and Mette Bech Risør. 2017. 'Sensations, symptoms and healthcare seeking', *Anthropology in Action* 24(1): 1–5. https://doi.org/10.3167/aia.2017.240101.

Bakah, May and Dennis Raphael. 2017. 'New hypotheses regarding the Danish health puzzle', *Scandinavian Journal of Public Health* 45(8): 799–808. https://doi.org/10.1177/1403494817698889.

Biehl, João, Byron J. Good and Arthur Kleinman. 2007. *Subjectivity: Ethnographic investigations*. Berkeley: University of California Press.

Brønnum-Hansen, Henrik and Mikkel Baadsgaard. 2008. 'Increase in social inequality in health expectancy in Denmark', *Scandinavian Journal of Public Health* 36(1): 44–51. https://doi.org/10.1177/1403494807085193.

Dalton, Susanne Oksbjerg, Maja Halgren Olsen, Christoffer Johansen, Jørgen H. Olsen and Kaae Klaus Andersen. 2019. 'Socioeconomic inequality in cancer survival – changes over time: A population-based study, Denmark, 1987–2013', *Acta Oncologica* 58(5): 737–744. https://doi.org/10.1080/0284186X.2019.1566772.

Davies, Hilary, Afrodita Marcu, Peter Vedsted and Katriina L. Whitaker. 2018. 'Is lower symptom recognition associated with socioeconomic inequalities in help-seeking for potential breast cancer symptoms?' *Psycho-Oncology* 27(2): 626–632. https://doi.org/10.1002/pon.4557.

Dencker-Larsen, Sofie and Kjetil G. Lundberg. 2016. 'Depicted welfare-recipient stereotypes in Norway and Denmark: A photo-elicitation study', *Nordic Journal of Social Research* 7: 1–15. https://doi.org/10.15845/njsr.v7i0.866.

Farmer, Paul. 1999. *Infections and Inequalities: The modern plagues*. Berkeley: University of California Press.

Foucault, Michel. 1994. *The Birth of the Clinic: An archaeology of medical perception*. New York: Pantheon Books.

Frank, Arthur. 1995. *The Wounded Storyteller: Body, illness, and ethics*. Chicago: University of Chicago Press.

Hamilton, William. 2009. 'The CAPER studies: Five case-control studies aimed at identifying and quantifying the risk of cancer in symptomatic primary care patients', *British Journal of Cancer* 101(2): S80–86. https://doi.org/10.1038/sj.bjc.6605396.

Hamilton, William. 2010. 'Cancer diagnosis in primary care', *British Journal of General Practice* 60(571): 121–128. https://doi.org/10.3399/bjgp10X483175.

Hay, M. Cameron. 2010. 'Suffering in a productive world: Chronic illness, visibility, and the space beyond agency', *American Ethnologist* 37(2): 259–274. https://doi.org/10.1111/j.1548-1425.2010.01254.x.

Hinton, Devon E. and Byron Good, eds. 2009. *Culture and Panic Disorder*. Stanford, CA: Stanford University Press.

Hinton, Devon and Susan Hinton. 2002. 'Panic disorder, somatization, and the new cross-cultural psychiatry: The seven bodies of a medical anthropology of panic', *Culture, Medicine and Psychiatry* 26(2): 155–178.

Hinton, Devon, David Howes and Laurence Kirmayer. 2008. 'Toward a medical anthropology of sensations: Definitions and research agenda', *Transcultural Psychiatry* 45: 163–197. https://doi.org/10.1177/1363461508089763.

Hvidberg, Line, Christian Nielsen Wulff, Anette Fischer Pedersen and Peter Vedsted. 2015. 'Barriers to healthcare seeking, beliefs about cancer and the role of socio-economic position: A Danish population-based study', *Preventive Medicine* 71C: 107–113. https://doi.org/10.1016/j.ypmed.2014.12.007.

Ibfelt, Else Helene, Susanne Krüger Kjær, Claus Høgdall, Marianne Steding-Jessen, Troels Kjær, Merete Osler, Christoffer Johansen et al. 2013. 'Socioeconomic position and survival after cervical cancer: Influence of cancer stage, comorbidity and smoking among Danish women diagnosed between 2005 and 2010', *British Journal of Cancer* 109(9): 2489–2495. https://doi.org/10.1038/bjc.2013.558.

Jain, S. Lochlann. 2013. *Malignant: How cancer becomes us*. London: University of California Press.

Jensen, Annie, Jan Mainz and Jens Overgaard. 2002. 'Impact of delay on diagnosis and treatment of primary lung cancer', *Acta Oncologica* 41(2): 147–152. https://doi.org/10.1080/028418602753669517.

Jensen, Henry, Marie Louise Tørring and Peter Vedsted. 2017. 'Prognostic consequences of implementing cancer patient pathways in Denmark: A comparative cohort study of symptomatic cancer patients in primary care', *BMC Cancer* 17: 627. https://doi.org/10.1186/s12885-017-3623-8.

Jöhncke, Steffen. 2011. 'Integrating Denmark: The welfare state as a national(ist) accomplishment'. In *The Question of Integration: Immigration, exclusion and the Danish welfare state*, edited by Karen Fog Olwig and Karsten Pærregaard, 30–53. Newcastle upon Tyne: Cambridge Scholars.

Kleinman, Arthur and Joan Kleinman. 1994. 'How bodies remember: Social memory and bodily experience of criticism, resistance, and delegitimation following China's Cultural Revolution', *New Literary History* 25(3): 707–723. http://www.jstor.org/stable/469474.

Livingston, Julie. 2012. *Improvising Medicine: An African oncology ward in an emerging cancer epidemic*. Durham, NC: Duke University Press.

Lock, Margaret. 1993. *Encounters with Aging: Mythologies of menopause in Japan and North America*. Berkeley: University of California Press.

Lock, Margaret. 2018. 'Mutable environments and permeable human bodies', *Journal of the Royal Anthropological Institute* 24(3): 449–474. https://doi.org/10.1111/1467-9655.12855.

Lock, Margaret and Vinh-Kim Nguyen. 2010. *An Anthropology of Biomedicine*. Singapore: Wiley Blackwell.

Manderson, Lenore and Fiona C. Ross. 2020. 'Publics, technologies and interventions in reproduction and early life in South Africa', *Humanities and Social Sciences Communications* 7(40). https://doi.org/10.1057/s41599-020-0531-3.

Martinez-Hernandez, Angel. 2000. *What's Behind the Symptom? On psychiatric observation and anthropological understanding*. Abingdon: Routledge.

Meinert, Lotte and Susan Reynolds Whyte. 2017. 'Social sensations of symptoms: Embodied socialities of HIV and trauma in Uganda', *Anthropology in Action* 24(1): 20–26. https://doi.org/10.3167/aia.2017.240104.

Merleau-Ponty, Maurice. 2012. *Phenomenology of Perception*, translated by Donald A. Landes. Oxford and New York: Routledge.

Merrild, Camilla Hoffmann and Rikke Sand Andersen. 2019. 'Welfare transformations and expectations of sameness: Living on the margins in Denmark', *Nordic Journal of Social Research* 10(1): 66–84. https://doi.org/10.7577/njsr.2858.

Merrild, Camilla Hoffman, Peter Vedsted and Rikke Sand Andersen. 2017. 'Noisy lives, noisy bodies: Exploring the sensorial embodiment of class', *Anthropology in Action* 24(1): 13–19. https://doi.org/10.3167/aia.2017.240103.

Nguyen, Vinh-Kim and Karine Peschard. 2003. 'Anthropology, inequality and disease: A review', *Annual Review of Anthropology* 32(1): 447–474. https://doi.org/10.1146/annurev.anthro.32.061002.093412.

Nichter, Mark. 2008. 'Coming to our senses: Appreciating the sensorial in medical anthropology', *Transcultural Psychiatry* 45: 163–197. https://doi.org/10.1177/1363461508089764.

Offersen, Sara Marie Hebsgaard, Mette Bech Risør, Peter Vedsted and Rikke Sand Andersen. 2016. 'Am I fine? Exploring everyday life ambiguities and potentialities of embodied sensations in a Danish middle-class community', *Medicine Anthropology Theory* 3(3): 23–45.

Offersen, Sara Marie Hebsgaard, Mette Bech Risør, Peter Vedsted and Rikke Sand Andersen. 2018. 'Cancer-before-cancer: Mythologies of cancer in everyday life', *MAT Medicine Anthropology Theory* 5(5): 30–52. https://doi.org/10.17157/mat.5.5.540.

Ølholm, Anne M., Janne B. Christensen, Stine L. Kamionka, Mette L. Eriksen and Morten Sodemann. 2016. 'Hospital-based case management for migrant patients: A systematic review', *Public Health Panorama* 2(4): 515–526.

Olsen, Maja Halgren, Trille Kristina Kjær and Susanne Oksbjerg Dalton. 2019. *Hvidbog: Social Ulighed I Kræft i Danmark*. Copenhagen: Kræftens Bekæmpelse.

Rose, Niklas. 2007. *The Politics of Life Itself*. Oxford: Princeton University Press.

Rosenkrands, Hanna S., Maria Kristiansen, Amalie Lipczak Hansen and Marie Norredam. 2020. 'Providing targeted healthcare services for immigrants with complex health needs', *Danish Medical Journal* 67(10). Accessed 15 September 2022. https://ugeskriftet.dk/dmj/providing-targeted-healthcare-services-immigrants-complex-health-needs.

Rytter, Mikkel. 2019. 'Writing against integration: Danish imaginaries of culture, race and belonging', *Ethnos* 84(4): 678–697. https://doi.org/10.1080/00141844.2018.1458745.

Scheper-Hughes, Nancy and Margaret Lock. 1987. 'The mindful body: A prolegomenon to future work in medical anthropology', *Medical Anthropology Quarterly* 1(1): 6–41.

Seeberg, Jens and Lotte Meinert. 2015. 'Can epidemics be noncommunicable? Reflections on the spread of "noncommunicable" diseases', *Medicine Anthropology Theory* 2(2): 54–71. https://doi.org/10.17157/mat.2.2.171.

Sundhedsdatastyrelsen. 2020. 'Udvalgte nøgletal for praksisområdet 2009–2019'. Accessed 17 August 2021. https://sundhedsdatastyrelsen.dk/da/tal-og-analyser/analyser-og-rapporter/sundhedsvaesenet/noegletal-om-sundhedsvaesenet.

Tronto, Joan. 2012. 'Democratic care politics in an age of limits'. In *Global Variations in the Political and Social Economies of Care: Worlds apart*, edited by Shara Rahzavi and Silke Staab, 29–42. London: Routledge.

Udesen, Caroline Holt, Carina Skaarup, Maria Nivi Schmidt Petersen and Anette Kjær Ersbøll. 2020. *Social Ulighed i Sundhed og Sygdom*. Copenhagen: Sundhedsstyrelsen.

Vallgårda, Signild. 2019. *Hvordan Mindsker vi Uligheden i Sundhed*. Copenhagen: Informations Forlag.

Vilhelmsson, Andreas and Per Olaf Östergren. 2018. 'Reducing health inequalities with interventions targeting behavioral factors among individuals with low levels of education: A rapid review', *PLoS ONE* 13(4): e0195774. https://doi.org/10.1371/journal.pone.0195774.

White, Jarrod, Louise Newman, Glenn Melvin, Lenore Manderson and Katrina Simpson. 2017. 'Contextualizing posttraumatic stress disorder within culturally diverse groups: A comparison of Holocaust survivors and Sudanese refugees', *International Journal of Culture and Mental Health* 11(3): 321–331. https://doi.org/10.1080/17542863.2017.1377271.

WHO (World Health Organization). 2017. *Guide to Cancer Early Diagnosis*. Geneva: World Health Organization.

11
'Hard-to-reach'? Meanings at the margins of care and risk in cancer research

Kelly Fagan Robinson and
Ignacia Arteaga Pérez

It had taken us the better part of three hours by train, bus and foot to get to this community centre in a rural English village; it was even more difficult to reach a conversation like the one we were about to hear. The women spanning four generations who had agreed to talk repeatedly told us (the researchers) that they expected us 'to not get it'. One woman explained what it was like to be part of the community of Gypsy Roma Travellers – or 'GRTs' as they referred to themselves.[1] Her story came out in a steady stream and detached tone:

> My best friend is dying from bowel cancer. He is 43. Eighteen months ago he had rectal bleeding . . . He was told it was probably internal piles, but would be better for him to have the colonoscopy in order to know for sure. He never went. And he got iller and iller. Refusing to go and embarrassed about what was happening to him. By the time he went in it had metastasised. He's gone on the Facebook page to tell everyone his story. Dying has released him from the stigma [of cancer occurring in the community]. He saved the life of a 21-year-old girl who read his post and got the lump in her throat checked. But it's all been realised too late.

The woman paused and took a sip of her tea. Three other women who had introduced us to the service users at the drop-in GRT support hub ('the Hub') were listening, but the woman didn't seem to mind. She spoke as if recounting something from the deep past, already distant and completed. She brightened, wondering aloud how to manage her multiple roles in the community as childminder, lay church leader and housekeeper, just to make ends meet. 'Cancer' was like another country; not only did it mean long journeys to seek biomedical care from unknown towns, but cancer also went largely untold, only spoken of once finished. Cancer was bracketed off from everyday challenges in order to carry on living.

Another GRT woman, still mourning the death of her father from cancer, told us that when he was dying she did not accept help from nurses, because that was 'the family's responsibility'. She took care of him together with her other three siblings, receiving a hospital bed and some medical appliances from the National Health Service (NHS) 'but nothing else'. We naively asked: Why not? We were promptly scolded: 'We Roma people don't do that!' The woman's family would not admit her dying father into hospice. Cleaning his body, his care 'has to stay in the family!'

Discrimination was inherent in the experience of people in the GRT community of healthcare, particularly when accessing clinics and hospitals. This mistrust 'goes deep', the woman continued. The limited times they sought healthcare for their children when they had a high fever, GRT participants commented that they were turned away because of their lack of permanent residence. Other times, they felt embarrassed that they couldn't understand and be understood by clinicians. They were usually not allowed to bring their relatives – 'too many, too loud' – so they went alone and did not always feel able to ask questions. Others explained that GRT often try to deal with things themselves, sharing resources at hand and taking other people's medications rather than going to a clinic.

During our two-month field study on non-engagement in cancer screening, we were shown how 'cancer', 'care' and 'risk' are polysemic, informed by and situated within individual and local collectives' lived experiences. In this chapter, we ethnographically engage with the many different ways that collective and person-specific understandings of cancer affect healthcare research, particularly in attempts to engage groups whose lifeways are marginalised and underrepresented. We draw on relational understandings of care and risk as our interlocutors conceptualise and enact them (Gelsthorpe, Mody and Sloan 2020). We argue that differences in the value of knowledge-making practices may undermine effective connections between health researchers and the publics they seek to support. Ignoring these differences results in reproducing epistemic opacity, that is, remaining oblivious in our practices as researchers, so missing out the ways in which others create the knowledge required to manage health, illness and wellness in their everyday lives.

Health inequalities, cancer and risk in the United Kingdom

The United Kingdom is marked by inequalities in access to healthcare services and wellness outcomes. From epidemiological reports, we learn that residents of affluent areas in England live on average 9.3 (men) and 7.5 (women) years more, respectively, than those who live in the most deprived areas (Iacobucci 2019). The unequal distribution of cancer outcomes mirrors the social gradient of deprivation, with disproportionate incidences of disability and death affecting poorer populations. A report collecting evidence of the impact of health inequalities on cancer statistics in the United Kingdom demonstrated that higher economic deprivation rates are correlated with observations of higher cancer risks such as smoking and obesity,[2] higher rates of cancer diagnosed at emergency presentation or late-stage disease, worse quality of care and treatment and worse survival for people living in disadvantaged communities (CRUK 2020). Markers such as 'economic deprivation' inform genetic and environmental predispositions to cancer as they affect people's bodies, health-seeking practices, relationships with peers and healthcare services and ways of living.

In 2000 the Department of Health (DH) launched the NHS Cancer Plan, the first comprehensive national programme on cancer, which created a strategy to reduce inequalities and achieve survival rates that would compare with the best in Europe.[3] Fourteen years later, the NHS 5-Year Forward Plan set out to commence a paradigm shift in cancer diagnosis. The ambition was to change the diagnostic picture from one in which most patients were diagnosed when cancer had already advanced to other parts of the body ('emergency presentations' of metastasised cancers in acute care clinics) to a scenario where most patients are diagnosed when tumours are incipient and localised. This shift would be possible, the plan stipulated, through increased screening coverage free at the point of care and through improved referral pathways in primary care settings.

The promise of early cancer detection in the United Kingdom is underpinned by the idea that cancer is more treatable if diagnosed early, thus resulting in concern that access to detection programmes is available and ensuring that those most at risk engage with these services on time.

Here, diagnostic delays are understood with reference to the gap between symptom presentation and appropriate diagnosis (Andersen et al. 2009). This form of vigilant medicine – that is, medical attention which requires ongoing engagement both by clinicians and patients – reinforces the idea of populations as objects of biopolitical control, defined by normative expectations of prudence, watchfulness and responsibility (Lupton 1995).

In England, over 30 per cent of those invited to undergo cancer screening do not engage with the services offered by the NHS (Richards 2019). Applied health researchers in the United Kingdom (Marlow et al. 2017; Palmer et al. 2014; Smith et al. 2016) have identified patterns of non-engagement to cancer screening due to people's motivational and structural barriers. Previous attempts to tackle observed lack of engagement has been to rethink the procedures to approach eligible participants while counteracting the economic and language barriers of some groups so they can engage, as well as understanding the perceived benefits, knowledge base and attitudes towards screening from people who usually do not engage. This is done to promote services adequately and to 'help people make an informed choice'. The challenge in this context is getting to know the situated perceptions of cancer risk of underserved populations who do not engage with preventative programmes and so present to the clinic with symptoms late.

Anthropologists have contributed to this debate by drawing attention to shortcomings in mainstream approaches to health promotion in the community that reinforce dynamics of medical authority (Balshem 1993) and the differential effects of those messages across social groups (Manderson, Markovic and Quinn 2005). This scholarship outlines normative understandings of what is to be a good citizen based on sociomoral landscapes of action tied to personal responsibility. Increasing the presence of biomedicine in everyday lives, health promotion messages have shaped expectations about how people are supposed to engage with their bodies and make sense of bodily sensations (Offersen, Vedsted and Andersen 2017). Attempts to understand non-engagement with health services have deployed techniques of contextualisation, unpacking what is otherwise ring-fenced as 'awareness', looking instead at how sensations become symptoms through an interpretative and socially situated process of somatic modes of attention (Throop 2010). In other studies, the stunted temporality of lived experiences of those who can only struggle through the everyday, and are thus unable to engage in long-term planning, has also been highlighted (Desjarlais 1997), illustrating the temporal clashes between episodic times of biomedical interventions and biographical lifetimes (Aragón Martín 2017). Building on this scholarship, in this chapter we delve into the gaps observed in the uptake of cancer screening to unpack emic definitions of 'care' and 'risk' as articulated by people who, because of their social position, are 'at risk for negative health outcomes through their interface with socioeconomic, political and normative hierarchies' (Bourgois et al. 2017: 17).

Tackling epistemic opacities

Within the context of healthcare inequalities, structurally vulnerable populations are often deemed 'hard to reach'. This label is mostly used by epidemiologists and public health and health psychology researchers to describe tensions in the relationship between social groups and healthcare services to explain degrees of user engagement (Rockliffe et al. 2018). Cancer Research UK, the biggest charitable research organisation in the field, has defined it as the 'spectrum of different groups and communities across the UK who are not benefiting as much as the general population in terms of improved cancer outcomes' (CRUK 2014). As this definition attests, there is a tendency to see 'hard-to-reachness' as explaining the underrepresentation of certain groups in health research as well as their overrepresentation in mortality and morbidity statistics. The concept expresses both the challenges of including certain subjects in research and clinical landscapes and of improving health outcomes for them (Witham et al. 2020). Yet the use of this concept also reflects a desire for health services to innovatively engage with these social groups, based on the conviction that facilitating access to healthcare is beneficial (Raghavan et al. 2018).

The ambiguity with which the published and grey literature defines who belongs to a hard-to-reach or seldom-heard group is pervasive (Witham et al. 2020). Strathern's (2020) distinction between 'connections' and 'relations' is productive in this context. She writes that 'relations have an effect on – and pose problems for – actors far beyond the scope of their connections' (Strathern 2020: 8). Macrostructural determinants such as healthcare agendas, governmental dictums and geographic proximity may encourage grouping people together for demographic categorisation, when actually these persons have no knowledge of or social or physical connection with one another.

Categorical practices have methodological implications, leading us to propose that 'hard-to-reachness' stems from a problem of visibility from the point of view of public health initiatives. We can see the problem the other way around by recognising that the limitations that health researchers face might be reinforced by the unhelpful construction of 'at-risk' as framing some people as unknowledgeable or structurally limited, indirectly blaming them for 'opting out' of health promotion efforts (Freimuth and Mettger 1990; Minkler 1989). With interventions framed to fix adherence or compliance to medical mandates, Balshem (1993) shows that members of already marginalised US communities, when invited to participate in health promotion and prevention studies, often feel disenfranchised and patronised by the healthcare and behavioural mandates which focus on 'lifestyle choices', disregarding the environmental and structural issues that affect participants' lives. Considering this purview, in which 'talking about cancer translates into talk about other things' (Balshem 1993: 5), we realised that asking non-participants to articulate motivations and barriers concerning cancer screening would miss the opportunity to learn something far more pertinent: the practices through which people live and act on risks.

Our fieldwork focused on Cambridgeshire, representing former industrial centres, hubs of agribusiness and a university city. The local topography is flat and in some areas land lies below sea level, making its soil rich and fertile for agriculture (37 per cent of England's vegetables are grown here). The land is prone to severe flooding, discouraging public investment in transport infrastructure in more rural villages. Surrounded on all sides by countryside is Cambridge itself, where housing prices and incomes are significantly higher than in neighbouring towns. In the city, technological innovation and industry is increasing, sharply contrasting with the agricultural and manual work that is most prevalent around it. This region has one of the highest percentages of migrants in England. The university city claims over 40 per cent of its residents are in higher education. Meanwhile, the agribusinesses in the lowlands have historically employed a high number of seasonal migrant workers from minority ethnic communities, including GRT and contract labourers primarily from Eastern European countries. Uncertainty related to Brexit outcomes at the time of the fieldwork had left many workers, previously employed on longer-term seasonal agribusiness contracts, on short-term part-time contracts or out of work entirely. This had resulted in increased precarity and many had become homeless.

Koch and James (2022: 2) have argued that in a climate of ongoing economic austerity policies, which have at the time of writing been in place for over a decade in Britain, 'the state is today shedding its care responsibilities. The shift in public services delivery is both ideological and procedural.' Politics of care in the United Kingdom have been driven by the attrition of socialised welfare programmes and neoliberal practices of governance which are reliant on, and produce, particular kinds of British citizens. Infrastructural shift and technological innovation, key objectives in both the coalition government and the Conservative government which has succeeded it (Taylor Gooby 2017) assume a normative neoliberal subject: one with a stable home and family life, steady employment, knowledge of law and process, a bank account and easy access to the internet through which it can all be maintained (Robinson and Carroll, in press). Few of our research participants laid claim to all if any of these resources. When UK residents – particularly those who do not claim membership within the citizenry – cannot meet these expectations, they soon also find that the safety nets previously offered by the welfare state become very scarce. And yet 'expectations for welfare and support often outlast state-imposed cuts to welfare [. . .] they espouse and embrace "alternatives to austerity"' (Bear 2015; cited in Koch and James 2022: 11). Along these lines, innovations in the ways our interlocutors view care and how (and from whom) they sought support reflected new forms of found kinship and revised definitions of what 'care' and 'risk' meant in their lives.

With this complex backdrop in mind, we began by thinking strategically about the existing infrastructures through which we could most rapidly meet people from diverse ethnic and occupational backgrounds. With the support of six local service leaders who worked primarily in libraries and community centres rather than in more formalised state-institutional spaces, we participated in arts and therapy-based activities, visiting several groups multiple times; we took these interactions as a starting point for informal discussions about risk, cancer and care. In the space of eight weeks, we met 135 participants from 15 research sites. Participants could be characterised as people sleeping rough; people struggling with serious and long-term psychiatric and somatic conditions; people recovering from drug and alcohol addictions; elderly men and women living in rural and peri-urban areas; and people who self-identified as belonging to non-English, ethnic groups.

Several of these groups had grassroots support services which were led by and catered for specific collectives within the local community. These included the GRT Hub, 'the Centre', a space for people in various stages of recovery from addiction and 'the House', which supports homeless people. Service managers worked hard to connect their offerings with local council services and access to complementary health and well-being interventions. This was informed by a strong sense of 'clientship' (Reynolds Whyte, Meinert and Twebaze 2014: 56–69), cultivating strong social connection by offering services in exchange for service users' continued attendance and commitment. In each of these three settings, the service leaders had arranged for weekly clinics to increase access to biomedical care; these were keenly attended by many service users. However, at the time of writing, despite service managers' interest and attempts, none of these spaces were yet offering cancer screening. Service users tended to present at these clinics with suspected late-stage cancers or died before it was ever detected.

Like Luxardo's experience of fieldwork on cancer prevention among marginalised people in Argentina, we realised that, given people's circumstances, it was 'hardly relevant to these communities to continue asking questions about cancer' (Luxardo 2020: 4). Explaining the relevance of open-ended methodologies that incorporated the concerns that people have as research priorities, Luxardo sought to undo some of the cynicism about health researchers who come to the field, collect data on what they consider important and leave without impacting people's lives. Our ethnographic methods attempted to address how health researchers might avoid further undermining the low level of trust that members of underrepresented groups have on health research (Hunn 2017). We initially focused on 'care' and 'risk' as we participated in multiple arts-therapy initiatives which, on the basis of 'well-being', had attracted many local people from underrepresented groups. Seeking to avoid being solely extractive in our efforts to collect materials, we also followed guidelines from the National Institute of Health Research defining the need for compensation of participants' time and expertise. By bringing food and grocery vouchers and paying for the use of community resources we facilitated an 'economy of care' by which interlocutors felt encouraged to participate and to encourage their friends to come too, knowing that the incentive would directly address their most pressing needs.

In the section that follows, we analyse the ways that different life-ways give rise to unique communicative 'affordances' (Keane 2018), by which environments, education, affective responses and individual experiences inform a person's knowledge-making resources. We do so to better understand the ways that people come to define particular concepts, which in turn informs the questions researchers and health promotion campaigns ask and seek to answer. This requires understanding valuations of risk and care on our interlocutors' own terms.

Semiotics of care

Structural barriers consistently affected our research; transport cancellations, flooding and language barriers were chief amongst these.

Yet our greatest barrier to meaningful engagement was epistemic opacity – our inability to properly grasp what our interlocutors were telling us. For several weeks we failed to understand that 'care' meant intervention, coercion and exclusion to many participants. These experiences directly informed whether interlocutors engaged with cancer prevention programmes or not.

On our final day of fieldwork at 'the Centre' for drug and alcohol addiction recovery, a service user named Laura told us: 'If you've ever had social services involved, "care" will always mean people getting taken away.' Two other peer-mentors, Kris and James, agreed. The 'care' delivered by social services meant the perpetual risk of children being removed, or interventions in the form of incarceration, almost always resulting in families being demolished. However, more recently, the meaning of care in their lives had been shifting. For three years Laura, Kris and James had been up at 8 a.m. every morning just to come in to have something to do. Laura's consistency in attending had led her to become a 'service-user rep', supporting the Centre's peer mentors as they supported the other Centre service users during recovery. Engaging in recovery at the Centre was crucial for two reasons: first because Laura knew that if she wasn't 'clean' she would risk losing custody of her children; and secondly, it transformed what 'care' meant: from negative/nominative ('going into Care') to positive/transitive (a practice of flourishing).

As Canton and Dominey (2020: 15) contend, there is 'a dark side of care, when harm and oppression can be concealed behind pretensions to care'. This idea was foremost in the minds of many of our interlocutors. Faced with this interpretation, we had to step away from our own assumptions of 'care = positive' and map out the dimensions which were contributing to their perception of 'care = negative'. We ultimately broke the term down into three significant relations of care that we outline below. In these, we argue that structural barriers are not key to understanding low engagement of certain communities with cancer prevention, but, rather, concepts of 'care' are constructed through and entangled with these barriers to determine people's health status (Bourgois et al. 2017).

Care and regimes of harm/addiction

In addition to the interlocutors at the Centre, several people we met at the GRT Hub and the House for rough sleepers also experienced drug or alcohol addiction. In interlocutors' narratives, addiction recovery was less a 'journey' and more a framework on which elements of their lives were positioned. As Garcia (2008: 726) argued, 'the model of chronicity likens addiction to a lifelong disease. It is enduring and relapses are an expected occurrence.' Eating, exercise, sleep, (lack of) housing, socialising, relationships, childcare even television watching, contributed to the lived realities of ongoing recovery. Given that withdrawal can induce unpleasant and sometimes painful sensations including dizziness, nausea, tremors and cramps on top of biomedically recognised symptoms associated with maintenance treatment, the 'care' that addiction recovery represented in these interlocutors' lives was difficult and at times violent.

Stigma was a further problem, with the 'addict' label sticking long into recovery, making the idea of seeking clinical interventions for pain and illness less palatable. Service users consistently explained to us that in encounters with healthcare professionals they 'only ever feel treated like addicts'. James, Kris and Laura had all been clean for more than one year, but each time they entered a General Practice (GP) surgery they were confronted by what they perceived to be poor treatment and were frequently subjected to gross prejudice. One man explained he'd gone to a GP for a groin lump and pain that concerned him, but upon seeing him the practice receptionist said: 'We have no methadone.' This, he said, wasn't the kind of care he needed or wanted and so he left. Others at the Centre commented that this kind of prejudice was because their bodies still bore visible marks of previous using, including cracked and missing teeth and/or scars from needle use. Participants were uncomfortable about having to explain their stories to every treating physician, especially when suspicion about their deservingness as patients haunted the clinical encounters from the start.

In other conversations with interlocutors at the Centre and later with people at the House, a further concern was raised: people with addiction issues who are still regularly using tend to disengage with their bodies – the constant fatigue, dizziness, soreness, a lump or just a sense that something is 'off' – is either not felt or is not attended to. Though acting on those sensations might lead to earlier pursuit of medical attention and thus to earlier cancer detection,[4] the drugs used for recreation or therapy can produce a form of anaesthesia that lasts long periods of time,[5] masking discomfort, and may even be perceived as the most likely cause of the symptoms. One user summarised what many others intimated: 'You're much more likely to notice [something in] others before you notice yourself . . . you don't notice the pain.' Kris said that when people stopped methadone treatment 'they suddenly notice the pains they didn't have before', but James clarified 'they had them, they just couldn't feel them'. As a result people may notice the warning of tumours' presence only at very advanced stages, when there is nothing much that can be done.

Once off methadone, sensations of pain suddenly became meaningful and are interpreted as symptoms that warrant healthcare seeking because they interfere with daily living (Hay 2008). At the same time, their psychic pain was no longer muted by the chemical supports on which the person had previously relied, and so they were newly aware of their difficulties. Merrild, Vedsted and Andersen (2017; see also Chapter 10 by Andersen, Offersen and Merrild, this volume) show that underprivileged Danish citizens accessing primary care are considered to have noisy bodies with too many ailments that cannot be accommodated by the healthcare infrastructure. The unmasking of bodily sensations heralded for the service users that their bodies were also 'noisy', now generating more complex health problems. Manny explained that he'd suddenly noticed 'symptoms since I've come off drugs – heroin used to block pain [. . . Now I have an abscess] in my groin, I may look [clean] on the outside but I don't feel [that way] on the inside.' Experiences of discrimination within primary care settings, coupled with disconnected or unnoticed pain-full bodily sensations, over time rendered service users much less likely to visit their GP for preventative care, even if sometimes they were really frightened about something.

Coercive care

At least a third of the service users at the Centre, several people we met at the House and one person at the Hub had first-hand experiences of prison, wherein pain, hardship and deprivations were all aligned with 'care'. Laura, Kris and Paul explained that many interlocutors initially attended the Centre in response to a court-mandated requirement for parole. Care in this context assumed the shape of control over their bodies and minds, both while 'inside' and upon release in order to secure a future 'better life' via rehabilitation programmes. Weller (2013: 15) defines this as 'coercive care', the legal control-taking of someone's life and choices in anticipation of danger or harm; they are 'forms of state intervention that mandate benevolent medical and social intervention for the "person's own good"'.

Law enforcement institutions consistently reminded people that their own poor choices and behaviours had put them into prison. Choice itself was now countermanded by lack of options in terms of free movement, variety of activity and even healthcare access (Canton and Dominey 2020). For example, one man explained that while the constant arrests he and his acquaintances had experienced in the past were mostly triggered by drug use, domestic violence and theft, he had been introduced to hard drugs, particularly prescribed opioids, when he was in prison. Though this claim was unsubstantiated, service users also referred to the fact that healthcare professionals working in carceral institutions freely give tranquilisers to make prisoners more docile. Larry explained:

> In prison if you need to see a doctor – [it] takes weeks to get in there. [And then they're] giving painkillers at the prison – [you get into trouble] if you don't take them three times a day. In prison you can easily end up with other people who can drag you down. If anything [you] learn is to cut away from other people.

In a space where choices were institutionally limited, chosen disenfranchisement represented a form of care in which attempts to move away from relationships in prison (including health professionals in Larry's case), and away from some friends and relatives once out of custody, were techniques to care for oneself. This choice of social isolation was a key step for many interlocutors aiming to become both autonomous and well. People who would in most other contexts be expected to be figures of trust – siblings, parents or clinicians – in these cases represented threats as potential sources of addiction, violence or other well-being risks.

Larry's experience, and those of other service users, was that care was coercive and compulsory, limiting not only their choices but, by being medicated, inhibiting their ability to act in the world. This increased mistrust of healthcare institutions and workers and increased many interlocutors' sense of self-reliance. This reminded us of the GRT response to illness, a striving to avoid institutional care and 'get by without' even if they were in pain. 'We are not attention seekers', a middle-aged GRT women told us in the Hub. For these interlocutors, 'care' conducted via acts of removal and isolation was the only possible free choice. It facilitated reclamation of autonomy in their future decisions and directions by virtue of refusing what is offered. As Larry, who was GRT, explained, cutting off people also cuts out claims people can make on you; this, for him, was a clear act of self-care and independence.

Care and interventions of the state in families

The third definition of care as communicated by these interlocutors related to state intervention in the care of children. Parents feared that their own challenges (addiction, domestic violence, incarceration) would mean that their children would be damaged, whether by association or through negligence, leading to their sense that whether present or absent they were hurting their children. This led to feeling ashamed when, as a result of their own issues, they might not be able to be the primary carer of their children. These experiences converged for them with the word 'care', something which became apparent in our interlocutors' discussions of their fear of losing custody of their children if they were unable to provide for them in the way expected by different 'Care' institutions. An Irish Traveller woman in her mid-20s came to the Hub with her three-year-old son to seek support from the gatekeepers to apply for public benefits. She explained her fear of Care to us in relation to the educational system and visits to 'the site' if their children fail to attend school. 'They come to see us, and judge us based on the way we live. They see the children wearing dirty clothes as all children do, but don't see all the effort we make to provide them with something to eat so that they don't go hungry. They threaten us to take them away from us.' In cases like this, participants felt disempowered, with no opportunity to make any public protest to defend their position as their own children's guardians. This, the women at the Hub repeatedly told us, was why the greatest impediment to Travellers' engagement with healthcare was a lack of trust in non-Traveller people, particularly those connected to state institutions such as the NHS.

Due to breakdowns in their relationships with their partners pre- or post-incarceration, or because of past situations of domestic violence and economic scarcity, many research participants no longer lived full-time with their children. Their own difficult childhoods and experiences of physical, psychological and emotional abuse made them worry that their children might experience the same if subjected to the Care system, when they would be unable to protect them. Laura explained that she was always worried. One teenage daughter had learning difficulties and Laura could not be with her at all times: 'If she's got to do something, I cannot be there.' As Broadhurst and Mason (2017: 47–48) explained, relinquishment has emotional and psychological consequences: 'A major consequence of losing a child to public care or adoption is grief that is long lasting and difficult to resolve'. In this context, Care continues to wield painful potential in these interlocutors' lives.

Despite differences in the experiences of care reported by research participants at the Drug Recovery Centre, the GRT Hub and the House, concerns converged into the idea that moments of institutional care are concurrently coercive and corrosive. In the Centre, the House and the

Hub, interlocutors worried about being labelled 'addict' or 'Traveller' or 'homeless'. Because they felt pre-judged in clinical spaces, they often left before they even sat down in the waiting room. Experiences such as that of the man who was told there was no methadone reconfirmed fears of stigmatisation and its impact on cancer prevention: those who actually seek help retreat before it is provided. A logic emerges that institutional care is both painful and potentially inaccessible when actively sought. As a result those segments of the population (or their concerns) might not be visible to healthcare professionals. Compounding the resistance that informs participants' mistrust on institutional approaches to care, participants also struggle with the effort to access formal healthcare.

Situated risk hierarchies

The final ethnographic lesson we learned took place while visiting 'the House', a day centre for rough sleepers located in the centre of a post-industrial town. During a morning meeting, we brought fudge cake and talked with a group that grew over two hours to 15 participants and volunteers. As we spoke with the guests, it became clear that while survival was their top priority, it wasn't accurate to say that they disregarded cancer. Rather, prioritisation involved weighing one risk over another, with resources allocated accordingly. Vito, a GRT guest in his late 20s, explained simply that he had always been a risk taker, 'I gamble my life. There is no point in living your life otherwise. But cancer is already in each of us, it only needs something to be triggered.' The stress of precarity could trigger cancer as well, he said, because 'everybody is born with it'.

    The priority was most often to stay safe on the streets by getting closer to some people and avoiding others conceived as dangerous. Peter (British), Matteo (Moroccan) and John (Portuguese), men in their mid-40s, navigated life on the streets together. They emphasised their friendship as an example of the kind of 'care you make' while sleeping on the streets. This support network was essential for them to survive and this sometimes included encouraging others to seek biomedical care. They made sure to point out when someone was looking unwell. On the day of that visit, Peter had been encouraged by the others to schedule an appointment for a lung scan to find out the cause of pain on his chest and a persistent tickling cough. The GP who volunteers once a week at the House had made the referral, but Peter admitted he was scared. Having lost his mum and sister to cancer he knew it could be 'his turn'.

Nevertheless, we learned the following week that he did not go to the scan because a friend had overdosed and 'there's nothing to be done anyway'. Dom also explained to us that cancer was a persistent fear for him because he'd lost 'Nan, Grandad and Nanny' to different cancers. He perceived cancer as inevitable; addressing hunger and exposure were things which could impact on his life for the better. Manny nodded and said: 'The number of people in this room, 50 per cent will get cancer.' Rather than a problem of lacking awareness of warning symptoms, cancer threats were backgrounded in participants' lives. Cancer and care for them was described as an 'add on', something you could only address after meeting basic needs – food, shelter, safety.

Alongside the situated and complex nature of 'care', 'risk' emerged as fluid concept structured in relation to current needs or concerns. Many of the practices we as researchers might assume to be risky were not appraised that way by research participants, for example the removal of oneself from friends, family and healthcare in favour of friends on the street. Cancer risk was not an extraneous, ignorable risk. Research participants included it when possible in their prioritisation of matters of concern, depending on their available resources. As one interlocutor pointed out, 'seeing your sleeping bag set on fire' will always be the immediate and therefore most dominant concern. As Manderson, Markovic and Quinn (2005: 324) have argued, establishing a credible narrative to make sense of the presence of cancer in and around their lives was part 'of the process of establishing agency'; embedded in those narratives, we can understand 'people's attitudes to their [in]ability to prevent cancer' as something that was perceived as out of their control. In Vito's, Peter's and Vana's cases, cancer was approached as a 'minion of fate . . . at the same time "with us all" and "all around"' (Balshem 1993: 121).

In addition to risk prioritisation and a perceived sense of self-efficacy, participants dealt with knowledge about cancer in varied ways. Manderson (2011: 327) writes that '[l]ocal cosmologies contribute to lay etiologies of disease . . . These explanations are offered in conjunction with biomedical explanations as underlying more proximate reasons for disease.' We saw evidence of this during a group chat at the Centre: Kris insisted he never thought about cancer, but he was worried about a lump in his testicles. He initiated a conversation about cancer early diagnosis, cited some NHS leaflets he'd read and asked the group what we knew about self-checks. Another service user had recently found a lump and went to the clinic to have it checked. He gave a thorough explanation of when and where he went and even provided a demonstration with a clementine about how to palpate for lumps, making biomedical interventions newly relevant to Kris. He then encouraged Kris to go to the GP because 'you have plenty to worry about as it is'. To this point, many service users at the Centre and all the guests visiting the House were either sleeping rough or were in temporary accommodation. Many GRT interlocutors were still living primarily off-grid, with some Traveller sites lacking plumbing and sewers or reliable electricity. For these interlocutors, finding out where their next meal, bed or shower was coming from was an immediate priority which informed how they navigated their everyday lives (Arteaga Pérez, Robinson and McDonald 2020). It wasn't that cancer was silent; it was ongoing white noise in a landscape of sonic booms.

Ultimately, interlocutors only engaged with things that threatened their safety and could be addressed with some kind of action. This relational nature of risk, in which something poses a threat to an attribute that is personally valued, emerges through the situated circumstance of every person (Boholm 2003). This foregrounds the significance of understanding non-normative temporalities, those which do not obey the mandated timeframes of cancer screenings, medical appointments and other biomedical interventions, informing health professionals' perception of these social groups as ill-timed patients (Aragón Martín 2017). The ways in which people living in precarious situations experience their bodies and seek care does not necessarily fit neatly within the expected symptom awareness and timeliness represented by institutionalised healthcare (Merrild and Anderson 2019). Diverging temporalities challenge preconceived messages of health promotion, whereby awareness of the threat of cancer is attached to the imperative to seek healthcare as a sign of personal responsibility. Peter's, Dom's and Vana's examples of witnessing close kin dying of the disease show that many participants were well aware of the risk that cancer posed to their lives.

Overcoming epistemic opacity: where to go from here?

Concepts such as care and risk are essential to public programmes that aim to support healthful living. However, the impact of these programmes is undermined by the persistent exclusion of the realities that so-called hard-to-reach people face. Through unpacking our encounters with research participants at the Hub, the Centre and the House, we begin to better understand the difficulties that they faced every day, their relationship to institutional forms of care and the role cancer plays amid a host of other concerns. Here, our contribution is a glimpse not of further structural barriers, but offers a means of troubling some of the basic definitional assumptions which undergird early detection research. Such assumptions need to be challenged in order to foster trust and widen uptake of preventative healthcare agendas. Multiple interlocutors insisted that care was not always good; at times it felt coercive. We have analysed this as an instance of epistemic opacity, a degree of unwarranted certainty that our form of knowledge is the only way to apprehend the world (Jugov and Ypi 2019). While we as researchers set up the pilot with open minds and an aspiration for full inclusivity of a highly diverse participant base, we persisted in the misapprehension that care could only be positive and that all risk must be negative. Through the moral assumptions with which we approached care and risk we initially missed key information about and failed to empathise with the pernicious role that care sometimes played in our interlocutors' lives. Such empathy failure is not uncommon and can wield both positive and negative effects. It therefore follows that if human empathy is constantly directed within varied moral and socially specific valences, then care – and risk – can be viewed as equally variable, subject to previous experiences, education, available resources and relevant relationships with family and chosen kin as well as with institutions and their officers.

Moving against the intentions of much applied health research, researchers struggle to design studies that enable true recursivity. The questions we ask are filtered through our own perceptions of the terms we use, which directly impact the data we are able to identify and collate. As Groark (2008: 430) argues, in order to apply an empathetic stance we must take into account the experiences of our interlocutors and reshape our terms to fit their definitions, rather than our own. Following Bryson and Stacey (2013: 197), we could argue that an inability to design research in this way can create 'irremediable opacity at the very core of language . . . knowledge practices that are incommensurable with canonical forms'. Such epistemic opacity makes the collection of field materials challenging and potentially undermines the value of any resulting analysis. Once we understood that definitions of care and risk were situated through the ways in which specific 'resources' were valued by our interlocutors, we began to transform our own definitions. How much food, money and housing were at hand and apportioned at a given time was paramount. This was of much higher priority than any longer-term concern, including regarding personal health.

The health concerns that research participants have, and the reasons why they did or did not attend clinical appointments, were obscured from our view until we became open to the reality of lives informed by a fluid and incessant assessment of hierarchies of risk.

Elements of risk included the expected dangers of drug use and the violence encountered while living on the streets, but also included institutions and actors such as social workers and healthcare professionals, which we had categorised as forms of 'care'; these people were often viewed by our interlocutors with mistrust. When past experiences with health services were marked by discrimination (whether directly or indirectly), interlocutors resisted attending preventative care programmes which they might otherwise have valued. The decision to seek clinical care contended with the potential risks posed by these settings and was contingent on whether participants believed that a particular action could avoid or postpone death or not.

In general, the level of knowledge among research participants exhibited about cancer, preventative care and available institutional provisions in their local area indicated an awareness of cancer risks. Peer demonstrations about how to self-check for symptoms of testicular cancer was an example of this. They also understood recommended actions for addressing those risks, refuting approaches from behavioural medicine that frame non-participation as ignorance, depicting participants as in need of more education (Balshem 1993). Lack of knowledge did not appear to be a significant barrier to seeking preventative care, but survival of the present did supersede potential future health. Though cancer does not happen between brackets but is an experience embedded in people's ongoing life-ways, if those life-ways are constrained by precarity, so too will be the engagement with cancer, alongside other commitments, limitations and aspirations. As a result, in participants' lives, the existence of cancer risk is evident but not medicalised. Practices of prioritisation were how they evaluated and acted on risks at any given time and this was clearly a means of keeping themselves as 'well' as possible.

Within conversations on health and well-being, epistemic hierarchies are noted as leading inevitably on from power differentials between figures of authority such as healthcare professionals and structurally vulnerable populations (Toren and Pina-Cabral 2009). As researchers, we found ourselves inadvertently replicating a hierarchical knowledge structure. Our own experiences informed our positive definitional notions of care and our negative understandings of risk. As Toren and Pina-Cabral (2009: 5–6) have reflected:

> Each of us lives the world as a function of his or her unique history, whose parameters each of us projects into the world with some confidence that we are right, only to come up against those of other people . . . making it the ethnographer's task to understand fully

that his or her character and personality structure are both the limiting and facilitating conditions of the ethnographic project itself.

In light of the complexity with which our interlocutors dealt with care and risk in their lives, and in their use of these terms according to experiences so divergent from our own, rather than the other way around, we now see that we were the ones facing barriers to their understanding and processes of knowledge formation.

Acknowledgements

We would like to thank our research participants, the experts who let us understand some aspects of their social worlds and lived realities. We also thank the editors of this book for their thoughtful comments that helped us to strengthen the argument of this chapter. Ethics approval for this research was obtained from the Faculty of Political and Social Sciences, University of Cambridge. The research leading to this publication was generously funded by the pump-priming award 'Elusive Risks' from the Cancer Research UK Cambridge Centre Early Detection Programme.

Notes

1. While we cannot definitively account for the origins of the usage of 'GRT', we can confirm that it is how the interlocutors from the Gypsy Roma Traveller community with whom we worked identified themselves and each other, especially when contrasting themselves from Irish Travellers with whom there had been conflicts in the local area. They would say things like 'GRTs do this because . . . etc.' It should be noted, however, that most of our GRT interlocutors had long worked as educators and liaisons with their local councils so the language they used was possibly linked to its institutional usage in those roles.
2. To measure health and other inequalities in England, the Ministry of Housing constructs 'Indices of Deprivation' per neighbourhood, weighting different domains like disability, income and education. Accessed 28 June 2021. https://assets.publishing.service.gov.uk/government/uploads/system/uploads/attachment_data/file/835115/IoD2019_Statistical_Release.pdf.
3. D H (Department of Health). 2000. 'The NHS Cancer Plan'. Accessed 25 May 2020. www.doh.gov.uk/cancer.
4. 'Be Clear on Cancer' was one of the public health campaigns mobilised nationally at the time of the fieldwork. It sought to educate the public about cancer red-flag symptoms, promoting 'increasing awareness' and 'early' care seeking. Accessed 28 June 2021. https://campaignresources.phe.gov.uk/resources/campaigns/16-be-clear-on-cancer/overview.
5. Maintenance is a form of addiction recovery which employs prescribed drugs such a methadone or diamorphine to avoid full withdrawal and prevent the patient from returning to street-based opiate usage. Accessed 28 June 2021. https://www.ncbi.nlm.nih.gov/pmc/articles/PMC4014029/.

References

Andersen, Rikke Sand, Peter Vedsted, Frede Olesen, Flemming Bro and Jens Sondergaard. 2009. 'Patient delay in cancer studies: A discussion of methods and measures', *BMC Health Service Research* 9(189). https://doi.org/10.1186/1472-6963-9-189.

Aragón Martín, Beatriz. 2017. 'Ill-timed patients: Gitanos, cultural difference and primary health care in a time of crisis'. PhD dissertation. University College London. https://discovery.ucl.ac.uk/id/eprint/10033930.

Arteaga Pérez, Ignacia, Kelly Fagan Robinson and Maryon McDonald. 2020. 'COVID-19 test and trace: Look for the super-locals to access "hard to reach" groups'. The BMJ Opinion, 10 September. Accessed 13 May 2021. https://blogs.bmj.com/bmj/2020/09/10/covid-19-test-and-trace-look-for-the-super-locals-to-access-hard-to-reach-groups/.

Balshem, Martha Levittan. 1993. *Cancer in the Community: Class and medical authority*. Washington, DC, and London: Smithsonian Scholarly Press.

Bear, Laura. 2015. *Navigating Austerity*. Redwood City, CA: Stanford University Press. https://doi.org/10.1515/9780804795548.

Boholm, Asa. 2003. 'The cultural nature of risk: Can there be an anthropology of uncertainty?' *Ethnos* 68 (2): 159–178. https://doi.org/10.1080/0014184032000097722.

Bourgois, Philippe, Seth M. Holmes, Kim Sue and James Quesada. 2017. 'Structural vulnerability: Operationalizing the concept to address health disparities in clinical care', *Academic Medicine* 92(3): 299–307. https://doi.org/10.1097/acm.0000000000001294.

Broadhurst, Karen and Claire Mason. 2017. 'Birth parents and the collateral consequences of court-ordered child removal', *International Journal of Law, Policy and the Family* 31(1): 41–59. https://doi.org/10.1093/lawfam/ebw013.

Bryson, Mary K. and Jackie Stacey. 2013. 'Cancer knowledge in the plural: Queering the biopolitics of narrative and affective mobilities', *Journal of Medical Humanities* 34(2): 197–212. https://doi.org/10.1007/s10912-013-9206-z.

Canton, Rob and Jane Dominey. 2020. 'Punishment and care reappraised'. In *Spaces of Care*, edited by Loraine Gelsthorpe, Perveez Mody and Brian Sloan, 15–38. London: Bloomsbury Publishing.

CRUK (Cancer Research UK). 2014. 'Cancer prevention in harder to reach groups'. Accessed 13 May 2021. https://www.cancerresearchuk.org/sites/default/files/cruk_bupa_foundation_innovation_workshop_2014_cancer_prevention_in_harder_to_reach_groups.

CRUK (Cancer Research UK). 2020. 'Cancer in the UK 2020: Socio-economic deprivation'. Accessed 13 May 2021. https://www.cancerresearchuk.org/sites/default/files/cancer_inequalities_in_the_uk.pdf.

Desjarlais, Robert. 1997. *Shelter Blues: Sanity and selfhood among the homeless*. Philadelphia: University of Pennsylvania Press.

Freimuth, Vicki S. and Wendy Mettger. 1990. 'Is there a hard-to-reach audience?' *Public Health Reports* 105(3): 232–238. http://www.jstor.org/stable/4628863.

Garcia, Angela. 2008. 'The elegiac addict: History, chronicity, and the melancholic subject', *Cultural Anthropology* 23(4): 718–746. https://doi.org/10.1111/j.1548-1360.2008.00024.x.

Gelsthorpe, Loraine, Perveez Mody and Brian Sloan. 2020. 'Spaces of care: Concepts, configurations, and challenges'. In *Spaces of Care*, edited by Loraine Gelsthorpe, Perveez Mody and Brian Sloan, 1–14. London: Hart Publishing.

Groark, Kevin P. 2008. 'Social opacity and the dynamics of empathic in-sight among the Tzotzil Maya of Chiapas, Mexico', *Ethos* 36(4): 427–448. https://doi.org/10.1111/j.1548-1352.2008.00025.x.

Hay, M. Cameron. 2008. 'Reading sensations: Understanding the process of distinguishing "fine" from "sick"', *Transcultural Psychiatry* 45(2): 198–229. https://doi.org/10.1177%2F1363461508089765.

Hunn, Amanda. 2017. 'Survey of the general public: Attitudes towards health research'. British Health Research Authority. Accessed 13 May 2021. https://s3.eu-west-2.amazonaws.com/www.hra.nhs.uk/media/documents/survey-general-public-attitudes-towards-health-research.pdf.

Iacobucci, Gareth. 2019. 'Life expectancy gap between rich and poor in England widens', *British Medical Journal* 364. https://doi.org/10.1136/bmj.l1492.

Jugov, Tamara and Lea Ypi. 2019. 'Structural injustice, epistemic opacity, and the responsibilities of the oppressed', *Journal of Social Psychology* 50(1): 7–27. https://doi.org/10.1111/josp.12268.

Keane, Webb. 2018. 'Perspectives on affordances, or the anthropologically real: The 2018 Daryll Forde Lecture', *HAU: Journal of Ethnographic Theory* 8(1–2): 27–38.
Koch, Insa and Deborah James. 2022. 'The state of the welfare state: Advice, governance and care in settings of austerity', *Ethnos* 87(1): 1–21. https://doi.org/10.1080/00141844.2019.1688371.
Lupton, Deborah. 1995. *The Imperative of Health: Public health and the regulated body*. London: SAGE.
Luxardo, Natalia. 2020. 'Research on cancer and hard to reach populations: What to learn from social sciences methodologies', *Clinics in Oncology* 5: 1730.
Manderson, Lenore. 2011. 'Anthropologies of cancer and risk, uncertainty and disruption'. In *A Companion to Medical Anthropology*, edited by Merrill Singer and Pamela I. Erickson, 323–338. London: Wiley Blackwell.
Manderson, Lenore, Milica Markovic and Michael Quinn. 2005. '"Like roulette": Australian women's explanations of gynecological cancers', *Social Science & Medicine* 61(2): 323–332. https://doi.org/10.1016/j.socscimed.2004.11.052.
Marlow, Laura A. V., Amanda J. Chorley, Jessica Haddrell, Rebecca Ferrer and Jo Waller. 2017. 'Understanding the heterogeneity of cervical cancer screening non-participants: Data from a national sample of British women', *European Journal of Cancer* 80: 30–38. https://doi.org/10.1016/j.ejca.2017.04.017.
Merrild, Camilla Hoffmann and Rikke Sand Andersen. 2019. 'Disengaging with the cancerous body', *Health* 25(1): 21–36. https://doi.org/10.1177/1363459319848049.
Merrild, Camilla Hoffman, Peter Vedsted and Rikke Sand Andersen. 2017. 'Noisy lives, noisy bodies: Exploring the sensorial embodiment of class', *Anthropology in Action* 24(1): 13–19. https://doi.org/10.3167/aia.2017.240103.
Minkler, Meredith. 1989. 'Health education, health promotion and the open society: An historical perspective', *Health Education Quarterly* 16(1): 17–30. https://www.jstor.org/stable/45049840.
Offersen, Sara Marie Hebsgaard, Peter Vedsted and Rikke Sand Andersen. 2017. '"The good citizen": Balancing moral possibilities in everyday life between sensation, symptom and healthcare seeking', *Anthropology in Action* 24(1): 6–12. https://doi.org/10.3167/aia.2017.240102.
Palmer, C. K., M. C. Thomas, C. von Wagner and R. Raine. 2014. 'Reasons for non-uptake and subsequent participation in the NHS Bowel Cancer Screening Programme: A qualitative study', *British Journal of Cancer* 110: 1705–1711. https://doi.org/10.1038/bjc.2014.125.
Raghavan, R., A. Farooqi, K. Jutlla, N. Patel, B. Desai and S. Uddin. 2018. 'Recruitment and research participation of black and ethnic minority citizens in health research in the UK: A toolkit for good practice', *European Journal of Public Health* 28(1). https://doi.org/10.1093/eurpub/cky047.059.
Reynolds Whyte, Susan, Lotte Meinert and Jenipher Twebaze. 2014. 'Clientship'. In *Second Chances: Surviving AIDS in Uganda*, edited by Susan Reynolds Whyte, 56–69. Durham, NC: Duke University Press.
Richards, Mike. 2019. *Report of the Independent Review of Adult Screening Programmes in England*. London: NHS England.
Robinson, Kelly Fagan and T. Carroll. In press. 'Material ecologies of policy failure: Ruptures of bodies and of state'. In *Routledge International Handbook of Failure*, edited by Adriana Mica, M. Pawlak, A. Horolets and P. Kublicki. Abingdon: Routledge.
Rockliffe, Lauren, Amanda J. Chorley, Laura A. V. Marlow and Alice S. Forster. 2018. 'It's hard to reach the "hard-to-reach": The challenges of recruiting people who do not access preventative healthcare services into interview studies', *International Journal of Qualitative Studies on Health and Well-Being* 13(1). https://doi.org/10.1080/17482631.2018.1479582.
Smith, S. G, L. M. McGregor, R. Raine, J. Wardle, C. von Wagner and K. A. Robb. 2016. 'Inequalities in cancer screening participation: Examining differences in perceived benefits and barriers', *Psycho-Oncology* 25(10): 1168–1174. https://doi.org/10.1002/pon.4195.
Strathern, Marilyn. 2020. *Relations: An anthropological account*. Durham, NC: Duke University Press.
Taylor-Gooby, Peter. 2017. 'Re-doubling the crises of the welfare state: The impact of Brexit on UK welfare politics', *Journal of Social Policy* 46(4): 815–835. https://doi.org/10.1017/S0047279417000538.
Throop, Jason. 2010. *Suffering and Sentiment*. Berkeley: University of California Press.

Toren, Christina and João de Pina-Cabral. 2009. 'What is happening to epistemology?' *Social Analysis* 53(2): 1–18. https://doi.org/10.3167/sa.2009.530201.

Weller, Penelope. 2013. 'Towards a genealogy of "coercive care"'. In *Coercive Care: Rights, Law and Policy*, edited by Bernadette McSherry and Ian Freckelton, 15–30. Abingdon: Routledge.

Witham, Miles D., Eleanor Anderson, Camille Carroll, Paul M. Dark, Kim Down, Alistair S. Hall, Joanna Knee et al. 2020. 'Developing a roadmap to improve trial delivery for underserved groups: Results from a UK multi-stakeholder process', *Trials* 21(694). https://doi.org/10.1186/s13063-020-04613-7.

12
Precarity and cancer among low-income populations in France: intractable inequalities

Laurence Kotobi and Carolyn Sargent

Vulnerable populations lacking national health coverage create strategies of care in the context of structural inequalities (Lombrail, Pascal and Lang 2004), which include constrained access to health services. We can best understand these structures of health inequality by analysing the politics of care at local, state and global levels. Political agendas shape health status and healthcare access for vulnerable populations in the global north and south. In France, health inequalities have been increasingly evident since the 1990s (Fassin 2000; Leclerc et al. 2000). However, to date, relatively few studies in France have explored how marginalised populations confront non-communicable illnesses such as cancer (Pian 2012; Sarradon-Eck 2009).

In this chapter, we explore how structurally vulnerable patients – immigrants in two regions of France – navigate bureaucracies, hospitals and other institutional conventions and struggle with diverse discourses of disease to confront potentially life-threatening diagnoses such as breast cancer. Immigrant patients who reside in France with serious health problems face not only the biological realities of disease but also the politics of care, which encompass the economic and social precarities associated with immigration. Care, in our usage, is thus a broad concept comprising not only health services but other sectors such as social services, available housing, home caretaking and voluntary association services for vulnerable populations (Larchanché 2020: 187–188). The politics of care directs our attention to global questions regarding those who have the legitimacy or perceived rights to make claims on healthcare institutions and the role of state policies and politics in determining these rights (Strong 2020: 196). Moving beyond social and cultural representations, recent ethnographic studies in France have examined the therapeutic itineraries of immigrant populations, highlighting their diverse healthcare-seeking routes as they battle legal, economic and political obstacles (Després 2013; Kotobi and Lemonnier 2015; Sargent and Cordell 2003).

In 2003, France identified cancer as a national priority. A fine-grained analysis of the incidence of heath inequalities indicates that differential cancer mortality rates continue to merit attention (Vuillermoz et al. 2016). In addition, during this same period, the French social security system was globally renowned for its egalitarian model, with specific benefits reserved for the most vulnerable populations. Yet a nuanced grasp of how those most at risk take advantage (or are unaware) of social benefits and rights would allow us to understand the everyday realities of clinical practice and patient decisions regarding the diagnosis and treatment of cancer. This, in turn, would facilitate more effective prevention approaches and strategies to reduce serious cancer disease and associated suffering.

Drawing on three research projects that used ethnographic approaches, conducted in Paris and Bordeaux, we examine access to care for structurally vulnerable and seriously ill migrants with cancer. We explore: (1) the ways in which those confronting serious chronic illnesses negotiate and embody subjectivities; and (2) the resources on which people affected by cancer draw, including kin, interpreters, non-government organisations (NGOs), clinicians, social workers and immigrant associations. France boasts an ideologically egalitarian national health system, a lynchpin of national identity that aims to ensure care for all. Structural inequalities, however, challenge and constrain this system, influencing how low-income immigrants manage cancer and other illnesses. Accordingly, we will argue that all healthcare, including cancer treatment, is politicised and that the distribution of care is the outcome of political decisions and policies.

Background

The evolution of immigration in France is often traced to the Trente Glorieuses, the 30 years post-World War II which were characterised by prosperity and a need for an increased labour force. During this period, male labour migrants, particularly from former colonies in West and

North Africa, were welcomed to France (Barou 2014; INSEE 2019).[1] By 1974, deteriorating economic conditions brought the guest labour system to a halt, but in 1980, family reunification policies introduced on humanitarian grounds had modified the demographic profile of the immigrant population as women and children were allowed to join husbands and other family members already living in France (Manchuelle 1997). In 2019, 9.9 per cent of the total population in France consisted of immigrants, of whom 51 per cent were women (INSEE 2019). Approximately 46 per cent of immigrants now living in France were born in Africa. Of these, 10.4 per cent emigrated from sub-Saharan Africa; the remainder originated in Algeria, Morocco and Tunisia. Newly arrived immigrants include increasing numbers from Central Africa (INSEE 2019) and asylum seekers from conflict zones such as Democratic Republic of Congo and Syria.

The guest labour immigrants initially arrived by boat and settled in the large urban centres of France: Paris, Marseille, Lyon, Bordeaux and other sites with industrial, shipping and service occupations amenable to hiring migrant workers. Initially, the question of where to house the primarily male population was solved by the construction of hostels, built by private entrepreneurs or with state financial support. These remain a source of lodging for men arriving from West and North Africa today. The Foyer Bara in the north-eastern Parisian suburb of Montreuil, no longer habitable, was known for its efforts to reproduce the features of an African community, with artisans, a mosque and meals prepared by a team of West African women, and internal spatial organisation based on family or village affiliations in Africa. Bordeaux also houses immigrants from diverse countries in worker hostels, but these lack the unique characteristics of some of the Paris hostels constructed to replicate aspects of 'home'.

With the arrival of immigrant families in France in the late 1970s, public and private financing supported the expansion of low-income public housing, the HLM (*habitations à loyer modéré*, also known as *cités*). Often constructed as high-rise buildings situated in suburbs of the major French urban centres such as Paris and Bordeaux, the *cités* receive regular media attention for gang violence, political unrest, unhealthy living conditions and poor maintenance. For those who are undocumented, an HLM apartment cannot be legally rented. However, many migrants live unofficially with relatives renting an HLM lodging. Those who are impoverished, sleeping on the street or identified by hospital social workers as at risk may access 'social hotels', but these lack space and privacy and are a short-term solution. The 'politics of care' is evident here in the policies and regulations that produce a lack of safe, habitable housing for marginalised populations. In the absence of alternative accommodation, each major urban area in France has 'squats', buildings in disrepair and not officially in use, where immigrants congregate until they are expelled by authorities. The majority of our Paris research was conducted in the largely immigrant north and north-eastern suburbs located in the *petite couronne*, a concentric ring of administrative departments situated north of the city limits. The greater Paris region has a large number of associations to provide support services for low-income individuals, especially immigrants. The organisation GRDR (Groupe de recherché et de realisations pour le developpement rural), for instance, is a non-profit association that addresses economic and health development in the Senegal River Valley and provides support for immigrant associations in Paris/Île-de-France. The organisations oversee several hundred immigrant associations which raise funds for development initiatives in home communities in West Africa.

Bordeaux is France's sixth-largest city, known for its wine industry in the neighbouring Medoc region and shipping, among other enterprises. Approximately 8.3 per cent of the population consists of immigrants; however, this does not include those who are undocumented, living in squats or seasonal workers employed in the vineyards (Louarn 2019). In the region surrounding Bordeaux, nine communes have been identified as ZUS or *zones urbaines sensibles*, politically sensitive urban areas with periodic civil unrest. Similar to Paris, Bordeaux has a diverse immigrant population, largely North and West Africans who arrived just after World War II, but now including South Asians, Turks, Portuguese, Eastern Europeans, of whom a substantial proportion are Romas, and diverse asylum seekers. As in Paris, numerous associations have been established to provide legal and social support for low-income immigrants; some aim to assist migrants from a particular region or have a focused objective.[2] In addition, the Union of Senegalese Workers engages in political initiatives in France and in Senegal, as well as in charitable endeavours.

Immigrant health: imagined and experienced

Since the post-war period, immigrants have been conceptualised in the public imaginary as 'diseased bodies', 'Others' suffering from infectious or exotic ailments (Bouchaud and Cohuet 2011; Sargent and Larchanché 2014). In reality, contemporary immigrant populations include middle-aged and elderly individuals subject to chronic, degenerative diseases such as cancer, diabetes and cardiovascular disorders, often with multiple co-morbidities related to living in situations of economic deprivation.

In reflecting on political and economic factors contributing to inequalities in cancer treatment and survival, we draw on data collected in three intersecting research projects conducted in Paris and Bordeaux. The first is a study of the delivery of serious diagnoses such as cancer and the role of interpreters (Kotobi, Larchanché and Kessar 2013), conducted for one year in 2011, in three northern Paris hospitals with a high proportion of patients with minimal or no French language. This research identified practices by professionals trying to manage translation for non-French speakers on a daily basis, often using stereotypical representations of this patient population (for example, one nurse manager stated authoritatively that African women speak French – they say 'oui' – but Chinese women never do).

A second research project centred on the therapeutic itineraries of female West African breast cancer patients undergoing treatment in Paris and how they and their families confronted diagnoses and treatment approaches (undertaken by Carolyn Sargent, Stéphanie Larchanché and Peter Benson over the 2014–2019 period). Data were collected in four public hospitals, two in the northern immigrant suburbs and two in central Paris. In addition to observing consultations with six oncologists weekly over a two-year period, we interviewed 34 patients in treatment, with initial contact in hospitals followed by home visits. We also met with leaders of 50 immigrant associations to discuss widely shared understandings of cancer in the West African immigrant population. Like Kotobi's 2013 project, the language constraints in clinical communication were identified and evaluated.

The third study (undertaken by Laurence Kotobi and colleagues over the 2017–2021 period) is underway in Bordeaux and Paris. The Premiers Pas (First Steps) project addresses undocumented immigrants' trajectories to access healthcare and health insurance from longitudinal and multidisciplinary perspectives. This was the first project to explore how undocumented immigrants use the state-funded health insurance known as AME (Aide Médicale d'Etat). The French health insurance system is extremely complex and underwent major modifications in 2016, although AME coverage was retained. The core of the current system is universal sickness protection, known as PUMA (Protection Universelle Maladie), for adults living legally in France with stable employment or residence. Undocumented immigrants do not have the right to PUMA coverage, a clear example of the politicising of access to care.

Immigrants in France have differential access to health insurance and to health services, determined by their legal status and their migratory history. A significant issue is that AME allows 100 per cent coverage for undocumented migrants without access to PUMA who can provide evidence that they have lived in France for three consecutive months. AME offers coverage for medical consultations and hospitalisation; 100 per cent reimbursement for medication, pregnancy, contraception and abortion; healthcare for children under age six; vaccinations, screening tests and laboratory examinations; and treatment for injuries and diseases classified as serious and chronic. Health professionals are required to accept AME beneficiaries. However, in our respective studies, we found that many immigrants were unaware of their right to access AME.[3]

The samples from the three research projects on which we draw include patients, their kin, clinicians and members of immigrant associations in Paris and Bordeaux. While accompanying patients to hospital consultations, discussing these consultations with doctors and with the patient afterwards and interviewing interpreters, we concluded that translation problems were a recurrent issue, dramatically affecting patient understandings and treatment strategies. Lack of interpreters and subsequent limitations in comprehension exacerbate inequalities in care and may reduce the probability of survival for immigrants who fail to complete treatment (Lombrail, Pascal and Lang 2004). State cuts to the national health service budgets for interpreters since 2008 have progressively lessened the availability of trained interpreters in clinical settings.

Inequalities, breast cancer and migration: structural invisibilities in France

At the national level, the inequalities confronting diverse populations with cancer were addressed in the 2012 annual report of the National Cancer Institute (INCa). Reduction of health inequalities subsequently became the guiding theme of the Third Cancer Plan (2014–2019). Although the issue of poor access to preventive cancer services for women had been identified by the Council of Equality (Conseil à l'Egalité) in 2010, the question of cancer prevention among immigrant women remained invisible in policy and research agendas. A notable reason for this lack of attention is the state's resistance to collecting data measuring features of identity, such as the health status of immigrants or disease prevalence. Disease and death registries may only obtain state authorisation to collect statistics on ethnicity by petitioning the CNIL (Commission Nationale de l'Informatique et des libertés, and/or the Comité National d'Ethique), providing assurance of full anonymity and providing evidence that the data on race or ethnicity would supersede the potential harm of disclosing such data (Simon, Beauchemin and Hamel 2015; Vuillermoz et al. 2016; Wittwer et al. 2019).

In a national programme developed in 2004 to increase mammography screening,[4] immigrant women from 50 to 74 years of age are underrepresented. The implementation and patient recruitment strategies of the Santé Publique France programme are ill adapted to the life conditions of certain target populations, such as those without stable housing. Some humanitarian and state-sponsored associations, for a small fee, offer a home address for bureaucratic purposes. This serves those living in squats, on the streets, in social service 'hotels' or co-lodging with family without the formal status of renter or owner (thus having no known address). Similarly, the national cancer plan proposes a Pap smear biannually for early diagnosis of cervical cancer,[5] but cervical cancer screening has failed to reach vulnerable populations such as immigrant women for the same reasons.

Migratory trajectories and conditions affecting access to rights in the host country

Social protection measures may fail in various circumstances. For example, refugees seeking asylum and with PUMA insurance lose this coverage if their asylum plea is rejected. They then must wait three months for authorisation to request AME coverage. This gap in coverage generates uncertainty that prevents many from imagining and advancing plans for the future. The social protection system is complex for most users (Lafore 2017), having both insurance and social welfare benefits components. It is particularly difficult to navigate for those who are illiterate, speak limited French and lack a stable social network. The populations we report on include the many immigrant women living in precarity who confront the anguish of a cancer diagnosis and must then negotiate the bureaucratic and clinical complexities associated with obtaining appropriate treatment.

We illustrate these constraints affecting the distribution of care in the context of structural inequalities and vulnerability, though the narratives of Mariam and Oumou.

Mariam

An oncology nurse at one of the public hospitals introduced Mariam to our research team in 2016, expressing concern about her marginality: she was undocumented, with transient living conditions, precarious health status and lack of stable employment. She was classified at the hospital as 'homeless' because, after arriving in France, she lived on the street by the Gare du Nord while searching for a place to live.[6]

She initially presented at the Emergency Department for breast pain and swelling. Following a mammogram, biopsy and MRI, she met with the oncology surgeon, a gynaecologist, to receive the 'announcement' of her diagnosis and to plan her treatment trajectory. In what was to become a series of mishaps, Mariam began chemotherapy at a different hospital, very far from where she lived. No one could explain how referral to a distant location occurred. Mariam was so exhausted from the chemotherapy that she spent several days in hospital. In principle, she had the right to a taxi service to and from the hospital for treatment, but staff had neglected to request a taxi for her.

Martine, one of our ethnographers who is a retired midwife, went to visit Mariam at the residence where she undertook household chores in exchange for a place to sleep. She explained to Martine that after arriving in Paris, she encountered a man on the streets near the Gare du Nord who took her to the humanitarian organisation, Médecins du Monde (Doctors of the World). Mariam said: 'A woman met me there and offered to house me for a while. But when she learned the diagnosis, she said that I would not be able to stay with her for the time treatment would require.'

During three years of accompanying Mariam to medical consultations and the pharmacy, sitting with her in hospital during chemotherapy and after surgery and chatting with her over lunch, we learned that she had no health insurance, no friends and was deeply anxious. Although she wanted to find a job, she suffered side-effects from chemotherapy that were slow to dissipate, a cardiac problem newly diagnosed and lymphoedema, for which she was hospitalised. As Martine, Mariam and I (CS) sat in a small Turkish restaurant drinking tea Mariam told me (CS) she felt like crying. The only positive aspect of her life was having Martine as her companion at the hospital. We took the subway together and while waiting, she asked,

> Cancer is a disease that cannot be cured, I'm right, aren't I?
> (*Le cancer c'est une maladie qui ne se guérit pas, j'ai raison, non?*)
> What will become of me? I have no papers, no money, and I do not

know what to do. Any day I could end up on the street. And this sickness, why me?

Although she came to France from Conakry, the capital of Guinea, her family lived in a remote rural area, where she grew up. She expressed her regret that cancer not only threatened her life but also prevented her from achieving her goal as a migrant: to send money 'home'.

Mariam spoke good conversational French, having completed most of secondary school in Guinea where French is the language of instruction after primary school. Conversational French is not necessarily adequate for clinical communication, however. Mariam easily conversed about the prices of groceries, but she did not follow her physician's explanations about oestrogen receptors, lymphoedema and mastectomy. She relied on Martine to explain advice from the physician during or after every clinical encounter or meeting with a social worker. Between August and December 2016, Martine helped her apply for and obtain AME coverage, with which Mariam was not familiar. Because Mariam had no telephone, she relied on neighbours to pass messages to her. Doctors, in turn, relied on Martine to track down Mariam via these neighbours, to give her an injection at home intended to increase production of white blood cells and to remind her of appointments.

Currently, Mariam has recovered from a partial mastectomy,[7] lymphoedema and heart problems. But in the process, she has been shunted among oncologists, surgeons, social workers and social service associations, criticised for not following the rules regarding diagnostic testing and warned about the risk of not losing weight and exercising. She has also received a one-year renewable residence card because of her ongoing healthcare for a 'serious condition'. She is in remission and feeling well, in spite of the worries of everyday life. She left the home of 'the woman' and moved in with 'a man who knew her sister back home'. As she observed, 'You know, Martine, in the situation I'm in, I'm obliged to do things that I would rather not do.'

Oumou

Oumou was a 51-year-old woman from Guinea-Conakry who had been living in Bordeaux since 2016 and was being treated for breast cancer when she was interviewed by Faye, Kotobi's graduate student and a research assistant on Sargent's project.

Oumou was diagnosed with breast cancer in Guinea. In her own words, 'the sickness caught me in Guinea, and treatment there is very expensive'. Although chemotherapy is sometimes available in Conakry, cancer patients are usually directed to Senegal for radiation. However, when Oumou commenced treatment, the radiotherapy equipment in Senegal was not functioning and she would have needed to travel to Morocco.

Her brother, living in France with French citizenship, advised her on treatment options. He pointed out that financially and logistically it would be more efficient to come to France than Morocco. Following French immigration regulations, he wrote his sister a declaration of residence to confirm that she would have a place to stay in France. Rather than apply for a visa to seek healthcare, which is almost impossible to obtain, she requested a short-term tourist visit, which she received. She pointed out that it was important not to indicate that she was sick, but rather to convey that she was travelling to visit family. In reality, her objective was healthcare and upon her arrival her brother took her directly to a hospital. There, she explained that she was a tourist who had previously been diagnosed with breast cancer in Conakry. Beginning the first day and throughout her treatment trajectory, her brother supported her financially, she lived with his family in their state-subsidised apartment and he translated her interactions with clinical staff.

At the Emergency Department, staff asked for Oumou's medical reports to document tests already done in Guinea. She had not brought them with her. She brought only one document and she explained that the doctors did not exactly understand what was written on that paper. So she began again with diagnostic procedures – a mammogram, biopsy, scans then treatment anew – chemotherapy. For a year and a half, she lived at her brother's home and continued treatment.

Reflecting on the discovery of her breast cancer, Oumou said that she found a sore on her breast but she had no idea it was serious. She thought it was just an abscess or a sore. Considering why it never occurred to her that it could be a tumour, she pointed out that it was normal that she did not know because she hardly ever watched television (where she might have seen some publicity about cancer). Her husband was unemployed; she cared for her children and worked as a vendor of prepared foods, which she sold until midnight. She had no time for leisure activities such as television. As the household head, while her husband was unemployed, she also had no time to focus on her breast as it became more painful and swollen. Eventually, her husband insisted that she go to the hospital in Conakry, where she was diagnosed with cancer.

Oumou showed her breast to some of her friends. This is a subject women talk about together, she told us. They reminded her that there are certain breast ailments that make the breast swell and cause pain but are not necessarily fatal. Local healers have medications for these conditions (known as *lengue* or *khountougni* in the Malinke language, meaning breast pain or abscess). Periodically, she consulted an herbalist or a spiritual healer, but their therapies did not work and the symptoms continued. Her brother in France encouraged her to begin hospital treatment. Without him, the treatment in Conakry and in France would have been impossible.

Oumou's case illustrates how a network of kin and friends can make possible healthcare interventions that might otherwise be unattainable. She itemised the specific costs of each treatment phase and recounted with precision each intervention she had undergone. Oumou financed her treatment in Conakry and her plane ticket to France with funds from her brother and her brother helped her navigate the bureaucratic and hospital systems to obtain medical coverage and extend her visa. In addition to her brother's financial support, she eventually found an apartment in Paris with the help of the international organisation SOS Social Services (Groupe SOS social services).

Oumou proposed possible causes of why she had cancer. First, a large, heavy box fell off a shelf and hit her on the chest; this blow could have been responsible for her illness. More likely, the suffering and misery she experienced in her marriage, her work and with the death of her daughter led her to contract cancer. Ultimately, she concluded, she is in remission because of the will of God in response to her prayers. 'Cancer', she said, 'is a fatal sickness, a sickness that will reduce you to poverty, and if you have no resources, or someone to support you, your risk of death is even greater. In Guinea, people think cancer is a disease of the wealthy. However, for the poor, it is even worse.' Cancer changed Oumou's life in every way, separating her from family and home, making her an immigrant for life. Yet she finally feels hopeful that a cure is possible. 'Now I am feeling better', she said, 'thanks be to God.'

Administrative measures and health service access

The complexity of accessing the national health system challenges many potential patients. We found it common for those who are eligible to be unaware of the options available to them. The women with whom we worked had lived in France for more than a decade. They had no idea they were eligible for benefits such as AME health insurance, for special assistance such as taxi rides to treatment associated with the serious and chronic illness list, the right to time off work if they were employed or for childcare during treatment phases. In the greater Paris region, until recently, numerous state-subsidised and private humanitarian associations were active in supporting women needing legal aid, translation, housing, work and healthcare (Sargent and Kotobi 2017). Since the 2010s, however, austerity measures undertaken by the state in conjunction with EU policies have reduced subsidies for these associations. Many have since closed. One Paris association, which offered an array of support services primarily to immigrant women with serious illnesses, closed under duress with a backlog of over 1,000 patients in 2018. Bordeaux, which has fewer physicians and healthcare facilities, also lacks the strong network of associations that had been a vital source of support for low-income and undocumented patients in the Paris region.

Among the valuable services offered by associations is information regarding mammography. Immigrant women who experience breast symptoms while in their country of origin may be familiar with the concept of the mammogram if they had resided in the capital. But for West African women, even in larger cities in Mali, Senegal, Guinea or the Ivory Coast, access to mammography is erratic and, although mammograms are publicised in urban areas, equipment is not always accessible and functional. It is costly (USD 50–100), not widely accessed by women and is rarely the first resort for addressing breast anomalies (Black and Richmond 2019; Dano et al. 2019). Women with breast pain or swelling are likely to consult first with a local healer, a herbalist or a ritual specialist, likely leading to a delay in diagnosis. Women eventually went to a public hospital at the advice of family members.

Raima, whom we followed for two years, first consulted a Malian herbalist in Paris who gave her leaves to stew and use to bathe her breast. A year later, when her breast was so painful that she could not sleep, Raima went to the maternity clinic where a midwife who had assisted her during childbirth examined her breast. The midwife immediately sent her to one of the public hospitals that targets immigrant populations. By the time she had a biopsy and began treatment her oncologist expressed regret that her choice to consult a healer had lowered the probability of a positive outcome. Raima spoke little French and asked questions of our researchers with the help of multilingual friends. Hospital secretaries complained about Raima, observing that she missed appointments or was often late. To them she seemed incapable of following instructions. We learned from Raima that she had to collect her daughter at preschool at the time the secretaries regularly set her appointment. The situation only changed when one of us intervened with the secretary in charge.

Raima's oncologist was disturbed that she missed several chemotherapy sessions because of time conflicts. In an attempt to shock her into attending her chemotherapy sessions, he told her she would die if she refused to do what she was told. Such a direct prognosis was unspeakable from the perspective of Raima and other breast cancer patients we encountered. The consequence of this exchange was that Raima was terrified and stopped coming altogether. Her oncologist asked us if we could arrange a meeting with an interpreter. We brought two Malian friends, older women who had worked as interpreters in the past, and we collectively negotiated Raima's return to chemotherapy. One of the interpreters, Bintou, argued persuasively, 'You are a lucky woman. God and your husband both want you to continue with treatment!'

Unlike Raima, others with close relatives living in France, like Oumou, might be fortunate enough to obtain sufficient financial support and bureaucratic advice to manage the complex French national health system and immigration policies (Lafore 2017). Without her brother's intervention, Oumou would not have been able to afford the airfare to France or housing in France, nor would she have understood her rights as a seriously ill immigrant.

Whereas government mandates in France informed women over 50 years old of their right to a free mammography every two years, many African women live with relatives, are undocumented or have no formal address. They are therefore unlikely to receive a notification concerning their right to screening. For those seeking treatment in France, a mammogram usually begins to play a role in the process of diagnosis and treatment after a woman has felt a lump, has a breast abscess or a midwife has examined her in the course of prenatal or postnatal care. The concept of 'prevention' certainly has meaning for West African women we interviewed. However, women speculate that breast cancer is a 'sent illness', in other words, the result of ritual harmful acts, often from another woman, and, in this context, prevention is likely to involve ritual means of protection.

Mammography, we found in conversations with women in Paris immigrant associations, is often misunderstood and sometimes feared. The rumour that mammograms may be life-threatening sometimes overrides the presumption that it is a useful means of early breast cancer detection. As we heard from women in group discussions at several immigrant associations in Paris, a mammogram makes visible that which is otherwise invisible. For some, this implies causation. As one woman said, choosing to get a mammogram is 'walking towards death'. Other women expressed their discomfort with mammograms because of pain or discomfort and because upper body nudity is required; male partners or women themselves make decisions on this basis.[8]

Representations of difference in the production of inequality

In his reflections on immigrant health in France, Fassin (2000, 2007) underscored how cancer and other chronic illnesses escape the representational models dominant in medicine. These models associate 'foreigners' (immigrants, those without French nationality or not considered 'French French' in the public imaginary) with 'pathologies of importation', acquisition or adaptation rather than illnesses of aging, environmental risk or poverty. Accordingly, researchers have noted a delay in cancer treatment for immigrants on racial grounds. Assumptions about ethnic origin and probable affliction affect differential diagnosis. In contrast to HIV/AIDS, a disease linked to culture and sexuality by French clinicians who work with sub-Saharan Africans (Fassin 2000), cancer was long perceived by clinicians as a disease of modernity, rarely associated with migrants from resource-poor countries. Indeed, a video made by a French NGO focused on four West African women and their perspectives on 'what is breast cancer?' The speakers proposed such possible causes of breast cancer as colonialism, modernity, insufficient breastfeeding duration and living in France. They seem to echo Fassin's contention that clinicians may neglect the diagnostic possibility of cancer in African immigrant populations, perceiving it as a disease of modernity. Yet recently, oncologists working in French public hospitals serving immigrant populations have observed the unusually young age at onset and the high mortality rates of West African women presenting with breast cancer. The reality of cancer risk for immigrants, who were once considered threatening vectors of infectious disease, is increasingly incontrovertible.

In semi-structured interviews with 90 members of immigrant associations in Paris, a uniform perspective on cancer emerged: breast cancer was identified as the principle type of cancer 'in the world'. A few women also mentioned cervical cancer, not surprisingly, given the growing publicity by the INCa encouraging women to regularly schedule Pap smears. The concerns that women express about mammography are multiplied with cervical cancer screening, which requires removing undergarments in the presence of a physician (possibly male). One recent study of cervical cancer screening in Bordeaux suggested that clinicians are less likely to propose a free screening test for cervical cancer to non-Francophone or immigrant women. It was only recently, in the 2014–2019 National Cancer Plan, that screening for cervical cancer began to include a focus on cancer prevention in 'vulnerable' populations (La Ligue Contre le Cancer Comité Gironde 2017). This terminology is a euphemistic reference to immigrants, to avoid language widely considered politically incorrect and discriminatory.

Urrutia's (2017) research with humanitarian health associations suggests the need for enhanced attention in cervical cancer screening to be paid to the presence of an interpreter. The interpreter may be useful or intrusive depending on context. For instance, screening is more likely to be accepted with careful consideration of gender in matching patients, doctors and interpreters and in selecting an interpreter who speaks the patient's first language.[9] Other issues include differences in acceptability of undressing in the presence of a doctor or nurse. The sensitivity of North African women to the partial or total nudity expected during consultations is now well known, although not always addressed in clinical settings. West African patients have similar concerns, as we note, but these are less often recognised. Kotobi and Lkhadir's (2016) research on modesty (*pudeur*) in clinical settings suggests that one reassuring approach for patients uncomfortable with removing clothing is to allow sufficient consultation time to discuss the cervical cancer screening process and to ensure awareness of the intimacy inherent in this screening. This is only a first step in encouraging immigrant women to accept breast and cervical cancer screening, but nonetheless valuable in establishing rapport.

Interpreters and mediation

As the examples of breast and cervical cancer screening indicate, clinicians face daily constraints when communicating with patients who have limited language proficiency. The absence of interpreters is directly related to national political objectives to prioritise immigrants who speak adequate and preferably fluent French. In addition, oncologists and immigrant patients often do not share disease constructs or conventions of appropriate dress or behaviour (Kotobi, Larchanché and Kessar 2013). The subsequent miscommunication on the part of clinicians and patients contributes to burying awareness of health inequalities. The resulting limitations, which constrain patients from understanding their disease process and prognosis, pose serious ethical questions in terms of access to patient rights and consequences for survival. Limited comprehension among patients may thus contribute to the unequal distribution of mortality from breast cancer across populations (Kotobi 2017).

Interpreters reported particular difficulties translating for oncologists, given the absence of relevant vocabulary and concepts in patients' local languages. In the oncology waiting area, for example, women speaking in one of the West African languages, usually Soninke, Bambara, Wolof or Pulaar, would suddenly insert the word 'cancer', in French, into their sentence. This observation led us to ask our respondents whether there is a word equivalent to cancer in their primary language. This question provoked amusement, but also acknowledgement that there are many words – however, they do not translate well. Mystical attribution of breast cancer, for example, is difficult to convey in French, although symptoms such as swelling or pain can be translated easily.

Some caregivers and hospital staff interpret because they speak a language useful to hospital personnel. However, they often feel inadequate when translating a diagnosis, a poor prognosis or explaining the treatment modalities (Kotobi and Lkhadir 2016). Professional interpreters, as well as caregivers and staff not trained in translation, may have difficulty finding accurate or meaningful language to explain concepts without an equivalent expression in the first languages of patients.

In their research in several hospitals in northern Paris, Kotobi, Larchanché and Kessar (2013) showed that the system of action was rather that of 'making do' (*se débrouiller*) and of bricolage, in order to translate for patients or information on a case-by-case basis. Clinicians and hospital staff had, in addition, little prior knowledge of the concrete possibilities of recourse to trained and salaried interpreters. For cancer patients, the network OncoNord has funded interpreters dedicated to this population, but this service remains underutilised. Physicians valued the mode of telephone translation for its low cost, in spite of its limitations in communicating meanings.

Immigrants in need of care, whether health or social services, but without insurance often have consultations at the NGO Médecins du Monde or at PASS clinics (*permanences d'accès aux soins*) located in public hospitals across Paris, Bordeaux and other major urban areas. PASS clinics are intended to serve impoverished patients and to ensure greater access to vulnerable populations such as immigrants with serious illnesses in need of multiple forms of support. In principle, PASS clinics value interpreters but, in reality, rarely engage them. This, in spite of directives from the Haute Autorité de Santé (HAS 2017) that made explicit the benefits of interpreters to best practices in medicine.

The HAS directives contain a list of required skills for interpreters, published in conjunction with a similar list for those working as health mediators who are trained to offer patients broader conceptual explanations of their conditions. These compilations of requisite competence document the variation in treatment engendered by the presence or absence of a professional interpreter. In the INCa research conducted by Kotobi, Larchanché and Kessar (2013), a medical oncologist described her habit of proposing to prostate cancer patients who are not fluent in French that they undergo surgical rather than medical (pharmaceutical) intervention. She reasoned that 'foreigners', especially homeless immigrants, displayed low compliance with treatment regimens. Although surgical complications were often serious and debilitating, this oncologist doubted that immigrants with little education or French language could follow instructions on medication usage.

Similarly, a majority of physicians, whose social status may distance them from their patients, shared biased representations of non-Francophone patients (Bretin and Kotobi 2016; Sargent 2005). The oncologist who doubted her patients' capacity to follow instructions is one of many clinicians we encountered who share this view. Some oncologists were genuinely interested in the lives of their patients and directed them to social workers, nurses and associations that might be of help. But they spoke of colleagues who were 'colonial' in their attitudes (for example, one nurse manager who spoke of the similarities between her West African patients and her servants at her husband's embassy home in the Ivory Coast). In one difficult exchange, the administrative assistant at a hospital where we interviewed breast cancer patients told us that African patients were taking advantage of the French healthcare system. 'They should go home, they can get excellent cancer treatment in places like Ouagadougou', she said angrily.

Issues of patient comfort, comprehension, rapport and profound anxiety, common among patients at the end of life, are often invisible in exchanges among many physicians and their patient populations. Characterisations of patients as illiterate, uninformed and unable to manage their medication or their appointments lead certain clinicians to justify making decisions on the patient's behalf, rather than to engage in difficult and uncomfortable interactions.

There are still few studies in France focusing on the experiences of seriously ill immigrants and those at the end of life (Pian 2012). Research exploring the implications of a life-threatening diagnosis, such as the cancer patients in this research experienced, is also lacking (but see

Sarradon-Eck 2009 and Sargent and Benson 2019 on cancer lived as a biographic rupture).

Professional interpreters, patients, family members and immigrant association members with or without cancer histories feared that it might be fatal to a patient to receive a frightening cancer diagnosis or a prognosis of limited life expectancy (Sargent and Benson 2019). Interviews with six interpreters of West African languages at a translation centre led to a discussion of how an interpreter might deal with a doctor's expectation that the interpreter will provide a direct translation and the interpreter's determination to avoid translating 'words that are not said'.[10] These include dire prognoses or speaking directly of imminent death. Five patients in our sample expressed outrage at their oncologist who had said explicitly, 'we have no more medicine for you. Have you made plans for your children or your household?' These women, interviewed individually, all said of the doctor: 'Who does he think he is? God?' As is often said in West African Muslim contexts, 'only God knows the hour of our death'.

Patients understand cancer, like other diseases, in relation to language comprehension, the subjective experience of sickness and understanding of therapeutic interventions. Serious illness also disrupts sociality among those residing in France but also among transnational family networks, reminding us of the global politics of care. Life-threatening sickness brings with it challenging questions of meaning and suffering, particularly salient with a cancer diagnosis. Increasing hospital budget cuts and new budget management systems render systematic use of interpreters even less probable in the near future. Communication constraints, both conceptual and linguistic, contribute to the production of health inequalities and also reflect them, as we have shown. Thus our research documents the extent to which chronic, life-threatening illness intersects with economic and social precarity at multiple levels – the individual, familial and institutional – to exacerbate ill health and further marginalise vulnerable populations. With regard to cancer, public health policies focus especially on curative procedures and on early detection rather than attending to the politics shaping care: structural inequalities upheld by economic interests at state and global levels, but often invisible to local populations in everyday life.

New cancer prevention initiatives by institutions such as INCa have turned to the principle of proportionate universalism, the resourcing and delivering of services at a scale and intensity proportionate to perceived demand. Proportionate universalism is conceived as both a universal strategy and targeted action that responds to the specific needs of particular populations. This concept may be seen as congruent with an anthropological approach, in which conceptualising the universal and the particular together may work to avoid essentialising interpretations of patients as 'Other' in clinical contexts.

The cost of specific clinical interventions or of translation services are rarely evaluated in relation to the clinical and social benefits generated by adapting strategies of prevention for populations at risk as well as assuring mutual comprehension of medical vocabulary and concepts of cancer causation and therapeutic trajectories. Access to the voices of immigrants with cancer, for example, might lead to more effective screening policies and management of cancer treatment for immigrant patients and enhance clinicians' understanding of the subjective experience of sickness among immigrants. Increasingly, there are indicators of a policy shift that addresses the needs of immigrant populations, as we see with the national cancer plans currently in place. From the collaboration between the prestigious private cancer hospital Institut Curie and Hôpital Delafontaine, the purpose is for clinicians at Curie to better understand the immigrant populations of the northern suburbs and for oncologists at Delafontaine to access the latest pharmaceuticals and procedures. In addition, as oncologists treating women from sub-Saharan Africa have remarked on the younger age at onset of breast cancer, they are stimulated to analyse the possible explanations – societies of origin, adaptation to the host society or features of modernity – as immigrants themselves have suggested. The politics of care are in flux, troubled by austerity measures throughout EU countries. French state policies need, nonetheless, to re-politicise immigrant women's health in the interest of a truly egalitarian society, one that attends to the needs of its most vulnerable populations.

Acknowledgements

This chapter draws on research led by both authors. Carolyn Sargent thanks the National Science Foundation for supporting the research (from 2014 to 2019) on which this chapter is based by means of grant no. 1354336, 'The Influence of Sociality in Cancer Treatment Decision Making' (PIs: Sargent, Benson and Larchanché). Laurence Kotobi draws on research supported by Agence Nationale de la Recherche (ANR), undertaken between 2017 and 2022 and entitled Premiers Pas (First Steps) (PIs: Kotobi, Wittwer and colleagues). They express their appreciation for this ANR grant. The research conducted in the Paris region was reviewed by the Washington University in St. Louis Institutional Review Board (IRB)/Human Subjects Review Board and approved 18 April 2014, no. 201403075. The research conducted in the Medoc region was approved by the University of Bordeaux and Institute for Public Health Research (IReSP), convention no. 2009SS06. Informed consent protocols were approved by the ethics committees or IRB of the respective institutions.

Notes

1. Immigration from West and North Africa to France has been traced to the nineteenth century and earlier; Bordeaux, for example, was a significant transit point for the trans-Atlantic slave trade. These earlier periods are important but beyond the scope of this chapter.
2. For example, La Cimade, an NGO to assist migrants to access rights (Asti de Bordeaux 2020) has a broad mandate to support immigrants with legal and social dilemmas, Union des Travailleurs Sénégalais de France represents the substantial population of Senegalese workers and families in the Bordeaux region, l'Association des Musulmans de Bordeaux addresses concerns of area for Muslims and Orchidées Rouges supports those with female genital-cutting issues.
3. Systematic observation and discussion at a legal aid association which specialised in assisting West African immigrants with bureaucratic problems provided Sargent with an understanding of the most common issues confronting immigrant clients. Lack of health insurance and difficulty navigating the healthcare system were such widespread problems that the association began to reserve certain days of the week for walk-in clients with a need for health coverage. These were almost always undocumented migrants to whom the association staff would provide information on 'rights' and how to access them. Primary among these rights was AME and the documentation needed to obtain it.
4. https://www.santepubliquefrance.fr/maladies-et-traumatismes/cancers/cancer-du-sein/articles/taux-de-participation-au-programme-de-depistage-organise-du-cancer-du-sein-2018-2019-et-evolution-depuis-2005. Accessed 16 September 2022.
5. In France, gynaecologists specialise in reproductive health, which includes the breast. Gynaecologists perform breast surgery as well as surgery on the uterus, ovaries and vagina for diverse conditions. Male patients with breast cancer, although statistically rare, may also be treated by gynaecologists.
6. The neighbourhood by the train station Gare du Nord is well known as a location where those who are homeless sleep (Kleinman 2012).
7. A partial mastectomy involves removal of the breast tumour and some surrounding tissue and may include removal of some lymph nodes.
8. The ENFAMS survey, carried out in 2013, showed that homeless women living with a partner did not have regular gynaecological follow-ups and were less likely to have had a mammogram, especially single mothers with children (Vuillermoz et al. 2016: 4–5, tables 1 and 2). This study identified 801 homeless families in 193 social service lodgings in the greater Paris region, who were interviewed in 17 languages. Of women interviewed 73.4 per cent were homeless with family members and beneficiaries of CMU or AME.
9. In the absence of full-time interpreters, clinicians may rely on family members, cleaning staff, nurse's aides or others who speak the language of the patient. Interpreters describe scenarios where they are asked to interpret a language in which they are not fully fluent, which is uncomfortable and unproductive for all parties involved.
10. Interpreter Workshop, Inter Service Migrants, Paris, July 2019.

References

Asti de Bordeaux. 2020. 'Historique'. Accessed 13 October 2020. http://astibordeaux.fr.
Barou, Jacques. 2014. 'Integration of immigrants in France: A historical perspective', *Identities* 21(6): 642–657. https://doi.org/10.1080/1070289X.2014.882840.

Black, Eleanor and Robyn Richmond. 2019. 'Improving early detection of breast cancer in sub-Saharan Africa: Why mammography may not be the way forward', *Global Health* 15(3). https://doi.org/10.1186/s12992-018-0446-6.

Bouchaud, Olivier and Sandra Cohuet. 2011. *Les Maladies du Voyage et d'Importation*. Paris: La Documentation Française.

Bretin, Hélène and Laurence Kotobi. 2016. 'Inégalités contraceptives au pays de la pilule', *Agone* 58: 123–134.

Dano, Domitille, Clémence Hénon, Ousseynou Sarr, Kanta Ka, Mouhamadou Ba, Awa Badiane, Ibrahima Thiam et al. 2019. 'Quality of life during chemotherapy for breast cancer in a West African population in Dakar, Senegal: A prospective study', *Journal of Global Oncology* 5: 1–9. http://ascopubs.org/doi/full/10.1200/JGO.19.00106.

Desprès, Caroline. 2013. 'Négocier ses besoins dans un univers contraint. Le renoncement aux soins en situation de précarité', *Anthropologie et Santé* 6. https://doi.org/10.4000/anthropologiesante.1078.

Fassin, Didier. 2000. 'Repenser les enjeux de santé autour de l'immigration', *Hommes et Migration* 1225: 5–12. https://doi.org/10.3406/homig.2000.3506.

Fassin, Didier. 2007. 'La santé des etrangères: une question politique', *La Santé de l'Homme* 392: 15–16.

HAS (Haute Autorité de Santé). 2017. 'Interprétariat dans le domaine de la santé'. Accessed 1 September 2020. https://www.has-sante.fr/upload/docs/application/pdf/2017-10/interpretariatdansledomainedelasante.

INSEE (Institut National de la Statistique et des Études Économiques). 2019. 'L'essentiel sur les immigrés et les étrangers'. Accessed 1 October 2020. https://www.insee.fr/fr/statistiques/3633212.

Kleinman, Julie. 2012. 'The Gare du Nord: Parisian topographies of exchange', *Ethnologie Française* 42: 567–576. https://doi.org/10.3917/ethn.123.0567.

Kotobi, Laurence. 2017. 'L'interprétariat médico-social: une exigence éthique', *La Santé en Action* 44: 15–17.

Kotobi, Laurence and Clara Lemonnier. 2015. 'Ethnographier les itinéraires thérapeutiques en santé reproductive pour mieux comprendre les recours aux soins: Le cas des femmes en difficulté dans le Médoc', *Sociologie Santé* 38: 199–233.

Kotobi, Laurence and Aïcha Lkhadir. 2016. 'Une enquête anthropologique hospitalière autour de la pudeur et de la diversité culturelle'. Bordeaux, France: Fondation de France, Centre Hospitalier Universitaire (CHU) de Bordeaux.

Kotobi, Laurence, Stéphanie Larchanché and Zahia Kessar. 2013. 'Enjeux et logiques de recours à l'interprétariat en milieu hospitalier: Une recherche-action autour de l'annonce d'une maladie grave', *Migrations santé*, 1 January: 146–147.

Lafore, Robert. 2017. 'Les caractéristiques du Système Français de Protection Sociale', *Cahiers français* 399: 9–15.

La Ligue Contre le Cancer Comité Gironde. 2017. 'Cancer du col de l'utérus. Formation-action d'étudiants-relais à la prévention du cancer du col de l'utérus'. Accessed 2 June 2017. http://www.ligue-cancer33.fr/prevenir/cancer-col-uterus.

Larchanché, Stéphanie. 2020. *Cultural Anxieties: Managing migrant suffering in France*. New Brunswick, NJ: Rutgers University Press.

Leclerc, Annette, Didier Fassin, Hélène Grandjean, Monique Kaminski and Thierry Lang. 2000. *Les Inégalités Sociales de Santé*. Paris: La Découverte.

Lombrail, Pierre, Jean Pascal and Thierry Lang. 2004. 'Inégalités sociales de santé', *Santé, Société, Solidarité* 2: 61–71.

Louarn, Anne-Diandra. 2019. 'Living from day to day in Bordeaux's migrant squats'. InfoMigrants. Accessed 13 December 2019. https://www.infomigrants.net/en/post/21478/living-from-day-to-day-in-bordeaux-s-migrant-squats.

Manchuelle, François. 1997. *Willing Migrants: Soninke labor diasporas 1848–1960*. Athens, OH: Ohio University Press.

Pian, Anaïk. 2012. 'De l'accès aux soins aux trajectoires du mourir. Les étrangers atteints de cancer face aux contraintes administratives', *REMI* 28: 101–127. https://doi.org/10.4000/remi.5915.

Sargent, Carolyn. 2005. 'Counseling contraception for Malian migrants in Paris: Global, state, and personal politics', *Human Organization* 64(2): 147–156. https://www.jstor.org/stable/44127250.

Sargent, Carolyn and Peter Benson. 2019. 'Cancer and precarity: Rights and vulnerabilities of West African immigrants in France'. In *Negotiating Structural Vulnerability in Cancer Control*, edited by Julie Armin, Nancy J. Burke and Laura Eichelberger, 21–47. Santa Fe, NM: School for Advanced Research Press.

Sargent, Carolyn and Dennis Cordell. 2003. 'Polygamy, reproduction and the state: Malian migrants in Paris, France', *Social Science & Medicine* 56(9): 1961–1972.

Sargent, Carolyn and Laurence Kotobi. 2017. 'Austerity and its implications for immigrants in France', *Social Science & Medicine* 187: 259–267. https://doi.org/10.1016/j.socscimed.2017.05.007.

Sargent, Carolyn and Stéphanie Larchanché. 2014. 'Disease, risk, and contagion: French colonial and postcolonial constructions of "African" bodies', *Journal of Bioethical Inquiry* 11(4): 455–466. https://doi.org/10.1007/s11673-014-9578-4.

Sarradon-Eck, Aline. 2009. 'Le cancer comme inscription d'une rupture biographique dans le corps'. In *Faire Face au Cancer. Image du Corps, Image de Soi*, edited by Florence Cousson-Gélie, Emmanuel Langlois and Marion Barrault, 285–311. Paris: Editions Tikinagan.

Simon, Patrick, Cris Beauchemin and Christelle Hamel. 2015. *Trajectoires et Origines. Enquête sur la Diversité des Populations en France*. Paris: Ined.

Strong, Adrienne. 2020. *Documenting Death: Maternal mortality and the ethics of care in Tanzania*. Berkeley: University of California Press.

Urrutia, Carla. 2017. 'Saisir la santé perçue des migrants: l'exemple des dépistages dans une grand ville en France'. Master's thesis. Bordeaux University.

Vuillermoz, Cécile, Stéphanie Vandentorren, Mathilde Roze, Claire Rondet and Pierre Chauvin. 2016. 'Cervical cancer screening among homeless women in the greater Paris area (France): Results of the ENFAMS survey', *European Journal of Cancer Prevention* 26(3): 240–248. https://doi.org/10.1097/CEJ.0000000000000225.

Wittwer, Jérôme, Denis Raynaud, Paul Dourgnon and Florence Jusot. 2019. 'Protéger la santé des personnes étrangères en situation irrégulière en France. L'Aide Médicale de l'État, une politique d'accès aux soins mal connue', *Questions d'Economie de la Santé* 243. Accessed 16 September 2022. https://www.irdes.fr/recherche/questions-d-economie-de-la-sante/243-proteger-la-sante-des-personnes-etrangeres-en-situation-irreguliere-en-france.pdf.

Index

advocacy 6, 19, 20
  for abortion 56
  for breast cancer 173
  for cervical cancer 120
  organisations 19
  pink advocacy 173
  and survivor testimonies 125
AIDS (acquired immunodeficiency syndrome) *see* HIV
American Cancer Society 94–95
Argentina 42–61
  Early Cervical Cancer Detection Subprogram 43
  National Cancer Institute 43
  National Cervical Cancer Program 44
  National Risk Factor Survey 45

Banerjee, Dwaipayan 13
Banfield, Edward 183
Bennett, Elizabeth 13
Botswana 9, 13
Bourdieu, Pierre 62, 67
brachytherapy *see* treatment
Brazil 23–41
  Agência Nacional de Saúde Suplementar (ANS – National Supplementary Health Agency) 27
  Agência Nacional de Vigilância Sanitária (ANVISA – National Agency of Sanitary Surveillance) 27
  Bahia 26–27, 29–30, 33
  Comissão Nacional de Incorporação de Tecnologias no Sistema Único de Saúde (CONITEC – National Commission for the Incorporation of Technologies) 28, 39
  Constitution 25, 33, 39
  National Cancer Institute 26
  Sistema Único de Saúde (SUS – Unified Health System) 25–30, 33, 36–39
  patients 27, 30, 39
  Supreme Court of Justice 37
breast cancer
  in Brazil 28, 30, 38
  in France 232–253
  in India 83–108
  in Italy 171–189
  prevalence 1

  survivors of 71
  in USA 62–65, 68–71, 74, 77
  see also screening; treatment
Butler, Judith 18

California 11, 62
Cancer Research UK 214
cancer therapies
  chemotherapy 26–27, 30, 66, 71, 117, 147, 150–151, 155–156, 158, 160–161, 163, 180–182, 184, 239, 241, 244
  gene panel screening 7, 23
  radiotherapy 29, 112, 155–156, 158, 184, 241
  targeted medications 7, 23
care
  capacities for care 4, 19, 123–126
  carers 5, 14, 59, 124, 137
  compassionate care/sentimental work 12–13, 168
  in Greece 159–170
  hierarchies of care 126
  nursing care 12, 163
  physical care 152
  relationality and care 9, 13–14, 19
  right to care 124–125
  self-care 13, 19, 59, 123, 126, 179, 185, 221
caste 10, 83, 85–93, 96, 99, 101, 104–105, 191
Catholic/Catholicism
  in Argentina 46
  in Indonesia 116
  in Italy 179
cervical cancer 8, 10–12, 30
  in Argentina 42–61
  in France 238, 245–246
  in India 48–108
  in Indonesia 109–129
  screening for cervical cancer 8, 46–47, 54, 58–59, 83, 113, 238, 245–246
  stigma and cervical cancer 109–110, 115, 126
  treatment for 112
chemotherapy *see* treatment
class 2, 10
  in Argentina 43, 46–48, 54, 56–58
  in Denmark 193, 199, 204

in India 83–87, 89, 96, 98–105
in Indonesia 109, 116, 119
in Italy 174–175, 177, 181, 185
colon cancer 196–197
containment, theory of 11, 24, 123, 126–127, 171–177, 179, 181–182, 185–187

Denmark 6, 14–15, 190–209
   Jutland 193, 194, 201
diagnosis of cancer 1, 3, 5, 6, 9, 11–14, 17–19
   in Argentina 44
   in Brazil 24, 28, 30, 32, 37
   in Denmark 190, 193, 195–197, 204–205
   diagnosis and stigma 109–110, 112–113
   diagnosis and temporality/delayed/early 113, 193, 224
   in Greece 159, 157
   in Indonesia 104–105, 109–110, 112–113, 114–118
   in Italy 172, 176–181, 183–184, 186
   in UK 212–213, 224, 233, 238–239, 243–249
   in USA 63, 65
diagnostics 6–7, 54, 190–209 see mammogram
disclosure/concealment
   disclosure candidates 144
   disclosure and capacity for care 124, 126
   disclosure of diagnosis 120
   disclosure of prognosis 147
   harsh disclosure 143
   non-disclosure 13, 134–147
   selective/limited disclosure 109–110, 117–118, 123–125
   soft truth 13
discrimination
   and access or barriers to health services 9, 11, 16
   and Brazilian Constitution 25
   class/caste discrimination 55, 58, 191
   and eugenics 55
   in/by health services 21, 58, 211, 227
   and intersectionality 9, 55
   and mistrust 16, 211, 227
   racial discrimination 55, 58
   and stigma 110
drug use 49, 221, 227
   Drug Recovery Centre 222
Duclos, Vincent and Tomas Sánchez Criado 137–138

end of life/palliative care 6, 14, 130, 134, 136–142, 144–145, 147, 248
European Medicines Agency 33

faith
   as a cultural tool 179
   'regime of hope' 131
   and support 179
family planning 87, 95, 97
   and consent 104
   interuterine device (IUD) 119
   sterilisation 95
Farmer, Paul 84
   structural violence 8, 47, 54, 191

fatalism 117, 179, 186
Food and Drug Administration (FDA) 33
Foucault, Michel 77, 195
France 232–253
   African immigrants 232–253
   Bordeaux 223–237, 240, 243, 245, 247
   Council of Equality (Conseil à l'Egalité) 237
   Institut Curie and Hôpital Delafontaine 250
   National Cancer Institute (INCa) 237
   National Cancer Plan 238, 246
   Paris 233–237, 239, 242–245, 247
   Protection Universelle Maladie (PUMA) 236
   statistics on ethnicity 238
   Third Cancer Plan 237
Frank, Arthur 199
Freeman, Harold 63

gender
   femininity 10, 90, 173
   gender-based violence 49
   gender norms 103
   gender roles 86, 186
   masculinity 181
global divides
   global north 1, 5, 174, 232
   global south 1, 5, 174, 232
   south-within-the-north 14, 171, 174–175
Goffman, Erving 110, 119, 121
Gramsci, Antonio 174
Greece 150–170
Grimen, Harald 167
Gypsy Roma Travellers (GRTs) 15, 16, 210

hard-to-reach groups 16, 210–231
health advocacy see advocacy
health insurance 7, 9
   Argentina 44
   Brazil 25–27, 30, 37
   France 236–237, 239–242
   Greece 155
   Indonesia 113–114
health promotion 6, 10, 19, 37, 105, 113, 205, 213–215, 217, 225
hegemonic masculinity 181
hepatitis 2, 12
   hepatitis B 132–134, 137, 146
   hepatitis C 132
HIV (human immunodeficiency virus)
   access to treatment for PLWH 29, 135
   causality 245
   stigma 98, 111
   testing camps 10
HPV (human papillomavirus) 2, 6, 10, 44, 47, 51, 94, 98–99, 104, 119, 126

improvisation 9, 13, 24, 34, 67
India 83–108
   Government of 99
   see also Tamil Nadu
Indonesia 109–129
inequality
   economic 13, 47
   gender 47, 85

social 2–3, 14, 54, 191, 193–194, 199, 205–207
structural 3, 5, 7, 10, 43, 58, 63, 105, 232, 233, 238, 249
International Agency for Research on Cancer (IARC) 2
Inter-American Development Bank 44
Italy 171–189
   geopolitical divisions 14, 171, 174–175
   Salento 175–177

judicialisation 7, 19, 27–31, 34–38

Kleinman, Arthur and Joan Kleinman
   on the body 198, 201, 205–206
   on care 111, 512, 154
   on structural vulnerability 191–192

laughter 62–82
   Laughing Guru Madan Kataria 66
   laughter therapy 67
   role of laughter in patient navigation 79
liver cancer 2, 12, 130–149
Livingston, Julie 4, 9, 12–13, 24, 34, 79, 150, 163, 168
Lock, Margaret 24, 52, 198–199, 206

mammogram 30, 52, 160, 178, 239, 241–244
marginalisation 3, 19, 43, 47–48
marriage
   child marriage 87, 93–95
   delayed marriage and cancer risk 10, 94, 100–101
   divorce 116, 124
   early marriage and cancer risk 10, 93–94
   extramarital sex 126
   ideal age of marriage 94
   marriage and gender roles 86, 90, 194–195, 100–102
mastectomy 178, 182, 184, 240
Médecins du Monde 239, 247
melanoma 24, 27, 34, 38
mental health 49
   anxiety 9, 15, 176, 206, 248
   depression 122, 202–203
   social isolation 13, 121, 168, 221
   suicidality 122
Mexico 123
migrants
   in Argentina 43, 46
   in France 233–235, 237, 245
   in UK 215
Mol, Annemarie 13, 111, 131, 136–138
morality 10, 11
   and cancer causality 19
   in India 83, 85, 98
   in Indonesia 109, 121, 125
   and stigma 121, 125

noisy bodies 15, 190–209

oncologists 7, 16, 23, 68–69, 115, 119, 136, 236, 240, 245–248, 250
   ethics 34–35, 38
   improvisational practices 13
   judicialisation 31–32, 34–36
   practices of care 13, 156
   tinkering 13
   treatment decisions and options 24, 30, 35–36, 250
oncology
   in Brazil 23–36, 28, 30, 36–37
   in France 239, 247
   in Greece 150–151, 154–155
   oncology nurse 239
   precision oncology 28, 35–37
   in USA 68–71

paan 87, 89, 98–99, 103–104
pain
   medication 136
   relief 4, 12, 141, 142
palliative care *see* end of life
Pan American Health Organization 44
Pap smear
   in Argentina 44–46, 51, 57
   in France 238
   in Indonesia 113
   see also screening
pathology/laboratory
   anatomical pathology 195
   laboratory services 29, 135, 155, 237
   reports 68, 75
   results 75
patient navigation 8, 14, 19
   in USA 62–82
personalised medicine 23
prevalence
   of child marriage 94
   disparities in cancer prevalence 1
   of HPV 104
   limits of prevalence data 238
   of liver cancer 142
   of sexual violence against women and girls 50
prevention 3, 6, 11–12, 19
   in Argentina 43–47, 54, 58–59
   in Brazil 24, 25, 32, 37, 42
   in France 233, 237, 244, 246, 249–250
   in India 83, 89, 92–105
   primary prevention *see* vaccination
   secondary prevention *see* screening; mammograms
   in Senegal 134, 137, 147
   in UK 217–218, 223
   in USA 64
Puig de la Bellacasa, Maria 131, 138, 157

quality of life (QOL) 2, 12–13, 24, 31–33, 36, 52, 67, 183

racism 3, 8, 17, 47, 55, 59, 194
   see also discrimination
radiotherapy *see* treatment
Remennick, Larissa 97
reproduction (human) 10, 57, 86, 94, 122
reproductive health 10, 44, 46, 54–55, 58, 89, 109
   women's experiences of reproductive healthcare/services 50, 52, 54–55
resilience 14, 17, 19, 59, 114

resistance
    acts of 43
    caste-based 104
    to HPV vaccination 99
    to institutional approaches to care 233
    pragmatic 57–58
    to screening 16
    state–based 237

Sanz, Camilo 131, 144
screening for cancers 6, 19
    access to 2, 30, 44, 113, 133, 155, 237–238, 246
    barriers to 11, 47, 55–56, 58, 104, 113, 213, 245–246
    for breast cancer 64, 83, 88, 101, 180, 238–244, 100–102
    camps 9–10, 83–108
    for cervical cancer 8, 46–47, 54, 58–60, 83–103, 238, 245–246
    disengagement/non-adherence/resistance to 2, 16, 18, 46–47, 51, 54, 179, 211, 213
    educational materials 84–85, 90–103
    failures of 8, 54, 217, 238
    gene panel screening 2, 23
    guidelines/policies/protocols 44, 157–158
    presentation for 5, 8, 180
    risk perception 120, 126, 214–215
    as secondary prevention see prevention
    stigma/shame 104–105, 113
    target groups 45, 113, 238, 246
    see also mammogram; Pap smear; visual inspection with acetic acid (VIA)
Senegal 6, 13, 13, 130–149
sexual health 72
sexuality 10, 57, 72, 75, 78, 83, 85–86, 90, 118, 125, 245
    promiscuity 104, 110, 111, 118–119, 121, 123–124
stigma/shame
    and addiction 219
    by association 109, 114, 119
    and avoidance of care 210
    and blame 103, 105, 118
    and capacities for care 4, 123–126
    and containment 109
    in Denmark 194, 199
    and diagnosis 104, 122–123
    enacted stigma 110, 118
    felt stigma 110, 121
    in India 83–108
    in Indonesia 109–129
    in Italy 174
    mediating/mitigating 110, 117, 119–120
    and morality 85, 110, 121, 125–126
    and non-disclosure 8, 9, 11, 13
    and sexuality 85, 122
    in UK 210
    see also disclosure
Strathern, Marilyn 214
stratified patienthood/patient stratification 23–41
support
    family support 9, 11
    financial support 116, 121, 234, 242, 244

social support 16, 125, 235
    see also care and support under survivors; patient navigation
survivors
    and advocacy 125
    care and support networks 12, 65, 120–121, 125
    invisibility of 115
    quality of life 67
    and stigma/shame 103, 115
    support for 71
Susan G. Komen Foundation 72

Tamil Nadu 9–10, 83–86, 90–97
    Cancer Institute 87–93
    Government Cancer Hospital 83, 88
    Mahatma Gandhi National Rural Employment Guarantee Act (MGNREGA) 88
    Rural Women's Social Education Centre (RUWSEC) 88
tobacco 10, 89, 98, 103
translation 199, 236–237, 243, 247, 249–250
    translators 16
treatment for cancer
    access to 2, 4, 6, 7, 11, 27, 29, 30, 85, 111, 118, 133, 136, 147, 237
    alternative treatments 72
    brachytherapy 112
    chemotherapy 26–27, 30, 66, 71, 75, 117, 147, 150–151, 155–156, 158, 160–161, 163, 180–182, 184, 239–241, 244
    choice/s 5, 30, 117, 120
    cost of/funding for 11, 28, 30–34, 64, 112, 114, 133, 155, 237, 241–242
    cross-border treatment 232–254
    delays in/waiting times 9, 18, 27, 37, 112, 113, 131–132, 138, 195–197, 245
    discontinuation/withdrawal from 9, 64, 248
    efficacy 33, 44, 133, 172
    endocrine 62
    ethics 17
    genomic biotechnologies 23
    and health literacy 16, 35
    inequalities in 24–26, 28, 37, 64, 84–85, 111, 113–114, 174, 212, 233, 236
    judicialisation 30–37
    navigation 63, 65, 69, 116, 143 see also patient navigation
    oncologists' views 23, 31, 32, 36 see also oncology
    outcomes 19, 84, 114
    pathways/plans/protocols 28, 31, 36, 38, 44, 54, 68, 117, 158, 239
    patient perceptions 111, 114, 184, 192, 219, 250
    post-treatment/new normal 172
    radiotherapy 29, 112, 115, 155–156, 158, 184, 241
    side effects 9, 114, 154
    support during 180, 240–242, 248
    symptomatic pain treatment 136, 142
    unnecessary treatment 144–146

United Kingdom 210–231
    Cambridgeshire 215
    National Health Service (NHS) 211–213, 222, 224, 237
    National Institute of Health Research 217
    NHS 5-Year Forward Plan 212
    NHS Cancer Plan 217
United States 23–41 *see also* California
    American College of Surgeons Commission on Cancer 64
    Breast Cancer Patient Navigation Program 64
    Congress 64
    Patient Navigation Outreach and Chronic Disease Prevention Act 64
    Patient Protection and Affordable Care Act 64

vaccination
    hepatitis B 132–134, 137–138, 146
    human papilloma virus (HPV) 20, 44, 51, 99, 126
    universal vaccination (child vaccination) 25
Venezuela 123

violence
    gender-based violence 49
    institutional 17, 48, 50, 54, 57
    interpersonal 50
    obstetric 48, 54–55
    sexual violence against women and girls 50
    structural 8, 19, 47–50, 54, 58–59, 191
visual inspection with acetic acid (VIA) 45, 84, 113
vulnerability 8, 9, 18–19, 47, 116, 181
    amplified vulnerability 59
    avoidance of 49
    biographies of vulnerability 114
    physical vulnerability and reliance on nurses 167–168
    resistance as protection from vulnerability 58
    structural 18, 238

welfare society *see* Denmark 190–209
World Bank 44, 84
World Health Organization (WHO) 33, 44, 205

Yates-Doerr, Emily 138

Lightning Source UK Ltd.
Milton Keynes UK
UKHW021256260123
416011UK00027B/289